Adverse Reactions
to Anaesthetic Drugs

VOLUME 8

Adverse Reactions to Anaesthetic Drugs

Edited by
J.A. Thornton

Department of Anaesthesiology
University of Sheffield Medical School
Beech Hill Road
Sheffield S10 2RX, U.K.

1981

Excerpta Medica/Elsevier North-Holland Biomedical Press
Amsterdam · Oxford · New York

Published by:

ELSEVIER/NORTH-HOLLAND BIOMEDICAL PRESS
335 JAN VAN GALENSTRAAT, P.O. BOX 211
AMSTERDAM, THE NETHERLANDS

Sole distributors for the U.S.A. and Canada:

ELSEVIER/NORTH-HOLLAND INC.
52 VANDERBILT AVENUE
NEW YORK, N.Y. 10017

ISBN–series: 0-444-80023-9
–volume 0-444-80213-4

Printed in The Netherlands

PREFACE

Since the introduction of general anaesthesia in the mid-19th century the development of anaesthetic practice has been associated with remarkable improvements in the standards and safety of patient care. Better training of anaesthetists, the more precise control of the depth of anaesthesia and cardio-respiratory function made possible by developments in anaesthetic apparatus and monitoring equipment, have all played a part in a reduction of the morbidity and mortality associated with anaesthesia. The relentless search for agents with wider margins of safety continues. Despite all these advances the patient may respond adversely and sometimes unpredictably to the drugs which are administered.

Recent experience and research has led to a better understanding of the fundamental mechanisms involved in adverse reactions.

It is the purpose of this book to focus attention on some of these problems. The topics covered in this book inevitably have a heavy bias towards reactions which may have a immunological relationship. The Editor makes no apology for this, and in an attempt to help those with a limited understanding of Immunology a Chapter and Glossary in Basic Immunology have been included in the text.

Acknowledgements and appreciation are not only due to the authors but also to Mrs. D. Broadhurst, Mrs. C. King and Mrs. Y. Jones, without whose help the preparation of this text would not have been possible.

J.A. Thornton
Sheffield
September 1980

LIST OF CONTRIBUTORS

H.C. CHURCHILL-DAVIDSON
  Department of Anaesthetics, St. Thomas' Hospital, London SE1 7EH, England
R.S.J. CLARK
  Department of Anaesthetics, The Queen's University of Belfast, Whitla Medical
  Building, 97 Lisburn Road, Belfast BT9 7BL, Ireland
A. DOENICKE
  Division of Experimental Surgery and Pathological Biochemistry, Department of
  Operative Medicine I, University of Marburg/Lahn, Robert-Koch-Strasse 8,
  D-3550 Marburg/Lahn, F.R.G.
J.W. DUNDEE
  Department of Anaesthetics, The Queen's University of Belfast, Whitla Medical
  Building, 97 Lisburn Road, Belfast BT9 7BL, Ireland
T.E.J. HEALY
  Reader in Anaesthesia, The University of Nottingham, Nottingham, England
M. LIM
  Department of Anaesthetics, St. Thomas' Hospital, London SE1 7EH, England
W. LORENZ
  Division of Experimental Surgery and Pathological Biochemistry, Department of
  Operative Medicine I, University of Marburg/Lahn, Robert-Koch-Strasse 8,
  D-3550 Marburg/Lahn, F.R.G.
E. NEUGEBAUER
  Division of Experimental Surgery and Pathological Biochemistry, Department of
  Operative Medicine I, University of Marburg/Lahn, Robert-Koch-Strasse 8,
  D-3550 Marburg/Lahn, F.R.G.
B. SCHÖNING
  Division of Experimental Surgery and Pathological Biochemistry, Department of
  Operative Medicine I, University of Marburg/Lahn, Robert-Koch-Strasse 8,
  D-3550 Marburg/Lahn, F.R.G.
J.A. THORNTON
  Department of Anaesthetics, University of Sheffield, Sheffield, England
B. WALTON
  Consultant Anaesthetist, London Hospital, Whitechapel, London E1 1BB,
  England

J. WATKINS
Department of Immunology, Hallamshire Hospital School, Sheffield S10 2RX, England
J.G. WHITWAM
Department of Anaesthetics, Royal Postgraduate Medical School, Hammersmith Hospital, Du Cane Road, London W.1.2.OH, England

CONTENTS

Thornton (ed.) Adverse Reactions of Anaesthetic Drugs
© Elsevier/North-Holland Biomedical Press, 1981

1

The effects of drug therapy on the response to anaesthetic agents

J.A. Thornton

INTRODUCTION

Increasing numbers of patients presenting for anaesthesia are being found to be receiving drug therapy. Some of these drugs can modify the patient's response to general and local anaesthetic agents, and, in some instances, the response may be such as to hazard the patient's life.

Prescott (1975) reported that as many as 20% of patients admitted to hospital may be there because of drug induced disease. Kyei-Mensah and Thornton (1974) reporting on the findings of a number of anaesthetic outpatient clinics emphasised the magnitude of this problem. Although most anaesthetists see their patients in the immediate preoperative period it is often not possible to adjust the medication in the time available, even though the nature of the therapy may be known. The development of the anaesthetic outpatient clinic is one way of avoiding this dilemma but current limitations required to develop this service make its widespread adoption unlikely. A drug history enquiry form sent to the patient's doctor some weeks prior to admission to hospital has proved to be of considerable value.

A prior knowledge of the drugs administered to the patient can alert the anaesthetist to possible hazards and permit him to modify therapy as appropriate. This chapter attempts to cover most of the adverse reactions that may be encountered but no attempt has been made to consider the increasing problem of drug abuse and addiction, nor the use of premedicant drugs routinely employed in the immediate preoperative period.

CARDIOVASCULAR DRUGS

Quinidine has been reported to aggravate or unmask myasthenia gravis (Weisman 1949; Kornfeld et al., 1976) and to cause delayed postoperative respiratory depression due to interaction with muscle relaxants (Grogono, 1963; Miller, Way and Katzung, 1967; Way, Katzung and Larson, 1967). The neuromuscular-blocking of its L-isomer quinine are well known, so much so that at one time it formed the basis of a provocative test for the diagnosis of myasthenia gravis.

Procainamide exerts a post synaptic curare-like effect, and, may aggravate myasthenia gravis (Drachman and Skom, 1965; Kornfeld et al., 1976). Procaine and lignocaine can cause a prolongation of the effect of suxamethonium (Usubiaga et al., 1967). This is thought to occur as a result of the local analgesics competing with suxamethonium for binding sites on plasma proteins or plasma cholinesterase (Hussar, 1967). A similar mode of action may account for the prolongation of neuromuscular blockade by non-depolarising agents (Harrah, Way and Katzung, 1970).

Certain agents used to induce hypotension during anaesthesia have been found to prolong the effect of neuromuscular blocking agents. Dale and Schroeder (1976) and Wilson et al. (1976) have found that trimetaphen when given intravenously caused a curare-like action. Tewfik (1957), Poulton, James and Lockridge (1979) have reported potentiation of succinylcholine by this drug. Sklar and Lanks (1977) have demonstrated that trimetaphan is a potent non competitive inhibitor of cholinesterase. Nitroglycerin has been noted as causing undue prolongation of pancuronium- induced blockade. In experiments using the cat sciatic gastrocnemius nerve-muscle preparation Glisson El-Etr and Lim (1979) have confirmed this clinical finding. Sklar and Lanks (1977) could find no inhibiting effect of nitroglycerin upon cholinesterase in vitro. Of the β-adrenergic blocking agents, propranolol, oxprenolol and practolol have been reported to induce a myasthenic syndrome or to unmask myasthenia gravis (Herishanu and Rosenberg, 1975; Hughes and Zacharias, 1976). Propranolol produces a post-synaptic curare-like effect in vitro at concentrations comparable to those reached during therapy and also a pre-synaptic-like action at higher concentrations. Wislicki and Rosenblaum (1967) have demonstrated that the neuromuscular block induced in cats by depolarizing drugs was intensified, and the effect of tubocurarine reduced by intravenous infusions of propranolol. However, there are no reports in the anaesthetic literature of problems arising from this potential adverse effect.

Theophylline has been reported to antagonise non-depolarizing neuromuscular block in animals (Dretchen et al., 1976) and man (Doll and Rosenberg, 1979). It is likely that such antagonsm is associated with doses of theophylline in excess of the normal therapeutic range. It is postulated that this action is probably associated with the inhibition of phosphodiesterase which is responsible for the degradation of cAMP to 5'-AMP. This in turn should lead to a rise in cAMP levels resulting in increased transmitter release and competitive inhibition of the non-depolarizing neuromuscular blocking agents.

The diuretics, acetazolamide, thiazides and frusemide may cause a loss of potassium from the body. The action of potassium at the neuro-muscular junction is similar to that of acetylcholine. When the serum potassium concentration has fallen below approximately 2.5 mmol $\cdot$ l^{-1} muscular weakness sometimes ensues. There are often associated cardiovascular changes which manifest themselves as bradycardia, dysrhythmias and even ventricular fibrillation. Miller, Sohn and Matteo (1976) reported an enhancement of the effect of d-tubocurarine in the hypokalaemic state. However, Hill et al. (1978) have demonstrated that potassium depletion induced by frusemide does not affect the action of neuro-muscular blocking drugs as the transmembrane potential remains unchanged. Feldman (1979) has confirmed this observation in man and animals. However, where potassium loss leads to a low serum potassium, particularly if this is associated with a metabolic alkalosis (hypokalaemic metabolic alkalosis), it would appear to be prudent to correct the hypokalaemia, and any associated electrolyte and acid-base disturbance, prior to the induction of anaesthesia, and to use a lower dose/body weight relationship of muscle relaxant in the first instance and then to augment this dose with small increments as required (Vaughan and Lunn, 1973).

Antihypertensive drugs

It has long been recognised that the hypertensive patient represents an increased anaesthetic risk. Associated coronary artery disease, myocardial ischaemia, left ventricular failure, renal and cerebral-vascular complications can compound themselves to add to this risk. Anaesthetic drugs all tend to produce varying degrees of myocardial depression and systemic vasodilation which in turn may lead to fall in blood pressure, coronary and cerebro-vascular perfusion. It was thought that patients on anti-hypertensive therapy increased this risk still further with a greater tendency to decapitation of the blood pressure particularly in association with intravenous induction agents and intermittent positive pressure ventilation (Dingle 1966). Those who subscribed to the view that anaesthesia in the patient on anti-hypertensive therapy represented a further increase in the risk advocated cessation of such therapy. Depending upon the particular drug this might take upwards to 3 weeks for the effect (methylopa and guanethidine) to fade, during which time the cardiovascular status of the patient might further deteriorate, the possible advantages of such being far outweighed by this deterioration.

Largely as a result of studies in patients with severe hypertension, Prys-Roberts and his colleagues (1971a,b, 1972; Foex, Meloche and Prys-Roberts, 1971) have advocated control of the hypertension prior to anaesthesia. They recommend that the preoperative assessment of the patient should include examination of the electrocardiogram with the patient at rest and during exercise with monitoring of the ECG operatively. Patients should have their blood pressures stabilized by anti-hypertensive therapy before anaesthesia. IPPV and normocapnia should be employed. Halothane and pressor amines should be avoided, blood pressure being controlled by intravenous fluid therapy with central venous monitoring. A neurolept technique using agents such as Droperidol and Fentanyl with N_2O O_2 has the least effect on myocardial function. Laryngocardiac reflexes leading to cardiac dysrhythmias can be minimised by prior administration of β-adrenergic receptor blocking agents. Simpson (1978) has suggested a rational approach to the selection of patients requiring anti-hypertensive therapy. A diastolic blood pressure in excess of 110 mm Hg in patients less than 40 years of age, 115 mm Hg or more between 40 and 59 years and over 120 in patients 60 years or more is an indication of treatment. Where the diastolic blood pressures are in excess of 100 mm Hg, 105 mm Hg, 110 mm Hg in the respective age groups such therapy is advisable, but influenced by other factors such as symptoms, ECG heart size etc.

STEROIDS

For many it was the routine practice to give additional steroid cover for any patient undergoing surgery who had received steroid therapy within the two years preceeding the intended operation (Slaney and Brooke, 1957; Haller and Kirch-hoff, 1963). The rationale behind this approach was that a number of cases of cardiovascular collapse had been reported in relation to surgery where the patient had a history of being exposed to steroid therapy. One case of collapse even occurred after a single dose of intra-articular steroids. It was argued tha the pituitary-adrenal exis had lost the ability to respond to stress by sensitivity cortisol because of supression of adrenal cortical activity.

In a series of papers (Plumpton, Besser and Cole, 1969a,b) evidence was presented that not only was the past practice unnecessary but it was positively harmful. These workers suggested that collapse from adreno-cortical suppression is very unlikely to occur more than 2 months after cessation of steroid therapy and that routine cover need only be considered in patients who have received steroids since that time. Such routine cover should take the form of 100 mg intramuscular hydrocortisone hemisuccinate 6 hourly. This regime should be continued for 3 days following major surgery. If there is any doubt as to the ability of the adrenal cortex to respond to stress when a challenge using the synthetic polypeptide Synacthen may be employed. A 3–4 fold increase of plasma cortisol 30 min following the intramuscular injection of 250 μg Synacthen is indicative of a normal response to stress (Wood et al., 1965).

The contraceptive pill

In 1970 Vessey and his colleagues suggested that there may be a 3–4 fold increase in the risk of post-operative thromboembolism in women using oral contraceptives prior to surgery in comparison with those not doing so. A study by Greene and Sartwell in 1972 had shown a similar risk. As a result of this increased risk it seems reasonable to withdraw oral contraceptives 4–6 weeks prior to elective surgery. However, each surgeon or doctor advising the patient should make up his mind in each individual case as to whether or not this is a reasonable course of action. If the patient can be relied on to use an alternative method of contraception after withdrawal of the pill, then it would seem to be correct to advise her to stop. If on the other hand the chances of her getting pregnant before arriving in hospital are high, it would probably be best not to suggest any change in contraceptive practices.

Regardless as to which course of action is taken, the incidence of post-operative pulmonary embolism may be reduced by such measures as subcutaneous heparin, intravenous dextrans, and massage to the legs during operation. Regular digestion of oral contraceptives may reduce the level of plasma cholinesterase (Robertson, 1967), but not to the extent of significantly prolonging the response to suxamethonium.

NARCOTICS, SEDATIVES AND TRANQUILLIZERS

Phenothiazines. There is some evidence that phenothiazines can effect neuromuscular function. Argov and Yaari (1979) have suggested that chlorpromazine interferes with calcium ion fluxes at the nerve terminal, an action similar to that of magnesium ions. This action may account for the exacerbation of myasthenic state in myasthenia gravis (McQuillan, Gross and Johns, 1963). Depolarizing muscle relaxants should be used with caution in patients taking promazine (Regan and Aldrete, 1967). Methotrimeprazine (Veractil) has been reported to prolong tubocurarine-induced relaxation to prolonging the action of suxamethonium.

Benzodiazepines. It has been demonstrated that Diazepam may modify the action of gallamine and suxamethonium (Feldman and Crawley, 1970). However, Dretchen, Ghoneim and Long (1971) have been unable to substantiate this claim.

Recently Bradshaw and Maddison (1979) have shown that the intravenous administration of 0.16 mg · kg^{-1} diazepam had no effect on the depth and recovery from the block produced by suxamethonium, tubocurarine, pancuronium, fazadinium and alcuronium.

An interesting inter-reaction between diazepam and the H$_2$ receptor antagonist (cimetidine) has recently been reported. The two substances are not infrequently given together in the management of peptic ulceration and other gastric hyperacidity states. An increase in plasmadiazepam levels is associated with the administration of cimetidine (Klotz, Antilla and Reimann, 1979).

Barbiturates

The ability of the barbiturates to induce livr microsomal enzymes is well recognised. Fortunately the routine prescription of barbiturates in the United Kingdom is actively discouraged. However, chronic exposure to this group of drugs can lead to increased biotransformation of many substances. In particular, the formation of free fluoride as a result of the biodegradation of methoxyflurane increases the potentiality of kidney damage (Jones, 1972; Son, Colella and Brown, 1973).

The concomitant administration of pethidine (meperidine) and phenobarbitone has been shown to enhance the production of the toxic metabolite nor-pethidine by the increase in N-demethylation of pethidine resulting from the chronic exposure to phenobarbitone (Stambaugh, Hemphill, Wainer and Schwartz, 1977). Nor-pethidine apart from being more toxic than pethidine is less effective as an analgesic (Miller and Anderson, 1954) and is thought to be responsible for fetal depression (Morrison, Wiser and Rosser, 1973).

Monoamine oxidase inhibitors

Though the monoamine oxidase inhibitors (MAOIs) appeared likely to be superceded by the tricyclic antidepressants recent developments would suggest that this is an overoptimistic assessment. MAO is an important enzyme which is responsible for breaking down monoamines such as noradrenalines, tyramine, dopamine and 5-hydroxy tryptamine. The inhibition of MAO in the gut removes the protective mechanism whereby such active amines fas tyramine (present in cheese) are destroyed. These amines behave as indirectly acting sympathomimetic amines releasing nor adrenaline and causing hypertension.

Some MAOIs such as tranylcypromine and phenelzine are structurally similar to amphetamine and thus have indirect sympathomimetic activity which may cause hypertension. MAOIs are known to interact with a variety of drugs including tricyclic antidepressants, sympathomimetic amines, levodopa and analgesics. Pethidine, morphine, pentazocine, and phenazocine have been shown to lead to adverse reactions in patients receiving MAOIs.

Unconsciousness, hypotension, hypertension, hyperpyrexia, respiratory depression and death have all been reported. Experimental studies in mice pretreated with iproniazid and tranyl-cypromine have showed the acute toxicity to pentazocine is increased. (Rogers and Thornton, 1969). Subsequent studies in rabbits treated with pargyline indicate that pentazocine is safer than pethidine or morphine (Penn and Rogers, 1971).

The action of barbiturates is prolonged by MAOIs (Stockley, 1974). Patients on phenelzine have been found to have low plasma cholinesterase levels which rose on cessation of the drug therapy. One patient receiving phenelzine has been reported as having prolonged apnoea following the administration of suxamethonium (Bodley, Halwax and Potts, 1969). The sleeping time with inhalational anaesthetics is prolonged by monoamine oxidase inhibitors. Vasoconstrictor drugs can cause a catastrophic hypertensive episode in a patient on MAOI therapy. However MAO is not in the direct alternative pathway for the biodegraduation of adrenaline and nor-adrenaline. As this is provided by (catechol-O-methyl-transferase, COMT) it would appear reasonable to administer low concentrations of these particular pressor substances (Boakes et al., 1973).

The anaesthetist faced with a patient receiving MAOIs can either arrange for the discontinuation of therapy, in which case at least 3 weeks must elapse before any of the drugs known to cause adverse reactions can be given, or, alternatively proceed along the following lines. Avoid all narcotic analgesics, vasoconstrictors and pressor agents, postoperative analgesia being provided by "Entonox", trichloroethylene or methoxyflurane. Churchill Davidson (1965) has suggested a test whereby the possible adverse effects of pethidine can be assessed by noting the pulse, blood pressure and ventilation in response to incremental doses of the analgesic. All epidural and regional local anaesthetic solutions should have no additional adrenaline, noradrenaline or other similar vasoconstrictor added. Octapressin, a synthetic polypeptide with vasoconstrictor properties can however be used.

Tricyclic antidepressants

In 1972 Moir and his colleagues suggested that dysrhythmias may be responsible for sudden unexplained deaths in patients with cardiac disease who are taking tricy-clic antidepressants. It was postulated that these dysrhythmias may be due to sympathetic dominance as a result of the anticholinergic action of these drugs and their ability to block cataecholamine uptake.

Plowman and Thomas (1974) drew attention to prolonged cardiac dysrhythmias during general anaesthesia for oral surgery in two patients who were receiving halothane anaesthesia and were on medication with tricyclic antidepressants. If it is not possible to discontinue therapy it is suggested that halothane anaesthesia is best avoided and the patients closely monitored.

The administration of adrenaline, noradrenaline and similar pressor amines, to patients receiving tricyclic antidepressants is absolutely contraindicated (Boakes et al., 1973). Such patients attending for dental treatment under local anaesthesia present a particular problem as dental surgeons are in the habit of using local anaesthetic solutions containing adrenaline.

Fenfluramine (Ponderax). Fenfluramine, like amphetamine, is a cogener of adrenaline, and as such it has replaced the amphetamines in the United Kingdom in the management of obesity. Fenfluramine has both an α- and a β-stimulant action on blood vessels which results in a net fall in peripheral resistance, with a very slight fall in blood pressure which may be accentuated in patients receiving concurrent anti-hypertensive therapy (Waal-Manning and Simpson, 1969). The chronotropic and inotropic effects on the heart are said to be extremely mild. However, Bennett and Eltringham (1977) drew attention to the possibility that an interaction may exist between agents such as halothane and fenfluramine which may give rise to altered heart activity. They suggest that therapy with fenfluramine should be discontinued for a week prior to anaesthesia.

Levodopa. The introduction of therapy with levodopa has transformed the management of Parkinsonism. The symptoms of akinesia, rigidity and tremor arise because of a deficiency of dopamine in the basal ganglia. Levodopa a naturally occurring aromatic amino acid is the immediate precursor of dopamine. Levodopa, which can cross the blood-brain interface, is converted into dopamine with an alleviation of symptoms. Whilst dopamine has transformed the lives of many patients its side effects can give rise to difficulties such as abnormal movements, psychic and cardiovascular disturbances. These are apparently the result of increased formation of catecholamines centrally and peripherally. Inhibition of peripheral decarboxylase with hydrazine derivatives makes levodopa more available to the central nervous system, reduces the dose needed, and attenuates some of the peripheral side-effects. The combination of levodopa with a traditional anticholinergic such as benzhexol, or with carbidopa may sometimes be necessary.

As anaesthetists are being presented with more and more ageing patients, the opportunities of encountering a patient on levodopa therapy are increasing. Clinical doses of levodopa (1–2 g) do not usually affect blood pressure or heart rate however, the β-adrenergic receptors in the heart are stimulated (Whitsett and

Goldberg, 1972) possibly leading to an increased incidence of arrhythmias under halothane anaesthesia (Katz, Lord and Eakins, 1967). Hypotension during anaesthesia is another possibility and for these reasons the anaesthetist is advised to modify the therapy with levodopa prior to anaesthesia (Goldberg, 1972). Fortunately it has a relatively short half-life and the duration of the positive inotropic effect would appear to be approximately 2 hours. Ngai (1972) recommends that surgical patients being treated with levodopa therapy should be continued until the night before operation and resumed as soon as possible postoperatively. Excessive salivation leading to postoperative pulmonary complications may arise if the patient is deprived of levodopa therapy beyond the limits suggested by Ngai (1972). The anaesthetist should be reminded that the butyrophenones (haloperidol and droperidol) (Ngai and Wikland, 1972) and some phenothiazines may give rise to excessive rigidity particularly in Parkinsonian patients. Although cyclopropane and halothane are not absolutely contra-indicated in patients receiving levodopa therapy, they are possibly best avoided. If arrhythmias occur the use of β-adrenergic receptor blockade should be considered.

ANTICHOLINESTERASES

Situations where plasma cholinesterase activity is depressed or modified are likely to give rise to prolonged neuro-muscular blockade with suxamethonium. Pharmacologically induced depression of cholinesterase activity ranges from exposure to organophosphorous insecticides, nerve gases, cytotoxic and immunosuppressive drugs to agents used by the anaesthetists such as propanidid and tetrahydroaminacrine.

Immunosuppressives

Vetten (1973) has reported reduction in the potency of curare in patients receiving immunosuppressive therapy with azathioprine. The mechanism of this action is not clearly understood.

Wang and Ross (1963), Wolff (1965), Hone and Mathia (1967) and Gorman (1972) have reported prolonged apnoea after the intravenous infusion of suxamethonium in patients receiving anti-cancer agents such as AB-132 or cyclophosphamide. An in vitro study conducted by Zsigmond and Robins reported in 1972 has demonstrated that triethylenemelamine (TEM), cyclophosphamide (Cytoxan), mechlorethamine (Nitrogen Mustard) and triethylene thiophosphoramide (Thiotepa) have a significant anticholinesterase effect, TEM being more potent in this respect than Thiotepa.

Hexafluorenium (Mylaxen) The combination of hexafluorenium and suxamethonium decreases the amount of suxamethonium required (Foldes, 1960). The mode of action appears to be prevention of the rapid hydrolysis of suxamethonium. The mixture is said to eliminate the undesirable side-effects of suxamethonium such as fasciculations, increased intraocular pressure, and increases in serum potassium concentration (Radnay et al., 1979).

Ecothiopate iodide

Ecothiopate iodide eye drops are used to produce pupil constriction in cases of narrow angle glaucoma and sometimes in the management of squint in small children. McGavin (1965) suggested that prolonged action of suxamethonium might occur following the use of the latter drug in patients treated with ecothiopate iodide. In 1966 two such cases were reported (Pantuck, 1966; Gesztes, 1966).

Suxamethonium should be avoided in cases known to be receiving ecothiopate iodine eye drops, (Cavallero, Kruperman and Kugler, 1968). Alternatively 3–4 weeks interval from cessation of therapy before anaesthesia should be allowed to enable the cholinesterase levels to rise to normal values (De Roeth et al., 1965).

Tetrahydroaminacrine (Tacrine) This agent has been used to extend the effect of suxamethonium in clinical anaesthesia and therefore reduce the total dose of suxamethonium therapy lessening the intensity of dual-block. (McCaul and Robinson, 1962; Barrow and Smethurst, 1963; Smart, 1964; Spiers, 1966).

Propanidid (Epontol) This induction agent has been found to prolong the action of suxamethonium (Clarke, Dundee and Hamilton, 1967, Monks and Norman, 1972). Propanidid is broken down by an esterase and plasma cholinesterase activity is reduced after its administration (Doenicke et al., 1968). Recently, Taussig, Stojak and Bennett (1979) investigated this interaction under in vitro conditions. Propanidid was found to inhibit plasma cholinesterase as did suxamethonium. The binding of these drugs to specific anionic sites is thought to result in stereochemical changes in the enzyme.

Aprotinin ("Trasylol") This polypeptide derived from bovine lung tissue, is sometimes used as an inhibitor of proteolytic enzymes in the treatment of hyperfibrinolysis, acute pancreatitis and fat embolism. There have been reports of apparent potentiation of muscle relaxants by this agent (Chasapakis and Dimas, 1966; Marcello and Porati, 1967). As a result of in vitro studies Doenicke et al. (1970) concluded that aprotinin could lead to a lowering below the critical threshold only in those patients who have a pathologically depressed cholinesterase level.

Both pancuronium (Stovner, Oftedal and Holmboe, 1975) and Ketamine (Schuh, 1975) have been found to inhibit cholinesterase and as a result may influence the duration of apnoea following suxamethonium (Foldes et al., 1956), particularly in the case of Ketamine (Bovill et al., 1971).

MAGNESIUM SULPHATE

Magnesium sulphate is widely used throughout the world for the treatment of pre-eclamptic and eclamptic toxaemias. Magnesium causes a neuromuscular block by decreasing the amount of acetylcholine liberated. The administration of calcium, although increasing the release of acetylcholine does not necessarily reverse the neuromuscular blocking effect of magnesium because the sensitivity of the end plate for the depolarizing action of acetylcholine and the excitability of the muscle membrane are decreased (Enbaek, 1952; Del Castillo and Enbaek, 1954).

Ghoneim and Long (1970) and De Silva (1973) have reported a prolongation of the neuromuscular block produced by d-tubocurarine in patients receiving intra muscular and intravenous magnesium sulphate. Studies on the rat phrenic nerve-diaphragm preparation suggest that magnesium will potentiate the neuromuscular blocking effect produced by d-tubocurarine, decamethonium and succinylcholine. (Giesecke, Morris, Dalton and Stephen, 1968; Ghoneim and Long, 1970).

Neostigmine only partially reverses the action of curare when the serum magnesium level is greater than 35 mmol/litre (Horton 1975). It is suggested that neuromuscular blocking agents should be avoided in patients who are receiving therapy with magnesium sulphate.

LITHIUM

This agent has been employed by psychiatrists for the management of manic-depressive states since 1949. Lithium is initially distributed in total body water, but shifts intracellularly against a concentration gradient. As a cation it will displace both sodium and potassium causing marked losses of these ions from the body. Toxic symptoms, such as nausea, vomiting, diarrhoea, abdominal pain, thirst, dazed feelings, muscle weakness and hand tremors occur with concentrations of 1.6 mmol/l to 2.0 mmol/l. Lithium carbonate reportedly unmasks myasthenia gravis (Neil, Himmelhoch and Licata, 1976).

In 1974 Jephcott and Kerry reported a potentiation of barbiturate anaesthesia in a patient with toxic levels of lithium in the blood. In the same year Borden, Clarke and Katz drew attention to a patient on lithium therapy in whom there was prolonged neuromuscular blockade following the administration of pancuronium, in this instance the blood lithium levels were not in the toxic range. In 1976 Hill, Wong and Hodges noted potentiation of succinylcholine neuromuscular blockade in a patient receiving lithium carbonate. Subsequent studies in dogs confirmed that the effect of suxamethonium could be extended particularly if the blood levels of lithium are in the toxic range. The precise mechanism of this action has yet to be determined, but the drug is thought to act mainly as a presynaptic agent substituting lithium ions for sodium ions at the nerve terminal. Männistö and Saarnivaara (1976) have demonstrated prolongation of sleeping time induced by thiopentone, methohexitone, diazepam in mice given lithium. Hill, Wong and Hodges (1977) in studies with dogs have demonstrated interactions between lithium, succinylcholine, decamethonium, gallamine, d-tubocurarine and pancuronium.

Havdala, Borison and Diamond (1979) suggest that when anaesthetics are to be electively given to patients on lithium therapy the last two doses prior to the procedure are to be withheld. As most psychiatrists now control lithium dosage on the basis of plasma assay, and as such lithium levels are relatively easy to carry out, it is possible that the plasma level should be ascertained prior to anaesthesia. An interesting interaction has been reported by Pakes (1979) who has noted that the withdrawal of concomittant phenothiazine therapy (chlorpromazine) is associated with a rise in the lithium levels. This phenomenon is attributed to the fact that lithium is excreted more rapidly during simultaneous treatment with chlorpromazine (Sletten, Pichardo, Korol and Gershon 1966).

ANTIBIOTICS

The drugs most frequently implicated in druginduced neuro-muscular blockade, giving rise to post-operative respiratory depression, are the amino-glycoside group (neomycin, gentamicin, streptomycin, dihydrostreptomycin and kanamycin). The effects usually manifest themselves as failure to recover spontaneous ventilation in the immediate post-operative period. When administered before or during operation these drugs may enhance neuromuscular blockade induced by muscle relaxants but they may also cause respiratory depression after inhalational anaesthesia. The neuro-muscular block varies even from one antibiotic group to another or within the same chemical group.

The possibility that the administration of antibiotics could lead to neuromuscular blockade was first drawn to the attention of anaesthetists in 1957, when Vital Brazil and Corrado reported on the curariform action of streptomycin. Since that date at least a dozen antibiotics have been incriminated as leading to a prolonged neuromuscular blockade in patients subjected to anaesthesia, especially in patients who have received a neuromuscular blocking agent (Burkitt et al 1979).

Table 1. lists the antibiotics which have been incriminated.

TABLE 1.

ANTIBIOTICS	
AMIKACIN	Finland Brumfitt and Kass 1976; Hashimoto et al., 1978; Singh, Marshall and Harvey, 1978
BACITRACIN	Small, 1964; Pittinger, Eryasa and Adamson, 1970.
CLINDAMYCIN	Fogdall and Miller, 1974a,b. Becker and Miller, 1976; Wright and Collier, 1976b; Rubo, Gergis and Sokoll, 1977.
COLISTIN/COLYMYCIN	Perkins, 1964; Paris and Kaplan, 1965 Zauder et al., 1966; Pittinger, Eryasa and Adamson, 1970, Eppens and Kleine, 1971; Chinyanga and Stoyka, 1974.
GENTAMICIN	Vital Brazil and Prado-Franceschi, 1969a,b; Warner and Sanders, 1971; Hall et al., 1972; Chinyanga and Stoyka, 1974.
KANAMYCIN	Corrado, 1963; Hashimoto et al., 1971; Chinyanga and Stoyka, 1974; Noble, 1976; Paradelis et al., 1977.
LINCOMYCIN	Straw et al., 1965; Hashimoto et al., 1971; Daubeck, Doughety and Petty, 1974; Samuelson et al., 1975; Sokoll, Cronnelly and Gergis, 1975; Wright and Collier, 1976b; Rubo, Gergis and Sokoll, 1977.
NEOMYCIN	Pridgen, 1956; Middleton, Morgan and Moyers, 1957; Foldes, 1958; Pittinger and Long, 1958; Pittinger, Long and Miller, 1958; Corrado, Romas and De EscoDar, 1959; Elmquist and Josefsson, 1962; Markalous, 1962; Emery, 1963; Stanley, Giesecke and Jenkins, 1969; Vital Brazil and Prado-Franceschi, 1969b; Flacke, 1972; Lee et al., 1976; Weinstein, McHenery and Gavan, 1977. Wright and Collier, 1977; Lee and DeSilva, 1979a,b,
POLYMYXIN B	Timmerson, Long and Pittinger, 1959; Adamson, Marshall and Long, 1960; Small, 1964; Naiman and Martin, 1967; Lindesmith et al., 1968; Pittinger, Eryasa and Adamson, 1970; Pittinger and Adamson, 1972; Hsuchen and Faringold, 1973; Fogdall and Miller, 1974a. Lee et al., 1976; Van Nyhuis, Miller and Fogdall, 1976; Lee, Chen and Nagel, 1977; DeSilva and Lee, 1978; Lee and DeSilva, 1979b; Lee, DeSilva and Katz, 1978.
STREPTOMYCIN	Vital Brazil and Corrado 1957; Loder and Walker, 1959; Bush, 1961; Benz, Lunn and Foldes, 1961; Fisk, 1961; Bodley and Brett, 1962; Corrado, 1963; Bennetts, 1964; Pittinger and Adamson, 1972; Dretchen et al., 1973; Wright and Collier, 1977.
TOBRAMYCIN	Griffiths et al., 1976; Waterman and Smith, 1977; Boliston and Ashman, 1978.

General reading: McQuillen, M.P., Cantor, M.E. and O'Rourke, J.R. (1966): Myasthenic syndrome associated with antibiotics. *Arch. Neurol. 18*, 402-415.

Streptomycin and dihydrostreptomycin

In 1959 Loder and Walker described muscular weakness responding to neostigmine following injection of streptomycin into three patients who were not under anaesthesia.

This report was followed in 1961 by the independent reports (Fisk, 1961; Bush, 1961; Benz, Lunn and Foldes, 1961), where large doses of streptomycin were placed in serous cavities (peritoneal and pleural). This administration was followed by progressive paralysis. In a case reported by Bennetts in 1964 1 g of streptomycin was introduced into the serous cavity of a 1.9 kg anaesthetised infant and, despite the fact that no neuromuscular blocking agents were employed, respiratory paralysis ensued.

Streptomycin may exacerbate previously stable myasthenia gravis or may unmask a latent myasthenia (Argov and Mastaglia, 1979).

Mode of action

In common with most of the amino-glycoside antibiotics, streptomycin exerts a combined pre-synaptic and post-synaptic effect (Elmqvist and Josefsson, 1962), and as such produces an effect similar to that found with magnesium (Vital Brazil and Prado-Franceschi, 1969a,b; Pittinger and Adamson, 1972; Singh, Marshall and Harrey, 1979). The prejunctional role of streptomycin in decreasing the output of transmitter is less dominant than the post-synaptic effect which reduces the muscle motor end-plate response to acetylcholine (Lee and DeSilva, 1979a). In contrast to neomycin prolonged exposure to streptomycin does not change the characteristics of the block (Lee and DeSilva, 1979a).

Management and treatment of block

Streptomycin and dihydrostreptomycin are poorly reversed by neostigmine alone but in combination with calcium reversal can reach nearly 80% (Singh, Harvey and Marshall, 1978).

Neomycin. In 1956 Pridgen reported respiratory arrest in a patient which was thought to be due to intraperitoneal neomycin. Since that time there have been many reports of paralysis related to the administration of this amino-glycoside which is normally poorly absorbed from the gastrointestinal tract and largely excreted by the kidney. Caution should be exercised when using the drugs where renal excretion is impaired and where there is an increased chance of absorption from the intestine (ileus and other damage to the bowel). It has been employed as a constituent of fluids used to irrigate the bladder and peritoneal cavity and it is in this latter situation that problems have arisen as a result of its absorption.

It has been variously suggested that the mechanisms by which neuromuscular block are produced may be chelation of calcium (Corrado, Ramos and DeEscobar, 1959; Elmqvist and Josefsson, 1962; Corrado, 1963; Adriani, 1968), competition with calcium (Elmqvist and Josefsson, 1962; Adriani, 1968; Vital Brazil and Prado-Franceschi, 1969b) and curare-like properties (Elmqvist and Josefsson 1962). Lee, Chen, Barnes and Katz (1976) consider that the neuromuscular block is unique, despite nearly complete blockade of the twitch, the tetanus is not blocked and does not fade. Anticholinesterases and calcium antagonise the block but this antagonism may not be complete. Neomycin, the most potent neuromuscular blocking amino-glycoside, appears to produce its effect by a pre-dominantly pre-junctional action, decreasing the influx of calcium ions into the motor nerve terminal which in turn decreases the output of acetylcholine (Lee and DeSilva, 1979a). Flacke (1972) demonstrated that the characteristics of neuromuscular block changed over a 48-h period, the unique characteristics of neomycin-induced neuromuscular block giving way to a pattern of block usually observed with tubocurarine. Despite the difference in mode of action compared with the most potent polypeptide Polymyxin B these two antibiotics are additive in their neuromuscular blocking effects (Lee and DeSilva, 1979b).

Amikacin. This antibiotic is structurally related to the aminoglycoside group of antibiotics which included gentamicin, kanamycin, dibekacin, streptomycin, dihy-drostreptomycin and tobramycin. Hashimoto et al. (1978) suggests that amikacin sulphate may produce neuromuscular blockade in circumstances of overdosage or excessive absorption in myasthenia gravis. Singh, Marshall and Harvey (1978) confirm that this antibiotic blocks neuromuscular transmission and that this is reversed by calcium, 4-aminopyridine, 3,4-diaminopyridine and partially by neostigmine and suggest that care should be exercised if curare is also administered to the patient.

Bacitracin. Small (1964) reported respiratory paralysis in a patient after a large intraperitoneal dose of polymyxin B and bacitracin. Such paralysis has since been noted by Pittinger, Eryasa and Adamson (1970).

Clindamycin. Fogdall and Miller (1974b) reported on the prolongation of pancuronium induced neuromuscular blockade by clindamycin, an antibiotic closely related chemically to lincomycin. Becker and Miller (1976) concluded from studies in the guinea pig that clindamycin may augment neuromuscular blockade in man and that antagonism by calcium and neostigmine may be incomplete. Rubbo, Gergis and Sokol (1977) suggest that clindamycin produces its effect by blocking post-synaptic transmission. It is possible that in addition to this effect clindamycin decreases muscle contractility (Singh, Marshall and Harvey, 1978), and produces a pre-synaptic local anaesthetic effect (Samuelson et al., 1975; Singh, Marshall and Harvey, 1979).

Colymycin. Chingyanga and Stoyka (1974) have demonstrated that this poly-peptide antibiotic, although less potent than gentamicin and kanamycin in producing neuromuscular blockade, nevertheless potentiates the effect of pan-curonium. This antibiotic, otherwise known as colisitin is polymyxin E. Colisti-methate is colistin sodium methane sulphonate. Perkins (1964), Paris and Kaplan (1965) and Zauder et al. (1966) noted neuromuscular blockade leading to apnoea in patients under treatment with this drug. This substance has also been incriminated in prolonging the action of curare (Gebbie, 1971). There is conflicting evidence as to the mode of action of colistin but it is likely that it produces its effect by a combined pre- and post-synaptic effect. Gebbie (1971) was unable to fully reverse its effects iwth neostigmine and calcium.

Gentamicin. In 1971 Eppens and Kleine, Warner and Sanders reported prolongation of the neuromuscular blocking effect by Gentamicin. A study by Chinyanga and Stoyka (1974) confirmed this action and demonstrated resistance to reversal of the neuromuscular blockade by both calcium and neostigmine suggesting the multifocal nature of the block. Subsequent studies by Singh Harvey and Marshall (1978) suggested a blockade similar to that experienced with magnesium in that it acts by inhibiting the carriage of calcium across the pre-synaptic membrane thus preventing the release of adequate acetylcholine. Contrary to the findings of Chinyanga and Stoyka (1974), Singh and Harvey found almost complete reversal with calcium and neostigmine. It is important to realize that the defect is one of calcium transport and not calcium depletion. For this reason it is not likely that calcium gluconate administration will always be successful in reversing block produced by gentamicin.

Kanamycin. Again in 1971 Eppens and Kleine and Hashimoto et al reported on the neuromuscular blocking action of kanamycin. Noble (1976) described a case of respiratory insufficiency incompletely reversed by calcium arising in a patient who had received an intraperitoneal dose of kanamycin. It would appear that its neuro-muscular blocking action is similar to that of the previously mentioned amino-glycoside gentamicin, in that calcium and neostigmide has a variable effect in reversing neuro-muscular blockade (Singh, Harvey and Marshall 1978).

Lincomycin. Neuromuscular blockade with lincomycin has been reported by Straw et al., 1965; Tang and Schroeder, 1968; Samuelson et al., 1975. Studies by Rubbo, Gergis and Sokoll in 1977 suggest that this block occurs through a pre-synaptic local anaesthetic action but at high concentrations lincomycin has a nerve terminal depressant effect. Singh, Marshall and Harvey (1979) suggest that it has greater postjunctional and less prejunctional activity relative to streptomycin.

Polymyxin B. This is the most potent of the polypeptide antibiotics and is notoriously difficult to reverse (Timmerman, Long and Pittinger, 1959; Adamson, Marshall and Long, 1960; Naiman and Martin, 1967; Fogdall and Miller, 1974a). There is conflicting evidence as to the mode of action of the neuromuscular block but it is possible that there is a combined pre- and post-synaptic affect although Rubbo, Gergis and Sokol (1977) take the view that post-synaptic block is the predominant effect. Like lincomycin, Singh, Marshall and Harvey (1979) conclude that polymixin has greater postjunctional and less prejunctional blocking activity relative to streptomycin. It has a synergistic effect with neomycin (Lee and DeSilva, 1979a,b). DeSilva and Lee (1978) found that prolonged exposure of cats to polymyxin B did not result in a change in the nature of the neuromuscular block as has been found with neomycin (Flacke, 1972). It can also produce a profound and protracted cardiovascular depression. In view of the fact that neostigmine further potentiates the neuromuscular blockade by polymyxin B (Nyhuis, Miller and Fogdall, 1976), the temptation to try anticholinesterase drugs should be resisted (Lee, Chen and Nagel, 1977). However, Lee, DeSilva and Katz (1978), on the basis of studies in the cat, suggest that 4-aminopyridine is an effective antidote to neuro-muscular blockade.

Tobramycin. Studies by Griffiths et al. (1976) and Boliston and Ashman (1978) in patients receiving intravenous tobramycin suggested that there is no evidence that tobramycin potentiates the effect of neuromuscular blocking agents. However, Waterman and Smith (1977) reported a case of recurarisation following intravenous tobramycin, this effect was reversed with neostigmine.

OTHER ANTIBIOTICS

Tetracyclines may produce a post-synaptic block (Rubbo, Gergis and Sokol, 1977). Oxytetracycline (Wullen, Kast and Buck, 1967) and rolitetracycline (Gibbels, 1967) may aggravate myasthenia gravis. Although ampicillin and erythromycin are generally accepted as safe in myasthenia gravis there is some electromyographic evidence that these drugs may interfere with neuromuscular transmission (Hersishanu and Taustein, 1971). D-penicillamine is sometimes employed in the long term management of rheumatoid arthritis. A clinically indistinguishable syndrome from classical myasthenia gravis has been reported (Buchnall, 1977). It is thought that this block is an immunologically mediated reaction against the motor end-plate by the production of specific antibiodies to the acetyl choline receptor.

The penicillins, cephalosporins, vancomycin, colstimethate, polymyxin and the aminoglycosides are almost entirely excreted via the kidneys. It is suggested however

(Noone et al., 1978) that, provided therapy is carefully monitored, they are affective and safe in patients with severely impaired renal function. Care should also be exercised when employing agents which are predominantly excreted via the liver (chloramphenicol, tetracyclines, lincomycin, erythromycin and rifamycin).

Cardiovascular effects of antibiotics

Antibiotics are being increasingly administered during anaesthesia as bolus injections and continuous infusions, particularly in association with emergency intestinal surgery.

Amino-glycoside antibiotics produce direct cardiac depression and potentiate the depression produced by halothane (Swain, Kiplinger and Brody, 1956; Cohen, Wechsler, Mitchell and Glick, 1970; Adams, 1975a,b; Adams, 1976; Sohn and Katz, 1977). Sohn and Katz (1978) have demonstrated a concentration dependent myocardial depression which can be reversed by calcium.

Streptomycin, neomycin, amikacin, gentamicin, and tobramycin produce dose-related blockade of sympathetic ganglia. Corrado (1958), Fisk (1961), Ramos et al. (1962), Pandey, Kumar and Badola (1964), Wright and Collier (1974), Brogden et al. (1975), Singh, Marshall and Harvey (1978) have demonstrated that the blocking effect of amikacin on sympathetic ganglia can be reversed by calcium.

Several cases of cardiac arrest have been reported as occurring in association with the administration of lincomycin (Waisbren, 1968; Daubeck, Daughety and Petty, 1974). The latter workers suggested from studies in dogs that the arrest was likely to result from a quinidine action on the myocardium Lee, Chen and Nagel (1977) have observed a profound and protracted cardio-vascular depression with polymyxin B in the cat and have subsequently reported partial reversal by 4-aminopyridine. (Lee, DeSilva and Katz, 1978). Sohn and Katz (1979) have attempted to ascertain the cause of this cardiovascular depression with polymixin. Studies on isolated rat heart muscle suggest that depression of the myocardium does not occur with clinical doses.

REFERENCES

Adams, H.R. (1975a): Cardiovascular depressant effects of the neomycin streptomycin group of antibiotics. *Amer. J. Vet. Res., 36*, 103-108.

Adams, H.R. (1975b): Direct myocardial depressant effects of gentamicin. *Europ J. Pharmacol., 30*, 272-279.

Adams, H.R. (1976): Antibiotic-induced alterations of cardiovascular reactivity. *Fed. Proc., 35*, 1148-1150.

Adams, H.R., Matthew, B.P., Teske, R.H. and Mercer, R.D. (1976): Neuromuscular blocking effects of aminoglycoside antibiotics on fast- and slow-contracting muscles of the cat. *Anesth. Analg. Curr. Res., 55*, 500-507.

Adamson, R.H., Marshall, F.N. and Long, J.P. (1960): Neuromuscular blocking properties of various polypeptide antibiotics. *Proc. Soc. exp. Biol. Med. 105*, 494-497.

Adriani, J. (1968): *Appraisal of Current Concepts in Anaesthesiology*. Mosby, St. Louis, p. 139.

Argov, Z. and Mastaglia, F.L. (1979): Disorder of neuromuscular transmission caused by drugs. *New Eng. J. Med. 301*, 409-413.

Argov, Z. and Yaari, Y. (1979): The action of chlorpromazine at an isolated cholinergic synapse. *Brain Res., 164*, 227-336.

Barrow, M.E.H. and Smethurst, J.R. (1963): Suxamethonium modified by tetrahydroaminacrine. *Brit. J. Anaesth. 35*, 465-472.

Becker, L.D. and Miller, R.D. (1976): Clindamycin enhances a non-depolarizing neuromuscular blockade. *Anesthesiology, 45*, 84-87.

Bennett, J.A. and Eltringham, R.J. (1977): Possible dangers of anaesthesia in patients receiving fenfluramine. Results of animal studies following a case of human cardiac arrest. *Anaesthesia, 32*, 8-13.

Bennetts, F.E. (1964): Muscular paralysis due to streptomycin following inhalation anaesthesia. *Anaesthesia, 19*, 93-95.

Benz, H.G., Lunn, J.N. and Foldes, F.F. (1961): Recurarisation by intraperitoneal antibiotics. *Brit. med. J., 2*, 241-242.

Boakes, A.J., Laurence, D.R., Teoh, P.C., Barar, F.S.K., Benedikter, L.T. and Prichard, B.N.C. (1973): Interactions between sympathomimetic amines and antidepressant agents in man. *Brit. med. J., 1*, 311-315.

Bodley, P.O., Brett, J.E. (1962): Postoperative respiratory inadequacy and the part played by antibiotics. *Anaesthesia, 17*, 438.

Bodley, P.O., Halwax, K. and Potts, L. (1969): Low serum pseudo cholinesterase levels complicating treatment with phenelzine. *Brit. med. J., 3*, 510-512.

Boliston, T.A. and Ashman, R. (1978): Tobramycin and neuromuscular blockade. *Anaesthesia, 33*, 552.

Borden, H., Clarke, M.T. and Katz, H. (1974): The use of pancuronium bromide in patients receiving lithium carbonate. *Canad. Anaesth. Soc. J., 21*, 79-82.

Bovill, J.G., Dundee, J.W., Coppel, D.C. and Moore, J. (1971): Current status of ketamine anaesthesia. *Lancet, 1*, 1285.

Bradshaw, E.G. and Maddison, S. (1979): Effect of diazepam at the neuromuscular junction. A clinical study. *Brit. J. Anaesth. 51*, 955-960.

Brogden, R.N., Pinder, R.M., Sawyer, P.R., Speight, T.M. and Avery, G.S. (1976): Tobramycin: A review of its antibacterial and pharmacokinetic properties and therapeutic use. *Drugs, 12*, 166-200.

Buchnall, R.C. (1977): Myasthenia associated with D-penicillamine therapy in rheumatoid arthritis. *Proc.Roy. Soc. Med., 70*. Suppl. 3, 114-117.

Burkitt, L., Bikhazi, G.B., Thomas, K.C., Rosenthal, D.A., Wirta, M.G. and Foldes, F.F. (1979): Mutual potentiation of the neuromuscular effects of antibiotics and relaxants. *Anesth. Analg. Curr. Res. 58*, 107-115.

Bush, G.H. (1961): Prolonged neuromuscular block due to intraperitoneal streptomycin. *Brit. med. J. 1*, 557-558.

Cavallero, R.J., Krumperman, L.W. and Kugler, F. (1968): Effect of ecothiopate therapy on the metabolism of succinylcholine in man. *Anesth. Analg. Curr. Res., 47*, 570-574.

Chasapakis, G. and Dimas, G. (1966): Possible interaction between muscle relaxants and the kallikrein-trypsin inactivator "Trasylol": Report of three cases. *Brit. J. Anaesth. 38*, 408-409.

Chinyanga, M.M. and Stoyka, W.W. (1974): The effect of Colymycin M, Gentamicin and Kanamycin on depression of neuromuscular transmission induced by pancuronium bromide. *Canad. Anaesth. Soc. J., 21*, 569-579.

Churchill-Davidson, H.C. (1965): Anaesthesia and mono-amine oxidase inhibitors. *Brit. med. J., 1*, 520.

Clarke, R.S.J., Dundee, J.W. and Hamilton, R.C. (1967): Interactions between induction agents and muscle relaxants: clinical observations. *Anaesthesia, 22*, 235-248.

Cohen, L.S., Wechsler, A.S., Mitchell, J.H. and Glick, G. (1970): Depression of cardiac function by streptomycin and other antimicrobial agents. *Amer. J. Cardiol., 26*, 505-511.

Corrado, A.P. (1958): Ganglioplegic action of streptomycin. *Arch. int. Pharmacodyn. Ther., 114*, 166.

Corrado, A.P. (1963): Respiratory depression due to antibiotics: Calcium in treatment. *Anesth. Analg. Curr. Res., 42*, 1-5.

Corrado, A.P. and Ramos, A.O. (1958): Neomycin – its curariform and ganglioplegic action. *Rev. Brasil. Biol., 18*, 81.

Corrado, A.P., Ramos, A.O. and DeEscobar, C.T. (1959): Neuromuscular blockade by neomycin: potentiation by ether anaesthesia and *d*-tubocurarine and antagonism by calcium and prostigmine. *Arch. int. Pharmacodyn. Ther., 12*, 380.

Dale, R.C. and Schroeder, E.T. (1976): Respiratory paralysis during treatment of hypertension with trimetaphan camsylate. *Arch. int. Med., 136*, 816-818.

Daubeck, J.L., Daughety, M.J. and Petty, C. (1974): Lincomycin-induced cardiac arrest: A case report and laboratory investigation. *Anesth. Analg. Curr. Res., 53*, 563-567.

Del Castillo, J. and Enbaek, L. (1954): The nature of neuromuscular block produced by magnesium. *J. Physiol., 124*, 370-384.

De Roetth, A., Dettbarn, W.D., Rosenberg, P., Wilensky, J.G. and Wong, A. (1965): Effect of phospholine iodide on blood cholinesterase levels of normal and glaucoma subjects. *Amer. J. Ophthalmol., 59*, 586-591.

DeSilva, A.J.C. (1973): Magnesium intoxication: an uncommon cause of prolonged curarization. *Brit. J. Anaesth. 45*, 1228-1229.

DeRosayro, M. and Healy, T.E.J. (1978): Tobramycin and neuromuscular transmission in the rat isolated phrenic nerve-diaphragm preparation. *Brit. J. Anaesth., 50*, 251-254.

DeSilva, A.J.C. and Lee, C. (1978): Neuromuscular and cardiovascular depression produced by prolonged exposure to polymixin B. *Canad. Anaesth. Soc. J. 25*, 303-306.

Dingle, H.R. (1966): Antihypertensive drugs and anaesthesia. *Anaesthesia, 21*, 151-172.

Doenicke, A., Krumey, I., Kugler, J. and Klempa, J. (1968): Experimental studies of the breakdown of epontol: determination of propanidid in human serum. *Brit. J. Anaesth. 40*, 415-429.

Doenicke, A., Gesing, H., Krumey, I. and Schmidinger, St. (1970): Influence of aprotinin (trasylol) on the action of suxamethonium. *Brit. J. Anaesth., 42*, 943-960.

Drachman, D.A. and Skom, J.H. (1965): Procainamide – a hazard in myasthenia gravis. *Arch. Neurol. 13*, 316-320.

Drachman, D.B., Angus, C.W., Adams, R.N., Michelson, J.D. and Hoffmann, C.J. (1978): Myasthenic antibodies cross-link acetylcholine receptors to accelerate degradation. *New Engl. med. J. Med., 298*, 116-1122.

Dretchen, K., Ghoneim, H.M. and Long, J.P. (1971): The interaction of diazepam with myoneural blocking agents. *Anesthesiology, 34*, 463-468.

Dretchen, K.L., Sokoll, M.D. and Gergis, S.D. (1973): Relative effects of streptomycin on motor nerve terminal and end plate. *Europ. J. Pharmacol. 22*, 10-16.

Dretchen, K.L., Morgenroth, V.H., Standaert, E.G. Walts, L.F. (1976): Azothioprine. Effects on neuromuscular transmission. *Anesthesiology, 45*, 604-609.

Doll, D.C. and Rosenberg, H. (1979): Antagonism of neuromuscular blockage by theophylline. *Anesth.
Analg. Curr. Res., 58*, 139-140.

Drury, P.J. and Healy, T.E.J. (1975): Neuromuscular transmission and gentamicin. In: *Recent Progress
in Anaesthesiology and Resuscitation. Proceedings of the IVth European Congress of Anaesthesiology. Madrid, September 5–11, 1974).* Excerpta Medica, Amsterdam, p. 276.

Elmqvist, D, and Josefsson, J.O. (1962): The nature of neuromuscular block produced by neomycin.
Acta Physiol. Scand., 54, 104.

Emery, E.R.J. (1963): Neuromuscular blocking properties of antibiotics as a cause of post-operative
apnoea. *Anaesthesia, 18*, -65.

Enbaek, L. (1952): The pharmacological actions of magnesium ions with particular reference to the
neuromuscular and cardiovascular system. *Pharmacol. Rev., 4*, 396.

Eppens, H. and Kleine, J.W. (1971): Antibiotics and muscle relaxants: a dangerous combination. *Arch.
Chir. Neerl., 23*, 421.

Feldman, S.A. (1963): Effect of changes in electrolytes, hydration and pH upon the reaction to muscle
relaxants. *Brit. J. Anaesth. 35*, 546-551.

Feldman, S.A. (1979): Acute and chronic changes in intra – and extra-cellular potassium and responses
to neuromuscular blocking agents. *Surv. Anesth. 23*, 227.

Feldman, S.A. and Crawley, B.E. (1970): Diazepam and muscle relaxants. *Brit. med. J., 1*, 691.

Finland, M., Brumfitt, W. and Kass, E.H. (1976): Advances in aminoglycoside therapy: amikacin. *J.
infect. Dis., 134*, (Suppl.) S.242.

Fisk, G.C. (1961): Respiratory paralysis after a large dose of streptomycin. *Brit. med. J., 1*, 556.

Flacke, W.E. (1972): Acute and subchronic effects of neomycin on neuromuscular transmission. *Fifth
Int. Congr. Pharmacol.* San Francisco, p. 69.

Fogdall, R.P. and Miller, R.D. (1974a): Prolongation of a pancuronium-induced neuromuscular blockade by clindamycin. *Anesthesiology, 41*, 407-408.

Fogdall, R.P. and Miller, R.D. (1974b): Prolongation of a pancuronium-induced neuromuscular blockade by polymixin B. *Anesthesiology, 40*, 84-87.

Foldes, F.F., Lipschitz, E., van Hees, G.R. and Spanor, S.P. (1956): The influence of liver disease on the
enzymatic hydrolysis of succinylcholine. *Anesthesiology, 17*, 550.

Foldes, F.F. (1958): Neomycin block. *Anaesthesia, 13*, 191.

Foldes, F.F. (1960): Remarks on the potentiation of succinylcholine by hexafluorenium. *Anesth. Analg.
Curr. Res. 39*, 47-49.

Föex, P., Meloche, R. and Prys-Roberts, C. (1971): Studies of anaesthesia in relation to hypertension.
III. Pulmonary gas exchange during spontaneous ventilation. *Brit. J. Anaesth. 43*, 644-661.

Gebbie, D. (1971): Colismethate and curare: a case report. *Anesth. Analg. Curr. Res. 50*, 109-111.

Gesztes, T. (1966): Prolonged apnoea after suxamethonium injection associated with eye drops containing anticholinesterase agent: a case report. *Brit. J. Anaesth. 38*, 408.

Ghoneim, M.M. and Long, J.P. (1970): The interaction between magnesium and other neuromuscular
blocking agents. *Anesthesiology, 32*, 23-27.

Gibbels, E. (1967): Beobachtungen zum Nebenwirkung intravenoser Reverin-Gaben bei Myasthenia
Gravis pseudoparalytica. *Dtsch. med. Wschr., 92*, 1153-1154.

Giesecke, A.H., Morris, R.E., Dalton, M.D. and Stephen, N.C.R. (1968): of magnesium, muscle relaxants, toxaemic parturients and cats. *Anesth. Analg. Curr. Res. 47*, 689-695.

Glisson, S.N., El-Etr, A.A. and Lim, R. (1979): Prolongation of pancuronium-induced neuromuscular
blockade by intravenous infusion of nitroglycerin. *Anesthesiology, 51*, 47-49.

Goldberg, L.I. (1962): Anesthetic management of patients treated with antihypertensive agents or levo-dopa. *Anesth. Analg. Curr. Res., 51*, 625-632.

Gorman, G.M. (1972): Prolonged apnea after succinylcholine in a case treated with cytostatics for cancer. *Anesth. Analg. Curr. Res., 51*, 761-765.

Greene, G.R. and Sartwell, P.E. (1972): Oral contraceptive use in patients with thromboembolism following surgery, trauma or infection. *Amer. J. publ. Health, 62*, 680-685.

Griffiths, D.A., Shorey, B.A., Simpson, R.A., Speller, D.C.E. and Williams, N.B. (1976): Single dose preoperative prophylaxis in gastro-intestinal surgery. *Lancet, 2*, 325-328.

Grogono, A.W. (1963): Anaesthesia for atrial defibrillation: effect to quinidine on muscular relaxation. *Lancet, 2*, 1039-1040.

Hall, D.R., McGibbon, D.H., Evans, C.C. and Meadows, G.A. (1972): Gentamicin, tubocurarine lignocaine and neuromuscular blockade. *Brit. J. Anaesth., 44*, 1329-1332.

Haller, J. and Kirchhoff, H. (1963): Post-operative collapse as a result of steroid induced adrenal gland insufficiency. *Zentbl. Gynek., 85*, 1283.

Harrah, M.D., Way, W.L. and Katzung, B.G. (1970): The interaction of *d*-tubocurarine with anti-arrhythmic drugs. *Anesthesiology, 33*, 406-410.

Hashimoto, Y., Iwatsuki, N. and Shima, T., (1971): Neuromuscular blocking properties of lincomycin and kanamycin in man. *Jap. J. Anesth. 20*, 407.

Hashimoto, Y., Shima, T., Masukawa, S. and Satou, M. (1978): A possible hazard of prolonged neuromuscular blockade by amikacin. *Anesthesiology, 49*, 219-220.

Havdala, H.S., Borison, R.L., Diamond, B.I. (1979): Potential hazards and application of lithium in anesthesiology. *Anesthesiology, 50*, 534-537.

Herishanu, Y. and Taustein, I. (1971): The electrocardiographic changes induced by antibiotics: a preliminary study. *Confin. Neurol., 33*, 41-45.

Herishanu, Y. and Rosenberg, P. 1975. Beta blockers and myasthenia gravis. *Ann. int. Med., 83*, 834-835.

Hill, G.E., Wong, K.C. and Hodges, M.P. (1976): Potentation of succinycholine neuromuscular blockade by lithium carbonate. *Anesthesiology, 44*, 439-442.

Hill, G.E., Wong, K.C. and Hodges, M.R. (1977): Lithium carbonate and neuromuscular blocking agents. *Anesthesiology, 46*, 122-126.

Hill, G.E., Wong, K.C., Shaw, C.L. and Blatnick, R.A. (1978): Acute and chronic changes in intra- and extra-cellular potassium and responses to neuromuscular blocking agents. *Anesth. Analg. Curr. Res., 57*, 417-421.

Horton, J.A.G. (1975): Drug interactions and anaesthesia. *Adv. Drug React. Bull.,* No. 50.

Hsuchen, C.C. and Faringold, D.S. (1973): The mechanism of polymixin B action and selectivity toward biologic membranes. *Biochemistry, 12*, 2105-2111.

Hughes, R.O. and Zacharias, F.J. (1976): Myasthenic syndrome during treatment with practolol. *Brit. med. J. 1*, 460-461.

Jephcott, G. and Kerry, R.J. (1974): Lithium: an anaesthetic risk. *Brit. J. Anaesth., 46*, 389-390.

Jones, N.O. (1972): Methoxyfluorane nephrotoxicity − a review and a case report. *Canad. Anaesth. Soc. J., 19*, 152.

Katz, R., Lord, C.O. and Eakins, K.E. (1967): Anesthetic-dopamine cardiac arrhythmias and their prevention by beta-adrenergic blockade. *J. Pharm. exp. Ther. 158*, 40-45

Klotz, U., Antilla, V.-J. and Reimann, I. (1979): Cimetidine/Diazepam interaction. *Lancet, 2*, 699.

Kornfeld, P., Horowitz, S.H., Genkins, G. (1976): *Myasthenia gravis* unmasked by antiarrhythmic agents. *Mount Sinai J. Med. N.Y., 43*, 10-14.

Kyei-Mensah, K. and Thornton, J.A. (1974): The incidence of medical disease in surgical patients. *Brit. J. Anaesth., 46*, 570-574.

Lee, C., Chen, D., Barnes, A. and Katz, R.L. (1976): Neuromuscular block by neomycin in the cat. *Canad. Anaesth. Soc. J., 23*, 527-533.

Lee, C., Chen, D. and Nagel, E.N. (1977): Neuromuscular block by antibiotics: Polymyxin B. *Anesth. Analg. Curr. Res., 56*, 373-377.

Lee, C. and DeSilva, A.J.C. (1979a): Acute and sub-chronic neuromuscular blocking characteristics of streptomycin: a comparison with neomycin. *Brit. J. Anaesth. 51*, 431-434.

Lee, C. and DeSilva, A.J.C. (1979b): Interaction of neuromuscular blocking effects of neomycin and polymixin B. *Anaesthesiology, 50*, 218-220.

Lee, C., DeSilva, A.J.C. and Katz, R.L. (1978): Antagonism of polymyxin B-induced neuromuscular and cardiovascular depression by 4-amidopyridine in the anaesthetized cat. *Anesthesiology, 49*, 256-259.

Lee, C., Ricker, S. and Katz, R.L. (1979): Autonomic block, cardiovascular depression and histamine release produced by Polymyxin B in the cat. *Canad. Anaesth. Soc. J. 26*, 191-200.

Lindesmith, L.A., Baines, R.D., Bigelow, D.B. and Petty, T.L. (1968): Reversible respiratory paralysis associated with polymyxin therapy. *Ann. int. Med., 68*, 318-327.

Loder, R.E. and Walker, G.F. (1959): Neuromuscular blocking action of streptomycin. *Lancet, 1*, 812-813.

Marcello, B. and Porati, N. (1967): Trasylol e blocc neuromuscalare. *Minerva anest. (Torino), 33*, 814.

McCaul, K. and Robinson, G.D. (1962): Suxamethonium "extension" by tetra hydroaminacrine. *Brit. J. Anaesth., 34*, 536-542.

McGavin, D.D.M. (1965): Depressed levels of serum-pseudocholinesterase with ecothiopate iodide eye-drops. *Lancet, 2*, 272.

McQuillen, M.P., Cantor, H.E. and O'Rourke, J.R. (1968): Myasthenic syndrome associated with antibiotics. *Arch. Neurol., 18*, 402-415.

McQuillen, M.P., Gross, M. and Johns, R.J. (1963): Chlorpromazine-induced weakness in myasthenia gravis. *Arch. Neurol. 8*, 286-290.

Mann, L.S. and Levin, M.J. (1960): Respiratory depression with intraperitoneal neomycin. *Arch. Surg., 81*, 690-698.

Männistö, P.T. and Saarnivaara, L. (1976): Effect of lithium and rubidium on the sleeping time caused by various intravenous anaesthetics in the mouse. *Brit. J. Anaesth., 48*, 185-189.

Markakous, P. (1962): Respiration and the intraperitoneal application of neomycin and neolymphin. *Anaesthesia, 17*, 427-437.

Middleton, W.H., Morgan, D.D. and Moyers, S.J. (1957): Neostigmine therapy for apnoea occurring after administration of neomycin. Report of a case. *J. Amer. med. Assoc., 165*, 2186-2187.

Miller, J.W. and Anderson, H.H. (1954): Effect of N-demethylation on certain pharmacologic actions of morphine, codeine and meperidine in the mouse. *J. Pharmacol. exp. Ther., 112*, 191-196.

Miller, R.D., Sohn, Y.J. and Matteo, R.S. (1976): Enhancement of d-tubocurarine neuromuscular block-ade by diuretics in man. *Anesthesiology, 45*, 442-445.

Miller, R.D., Way, W.K. and Katzung, B.G. (1967): Potentiation of neuromuscular blocking agents by quinidine. *Anesthesiology, 28*, 1036-1041.

Moir, D.C., Crooks, J., Cornwell, W.B., O'Malley, K., Dingwall-Fordyce, I., Turnbull, M.J. and Weir, R.D. (1972): Cardiotoxicity of amitripyline. *Lancet, 2*, 561-564.

Mone, J.G. and Mathie, W.E. (1967): Qualitative and quantitative defects of cholinesterase activity. *Anaesthesia, 22*, 55-68.

24

Monks, P.S. and Norman, J. (1972): Prolongation of suxamethoniuminduced paralysis by propanidide. *Brit. J. Anaesth., 44*, 1303-1305.

Morrison, J.C., Wiser, W.L. and Rosser, S.A., Gayden, J.O., Bucovaz, E.T., Whybrew, W.D. and Fish, S.A. (1973): Metabolites of meperidine related to fetal depression. *Amer. J. Obstet. Gyn., 115*, 1132.

Naiman, J.G. and Martin, J.D. (1967): Some aspects of neuromuscular block by polymixin B. *J. Surg. Res., 7*, 199-206.

Neill, J.F., Himmelhoch, J.M. and Licata, S.M. (1976): Emergence of myasthenia gravis during treatment with lithium carbonate. *Arch. gen. Psych., 33*, 1090-1092.

Noble, R.C. (1976): Respiratory insufficiency after intraperitoneal administration of kanamycin: Failure of calcium gluconate to reverse toxic effects. *Sth. med. J., 69*, 1212-1219.

Noone, P., Beale, D.F., Pollock, S.S., Perera, M.R., Amirak, I.D., Fernando, O.N. and Moorhead, J.F. 1978. Monitoring aminoglycoside use in patients with severely impaired renal function. *Brit. med. J., 2*, 470-473.

Ngai, S.H. (1972): Parkinsonism, Levodopa and Anaesthesia. *Anesthesiology, 37*, 344-351.

Ngai, S.H. and Wiklund, R.A. (1972): Levodopa and surgical anaesthesia. *Neurology, 22 (Suppl)*, 38-42.

Nyhuis, L.S. van., Miller R.D. and Fogdall, R.P. (1976): The interaction between d-Tubocurarine, pancuronium, Polymyxin B and neostigmine on neuromuscular function. *Anesth. Analg. Curr. Res., 55*, 224-228.

Pakes, G.E. (1979): Lithium toxicity with phenothiazine withdrawal. *Lancet, 2*, 701.

Pandey, K., and Kumar, S. and Badola, R.P. (1964): Neuromuscular blocking and hypotensive actions of streptomycin and their reversal. *Brit. J. Anaesth. 36*, 19-26.

Pantuck, E.J. (1966): Ecothiopate iodide eyedrops and prolonged response to suxamethonium: a case report. *Brit. J. Anaesth. 37*, 406.

Paradelis, A.G., Triantaphyllidis, C. and Markomichelakis, J.M. (1977): The neuromuscular blocking activity of aminodeocykanamycin as compared with that of other aminoglycoside antibiotics. *Arzneimittel-Forsch., 27*, 141-143.

Paris, A.F. and Kaplan, M.M. (1965): Apnoea during treatment with sodium colisimethate. *J. Amer. med. Assoc., 194*, 298-299.

Penn, R.G. and Rogers, K.J. (1971): Comparison of the effects of morphine, pethidine and pentazocine in rabbits pretreated with a MAOI. *Brit. J. Pharmacol., 42*, 485.

Perkins, R.L. (1964): Apnoea with intramuscular colistin therapy. *J. Amer. med. Assoc. 190*, 421-424.

Pittinger, C.B. and Long, J.P. (1958): Neuromuscular blocking action of neomycin sulphate. *Antibiot. Chemother., 8*, 198-203.

Pittinger, C.B., Long, J.P. and Miller, J.R. (1958): The neuromuscular blocking action of neomycin: a concern for the anesthesiologist. *Anesth. Analg. Curr. Res., 37*, 276-282.

Pittinger, C.P., Eryasa, Y. and Adamson, R. 1970. Antibiotic-induced paralysis. *Anesth. Analg. Curr. Res., 49*, 487-501.

Pittinger, R.C. and Adamson, R. (1972): Antibiotic blockade of neuromuscular function. *Ann. Rev. Pharmacol., 21*, 169-184.

Plowman, P.E. and Thomas, W.J.W. (1974): Tricyclic antidepressants and cardiac dysrhyrhtmias during dental anaesthesia. *Anaesthesia, 29*, 576-578.

Plumpton, F.S., Besser, G.M. and Cole, P.V. (1969a): Corticosteroid treatment and surgery. I. An investigation of the indications for steroid cover. *Anaesthesia, 24*, 3-11.

Plumpton, F.S., Besser, G.M. and Cole, P.V. (1969b): Corticosteroid treatment and surgery. 2. Corticosteroid treatment and surgery. *Anaesthesia, 24*, 12-18.

Poulton, T.JH., James, F.M. and Lockridge, O. (1979): Prolonged apnea following trimetaphan and succinylcholine. *Anesthesiology, 50*, 54-56.

Prescott, L.F. (1975): The development of drugs. In: *A Comparison to Medical Studies, Vol. 3, Chapter 61*. Editors: R. Passmore and J.S. Robson. Blackwell, Oxford.

Pridgen, J.E. (1956): Respiratory arrest thought to be due to intraperitoneal neomycin. *Surgery, 40*, 571.

Prys-Roberts, C., Meloche, R. and Foëx, P. (1971a): Studies of anaesthesia in relation to hypertension. Cardiovascular responses of treated and untreated patients. *Brit. J. Anaesth., 43*, 122-137.

Prys-Roberts, C., Greene, L.T., Meloche, R. and Foëx, P. (1971b): Studies of anaesthesia in relation to hypertension. II. Haemodynamic consequences of induction and endotracheal intubation. *Brit. J. Anaesth. 43*, 531-547.

Prys-Roberts, C., Foëx, P., Greene, L.T. and Waterhouse, T.D. (1972): Studies of anaesthesia in relation to hypertension. III. The effects of artificial ventilation on the circulation and pulmonary gas exchanges. *Brit. J. Anaesth. 44*, 335-349.

Radnay, P.A., Badola, R.P., Dalsania, A., El-Gaweer, E.I. and Duncalf, D. (1979): Prevention of suxamethonium-induced changes in serum potassium concentration by hexafluorenium. Is this combined use justifiable?. *Brit. J. Anaesth., 51*, 447-451.

Ramos, L., Bustos, R.E., Deluca, A.M. and Ramos, A.O. (1962): Comparative study of the pharmacological activity of antibiotics (Streptomycin, neomycin, kanamycin, and viomycin) on autonomic ganglia, myoneural function and smooth and cardiac muscles. *Rev. Brasil. Biol., 22*, 221.

Regan, A.G. and Aldrete, J.A. (1967): Prolonged apnoea after administration of promazine hydrochloride following succinylcholine infusion. *Anesth. Analg. Curr. Res., 46*, 315-318.

Robertson, G.S. (1967): Serum protein and cholinesterase changes in association with contraceptive pills. *Lancet, 1*, 232-235.

Rogers, K.J. and Thornton, J.A. (1969): Interaction between MAO inhibitors and narcotic analgesics in mice. *Brit. J. Pharmacol. 36*, 470.

Rubo, J.T., Gergis, S.R. and Sokoll, M.D. (1977): Comparative neuromuscular effects of lincomycin and clindamycin. *Anesth. Analg. Curr. Res., 56*, 329-332.

Sabawala, P.B. and Dillon, J.B. (1959): The action of some antibiotics on the human intercostal nerve muscle complex. *Anesthesiology, 20*, 659-668.

Samuelson, R.J., Giesecke, A.M., Kallus, F.T. and Stanley, V.F. (1975): Lincomycin-curare interaction. *Anesth. Analg. Curr. Res., 54*, 103-105.

Schuh, F.T. (1975): Influence of ketamine on human plasma cholinesterase. *Brit. J. Anaesth., 47*, 1315-1319.

Simpson, F.O. (1978): Hypertension. *Brit. med. J., 2*, 882-883.

Singh, Y.N., Marshall, I.G. and Harvey, A.L. (1978): Some effects of the aminoglycoside antibiotic amikacin on neuromuscular and autonomic transmission. *Brit. J. Anaesth., 50*, 109-117.

Singh, Y.N., Harvey, A.L. and Marshall, I.G. (1978): Antibiotic-induced paralysis of the mouse phrenic-nerve-diaphragm preparation and reversibility of calcium and neostigmine. *Anesthesiology, 48*, 418-424.

Sklar, G.S. and Lanks, K.W. (1977): Effects of trimetaphan and sodium nitroprusside on hydrolysis of succinylcholine in vitro. *Anesthesiology, 46*, 122-126.

Slaney, G. and Brooke, B.N. (1957): Postoperative collapse due to adrenal insufficiency following cortisone therapy. *Lancet, 1*, 1167-1170.

Sletten, I., Pichardo, J., Korol, B. and Gershon, S. (1966): The effect of chlorpromazine on lithium excretion in psychiatric subjects. *Curr. ther. Res., 8* , 441-446.

Small, G.A. (1964): Respiratory paralysis after a large dose of intraperitoneal polymixin and bacitracin. *Anesth. Analg. Curr. Res., 43*, 137-139.

Smart, J.F. (1964): Potentiation of suxamethonium by tacrine (Romotol). *Anaesthesia, 19*, 524-535.

Sokoll, M.D., Cronnelly, R. and Gergis, S.D. (1975): Neuromuscular blocking effects of lincomycin. *Pharmacologist, 7,* 247.

Son, S.L., Colella, J.R. and Brown, B.R. (1973): The effect of phenobarbitone on the metabolism of methoxyflurane to oxalic acid in the rat. *Brit. J. Anesth., 4,* 1224-1228.

Sohn, Y.-Z. and Katz, R.L. (1977): Interaction of halothane and antibiotics on isometric contractions on rat-heart muscle. *Anesth. Analg. Curr. Res., 56,* 515-521.

Spiers, I. (1966): The use of tacrine and suxamethonium in anaesthesia for Caesarean section. *Brit. J. Anaesth., 38,* 394-400.

Stambaugh, J.E., Hemphill, D.M., Wainer, I.W. and Schwartz, I. (1977): A potentially toxic drug interaction between pethidine (meperidine) and phenobarbitone. *Lancet, 1,* 398-399.

Stanley, V.F., Giesecke, A.H. and Jenkins, M.T. (1969): Neomycincurare neuromuscular block and reversal in cats. *Anesthesiology, 31,* 228.232.

Stockley, I. (1974): *"Monoamineoxidase Inhibitors – Drug Interactions and their Mechanisms".* Pharmaceutical Press, London, p. 60-62.

Stovner, J., Oftedal, N. and Holmboe, J. 1975. Inhibition of cholinesterases by pancuronium. *Brit. J. Anaesth. 47,* 949-954.

Straw, R.N., Hook, J.B., Williamson, H.E. (1965): Neuromuscular blocking properties of lincomycin. *J. pharmacol. Sci., 54,* 1814.

Swain, H.H., Kiplinger, G.F. and Brody, T.M. (1956): Action of certain antibiotics in isolated dog heart. *J. Pharmacol. exp. Ther. 117,* 151-159.

Timmerson, J.C., Long, J.P. and Gittinger, C.B. (1959). Neuromuscular blocking properties of various antibiotic agents. Toxicol. Appl. Pharmacol., 1, 299-304.

Usubiaga, J.E., Wikinski, J.A., Morales, R.L. and Usubiaga, L.E.J. (1967): Interaction of intravenously administered procaine, lidocaine and succinylcholine in anaesthetized subjects. *Anesth. Analg. Curr. Res., 46,* 39-45

Van Nyhuis, L.S., Miller, R.D. and Fogdall, R.P. (1976): The interaction between d-tubocurarine, pancuronium, polymyxin B and neostigmine on neuromuscular function. *Anesth. Analg. Curr. Res., 55.,* 224-228.

Vaughan, R.S. and Lunn, J.N. (1973): Potassium and the anaesthetist: a review. *Anaesthesia, 28,* 118-131.

Vessey, M.P., Doll, R., Fairbairn, A.S. and Glober, G. (1970): Postoperative thromboembolism and the use of oral contraceptives. *Brit. Med. J. 3,* 123-126.

Vetten, K.B. (1973): Immunosuppressive therapy and anaesthesia. *S. Afr. med. J., 47,* 767-770.

Vital Brazil, O. and Corrado, A.P. (1957): The curariform action of streptomycin. *J. Pharmacol. exp. Ther., 120,* 452.

Vital Brazil, O., and Prado-Franceschi, J. (1969a): The neuromuscular blocking action of gentamicin. *Arch. int. Pharmacodyn Thér., 179,* 65-77.

Vital Brazil, O. and Prado-Franceschi, J. (1969b). The nature of neuromuscular block produced by neomycin and gentamicin. *Arch. int. Pharmacodyn. Thér., 179,* 78-85.

Waal-Manning, H.J. and Simpson, F.O. (1969): Fenfluramine in obese patient on various anti-hypertensive drugs: doubleblind controlled trial. *Lancet, 2,* 1392-1395.

Waisbren, B.A. (1968): Lincomycin in larger doses. *J. Amer. med. Assoc., 206,* 2118.

Wang, R.I.H. and Ross, C.A. (1963): Prolonged apnea following succinylcholine in cancer patients receiving A.B.-132. *Anesthesiology, 24,* 363-367.

Warner, W.A. and Sanders, E. (1971): Neuromuscular blockade associated with gentamicin therapy. *J. Amer. med. Assoc., 215,* 1153-1154.

Waterman, R.M. and Smith, R.B. (1977): Tobramycin-curare interaction. *Anesth. Analg. Curr. Res.,* *56,* 587-588.

Way, W.L., Katzung, B.G. and Larson, C.P. (1967): Recurarization with quinidine. *J. Amer. med. Assoc., 200,* 153-154.

Webber, B.M. (1957): Respiratory arrest following intraperitoneal administration of neomycin. *Arch. Surg. 75,* 174-176.

Weinstein, A.J., McHenery, H.L. and Gavan, T.L. (1977): Systemic absorption of neomycin irrigating solution. *J. Amer. med. Assoc., 238,* 152-153.

Weisman, S.J. (1949): Masked myasthenia gravis. *J. Amer. med. Assoc., 141,* 917-918.

Whitsett, T.L. and Goldberg, L.I. (19727: Effects of levodopa on systolic pre-ejection period, blood pressure and heart rate during acute and chronic treatment of Parkinson's disease. *Circulation, 45,* 97-106.

Wilson, S.L., Miller, R.N., Wright, C. and Hasse, D. (1976): Prolonged neuromuscular blockade associated with trimetaphan: A case report. *Anesth. Analg. Curr. Res., 55,* 353-356.

Wislicki, L. and Rosenblaum, I. (1967): Effects of propranolol on the action of neuromuscular blocking drugs. *Brit. J. Anaesth., 39,* 939-942.

Wolff, H. (1965): The inhibition of serum cholinesterase by cyclophosphamid. *Klin. Med., 43,* 819.

Wood, J.B., Frankland, A.W., James, V.H.T. and Landon, J. (1965): A rapid test for adrenocortical function. Lancet, *1,* 243-245.

Wright, J.M. and Collier, B. (1974): Inhibition by neomycin of acetylcholine release and ^{45}Ca accumulation in the superior cervical ganglia. *Pharmacologist, 16,* 537.

Wright, J.M. and Collier, B. (1976a): The site of neuromuscular block produced by polymixin B and rolitetraceyline. *Canad. J. Physiol. Pharmacol., 54,* 926-936.

Wright, J.M. and Collier, B. (1976b): Characterization of the neuromuscular block produced by clindamycin and lincomycin. *Canad. J. Physiol. Pharmacol. 54,* 937.

Wright, J.M. and Collier, B. (1977): The effects of neomycin upon transmitter release and action. *J. Pharmacol. exp. Ther., 200,* 576.

Wullen, F., Kast, G. and Brick, A. (1967): Uben Nebenwirkungen bei Tetracyclin-Verabreichung an myastheniker. *Dtsch. Med. Wschr., 92,* 667-669.

Zauder, H.L., Barton, N., Bennett, E.J. and Lore, J. (1966): Colistimethate as a cause of postoperative apnoea. *Canad. Anaesth. Soc. J., 13,* 607-610.

Zsigmond, E.K. and Robins, G. (1972): The effect of a series of anti-cancer drugs on plasma cholinesterase activity. *Canad. Anaesth. Soc. J., 19,* 75-82.

Thornton (ed.) Adverse Reactions of Anaesthetic Drugs
© Elsevier/North-Holland Biomedical Press, 1981

2

Adverse reactions to intravenous induction agents

R.S.J. Clarke and J.W. Dundee

INTRODUCTION

Adverse responses to intravenous anaesthetic drugs have always been recognised but the type of reaction which is attracting attention has changed over the last 10 years. Hypotension following the administration of hexobarbitone and thiopentone caused many disasters in the early days of their usage and it was recognised in the nineteen-forties that both were potential myocardial depressants. Thiopentone also dilates peripheral arterioles, capillaries and larger veins and the resultant fall in arterial blood pressure at the same time as the skin becomes pink and warm are well known and the vasodilatation can even be useful to anaesthetists.

The introduction of methohexitone led to interest in a different kind of adverse drug effect — the involuntary muscle movement with or without hypertonus. This is rare with thiopentone but can occur with almost any intravenous anaesthetic agent, depending on the dose, the speed of injection and the premedication. The frequency in unpremedicated patients varies from 3–5 per cent with thiopentone to 25–40 per cent with etomidate. In general, opiates diminish the incidence and severity of the movements whereas hyoscine and some phenothiazines increase them. This also applies to the newer agents which are as excitatory in their properties as the barbiturates. Such movements occurring immediately after the injection of the intravenous agent and before the beginning of surgery must be regarded as a direct action of the drug although perhaps initiated by minor stimuli such as a full bladder or movement of the legs. They vary only slightly in type — from the small, frequent "twitches" with currently used babiturates and some steroids, to the more wide-spread activity with methylated thiobarbiturates and etomidate. Widespread convulsive movements may be described as an unexpected adverse reaction but do not really fit into the above description and they are totally unexplained so far. These have been seen with most drugs (even after recovery) (Galley, 1963; Gunner et al., 1965); Uppington, 1973) and, since they can be provoked rather than suppressed by the intravenous barbiturates, they are probably not manifestations of an epileptic focus, nor do they precede or follow a known epileptic history.

Respiratory upset, particularly hiccough is almost as common as involuntary muscle movements. It seems to be prevented by the antisialogogues (Haslett and Dundee, 1968) rather than by the opiates but it is difficult to explain its mechanism on this basis.

Other unexpected adverse reactions include the psychotomimetic phenomena during recovery from ketamine anaesthesia. Like those above-mentioned they are frequent in occurrence but equally obscure as regards mechanism.

The reaction described above have been accepted as inevitable side effects of intravenous anaesthetics because, although they upset the course of anaesthesia and may delay surgery they are not life-threatening. The particular type described below has resulted in several deaths and only our increasing understanding of emergency care in general has prevented more frequent disasters.

HYPERSENSITIVITY REACTIONS

This chapter is concerned principally with hypersensitivity or anaphylactoid reactions, that is reactions resembling the generalised effects of histamine liberation. The effects are therefore not those of an overdose of the drug concerned, whether this has been given or not. They involve most frequently the skin and cardiovascular system. Less commonly there is bronchospasm or other respiratory difficulty and rarely gastrointestinal symptoms.

Cutaneous reactions

Local histaminoid effects attributed to histamine liberation at the injection site or along the course of the vein are unimportant but, even if systemic, the effects of histamine are not uniform in distribution. The commonest sign is an erythematous flush most marked in the upper part of the body. However, such reactions occur not only with intravenous anaesthetics such as alphaxalone-alphadolone (Althesin) in 10–20 per cent of patients, but also with intravenous pethidine and more rarely with intramuscular atropine. They are also not uncommon following intravenous tubo-curarine (see Chapter 9), occurring in 40–60 per cent of patients. The effect lasts 5–15 min and is attended with no oedema or cardiovascular signs. It is presumably a manifestation of histamine release but this is due to a direct action of the drug rather than immune-mediated.

Following induction of anaesthesia, a smaller proportion of patients have, in addition, some degree of cutaneous oedema particularly of the eyelids and face and this can be quite widespread. It can also take the form of massive wheals (Davis, 1971). Widespread oedema results in loss of fluid from the circulation; a 1-mm layer of oedema throughout the body represents about 1.5 litres of fluid loss. This latter figure is very close to that calculated by Fisher (1977b) when measuring the degree of haemoconcentration in a group of patients after anaphylactoid reactions. Oedema can also affect the larynx and this may be the cause of the coughing and respiratory difficulty which has been frequently reported by anaesthetists. The actual skin colour in such patients begins as bright red but if there is any degree of circulatory failure or respiratory obstruction cyanosis follows rapidly.

Cardiovascular changes

The combination of vasodilatation with peripherol oedema is likely to be associated with hypotension and this is a feature of most reports. Some degree of hypotension occurs with most anaesthetic techniques but the association of hypotension with intense flushing or oedema suggests a hypersensitivity reaction. There is also a much greater tachycardia than is common with induction of anaesthesia.

Bronchospasm

Anaphylaxis in man is not invariably associated with bronchospasm and this feature is more prominent in certain species such as the guinea pig, where it is the principal cause of death. It has only been reported in about 50 per cent of patients with generalised reactions, though the combination of bronchospasm and cardiovascular collapse is more likely to be fatal than either on its own.

The term "bronchospasm" is often used to embrace all forms of respiratory difficulty, many of them iatrogenic and even if there is a true bronchiolar narrowing, it is certainly not synonymous with hypersensitivity. The two commonest causes of bronchospasm on induction of anaesthesia are aspiration of foreign material into the lower respiratory tract and irritation by a tracheal tube. It is difficult to rule out the former cause of bronchospasm, but aspiration is more likely to be responsible when the stomach is not empty, and when a myoneural blocker has been given. It is also unwise to regard bronchospasm following tracheal intubation as being due to hypersensitivity since it occurs mainly in patients with some form of asthma or bronchitis, is minimised by spraying the tracheal with lignocaine and aggravated by movement of the tube particularly if it is near the carina.

Other effects

Abdominal pain and vomiting are rare but do appear to be part of the anaphylactoid syndrome. These have been noted in about 5 per cent of reports of reactions and an persist for up to 12 hours.

Recovery

The majority of patients experiencing the typical flush, peripheral oedema and hypotension do not have a true "cardiac arrest" and a gradual return to normal in 10–30 min is to be expected. This is accellerated by the treatment to be discussed later but the recovery process is probably on its way before effective action can be taken. However, severe bronchospasm adding hypoxia to the circulatory depression is an additional factor in most of the deaths described. Analysis of many hundreds of case reports has yielded no clear picture of why some patients experience mainly hypotension and others bronchospasm. Return of consciousness after the anaesthetic will clearly be delayed if circulatory depression is rapid and prolonged but where respiratory difficulty is the main feature some patients have actually awakened before it was apparent. This situation will be more likely with rapidly metabolised anaesthetics such as propanidid and Althesin.

HISTORICAL SURVEY OF REACTIONS

Thiopentone has been in clinical use from 1934 but it was not until 1952 that the first case of a generalised hypersensitivity reaction occurred (Evans and Gould, 1952). In fact Hunter (1943) had described bulbous eruptions developing several days after thiopentone anaesthesia but these appear to be toxic manifestations akin to those occurring after barbitone overdosage. The first two case reports by Evans and Gould describe the typical erythema of face and arms, swelling of eyelids, hoarse voice and (in one case) abdominal colic. Rather surprisingly in one of the patients the problem recurred with two other administrations of thiopentone but not with hexobarbitone. Both patients had received thiopentone previously.

Dundee in his "Thiopentone and other Thioparbiturates" published in 1956 mentioned a transient urticarial rash on the upper chest, neck and face as being an occasional occurrence with thiobarbiturates. He accepted it as a true allergic response but until the nineteen seventies published reports of allergic or hypersensitivity reactions to thiopentone were very rare indeed. An analysis of published reactions 1952–1977 is given by Clarke (1979) and the reader is referred to the detailed tables in this publication for details.

Propanidid was introduced into clinical use in 1963 and the very first publications (Beck, 1965; Radnay, 1965; Zindler, 1965) mention hypersensitivity reactions to it. However the rarity of any previous reports of such reactions to any intravenous anaesthetic delayed our acceptance of them. Indeed, the hypotensive action of propanidid in high doses (Clarke and Dundee, 1970) and its depressant action on the myocardium (Soga et al, 1973) suggested overdosage as a more likely cause. However the review of thiopentone reactions by Clark and Cockburn (1971) and the number of reports of reactions to propanidid in 1969–1972 eventually convinced anaesthetists that these were a different effect from that of overdosage. Interest was further stimulated by the reports of reactions to Althesin (Avery and Evans, 1973), 65 of which were summarised by Clarke and his colleagues (1975). The pattern of reaction reports is clearly not due to any one anaesthetic agent thought it shows a preponderance of reports of reactions following Althesin.

The suggested causes of this rise in frequency of reaction reports during the seventies include cross-sensitisation by other drugs due to a rising drug intake by the population, the introduction of plastic syringes and the decline in usage of anti-histamine premedication. Communication with other anaesthetists and with the Committee on Safety of Medicines indicates that the occurrence of reactions is commoner than the graph shows. Alternatively, the apparent increase in frequency may merely show an increased enthusiasm for publication although still leaving the great majority unpublished and even unreported.

REACTIONS TO INDIVIDUAL AGENTS

Thiopentone

The 45 published reports of reactions to this drug up to the end of 1977 have been listed by Clarke (1979) and there do not appear to have been any specific case reports since then. However, reports of a further 35 reactions from 1974–1978, which appeared to be anaphylactoid in nature have reached the authors or been seen thanks to the courtesy of the Committee on Safety of Medicines. Clinical details are unfortunately very incomplete but the general features are listed in Table 2.1. The patient's past history must certainly be regarded as underestimating the incidence of atopy, allergies and previous thiopentone anaesthesia. However, the main interest of the table is to show that episodes are constantly occurring and that there have been 10 deaths which could be attributed to hypersensitivity reactions.

A problem of interpretation of these reactions is that in four of the cases faza-dinium had been given about the same time as the thiopentone while another patien had received pancuronium and another alcuronium. The number with fazadinium is greater than would have been expected from the limited usage of this drug and taken in conjunction with Fisher's findings on intradermal testing (Fisher, 1979) this raises the possibility that many reactions are attributed to the induction agent for which the muscle relaxant is responsible.

The incidence of reactions cannot be assessed from the figures discussed above but the "closed series" of Shaw (1974) in New Zealand and Evans and Keogh (1977) do give some basis for an estimation. The former paper suggests a figure of 1 in 36,000 and the latter 1 in 29,000, and even if both are underestimates the incidence of reactions following thiopentone is acceptably low.

The number of deaths amounts to 10 out of 80 reactions reported which is higher than with any other agent. This could be because the fatal reactions are selectively reported (or reach the CSM via the coroner) or it could result from the more prolonged duration of the reaction, compared with Althesin (Watkins et al., 1976a,b,c).

Other barbiturates

Reactions with other barbiturates are summarised in Table 2.1, though that reported by Shafto (1969) with methohexitone could be described as a simple faint. Some additional case have been reported to the Committee on Safety of Medicines and some to the author personally, but the total number remains small and no deaths have been attributed to these agents. In addition, over 12,000 well-documented methohexitone anaesthetics have been given in Belfast by members of the University Department and no reactions have occurred. On the whole one must agree with Whitwam (1978) that it is an extremely "safe" drug. The usage of thiamylal has always been relatively small in Britain but two reactions to this agent have been reported elsewhere. It is however unlikely to differ from thiopentone in incidence of reactions and their effects.

Propanidid

Reactions to propanidid have only been reported specifically in 52 publications, which is slightly more than the publications of alleged thiopentone reactions (Table 2.1; and Clarke, 1979) out of a much smaller usage of propanidid even at the height of its popularity. Danneman and Lubke (1970) give a reaction-incidence of 1 in 750 Kay (19727 gives an incidence of 1 in 1700 and Doenicke (1975) gives one of 1 in 540 which is 20–70 times more common than with thiopentone. Only four reports reached the authors in the survey conducted by Clarke and his co-workers (1975) and conversation with colleagues suggested that the drug had virtually passed out of routine use by anaesthetists. However, examination of the reports in the Committee on Safety of Medicines files indicates that the drug is still being used by dentists, and one reported 7 "severe anaphylactic reactions" in patients receiving the drug for the second time. It seems therefore that the frequency of reactions with this drug is unacceptably high and it is all the more surprising that it is still being used. It would appear from comments by anaesthetists or dentists who administered the propanidid that they were not aware of its dangers. There have been 4 deaths in the series listed, one of them in a dental surgery quite unprepared for treatment of a reaction whether involving bronchospasm or hypotension. Unless it is possible to restrict the use of propanidid to skilled personnel working in well equipped hospitals, the drug should probably be withdrawn from clinical use.

Althesin

Reactions to Althesin began to be reported almost as soon as the drug was clinically used (Avery and Evans, 1973) although there were no reactions during the extensive clinical trials between 1970 and 1973. This trial series included over 4000 documented anaesthetics given by members of the Belfast Department of Anaesthetics and covered a wide range of doses and premedicants and although most of the patients were classified as ASA grades 1 or 2 of physical fitness, it suggested that the drug would cause no unexpected problems. However 91 reports have appeared in print up to 1978 (Table 2.1) and 134 more unpublished reports have reached the author from other sources. Even this total is probably an underestimate so one must conclude that reactions to this drug are frequent.

Attempts to assess the incidence of reactions have inevitably produced a wide range. Clarke and his colleagues (1975) assessed 100 reported reactions and calculated from the number of "doses" sold that the reaction incidence was about 1 in 11,000. This incidence would be less if some of the reactions were due to a muscle relaxant given with the induction agent. However it could be much greater if many reactions were not reported, and this seems the likely explanation for the much higher incidence of 1 in 900 suggested by Watt (1975) and by Fisher (1976a) and the more recent figure of 1 in 1900 by Evans and Keogh (1977). These incidences were obtained in England, in New Zealand and in Wales and are sufficiently similar to indicate that Althesin like propanidid causes an unacceptably high incidence of hypersensitivity reactions.

The mortality attributable to Althesin still remains low – in fact, as a percentage of cases reported, it is lower than with any of the other induction agents. One of the patients reported by Avery and Evans (1973) was in poor health and it is difficult to say definitely that he died from a hypersensitivity reaction. Suxamethonium was also given in one of the other fatal cases and cannot be excluded as a causative agent. However even a non-fatal reaction presents a severe strain on the patient and on the anaesthetist's experitise and it would seem best to limit the use of Althesin to situations were its advantages of clear-headed recovery are useful. In addition, like propanidid, it should only be given where full facilities for resuscitation are available.

Cremophor EL

This is an organic solvent which is used to solubilise propanidid and the steroids alphaxalone and alphadolone acetate. These drugs are sparingly soluble in water and can only be administered in a reasonable volume by the use of a solubilising agent, or like diazepam, by administration in an organic solvent such as propylene glycol. Organic solvents are irritant to the veins and frequently cause both pain and subsequent thrombophlebitis. Cremophor EL has a high LD_{50} in the mouse (Child et al., 1971) and does not cause cardiovascular depression in man (Savege et al., 1973). There is no evidence of sensitivity to Cremophor EL on its own and it does not cause leucocyte degranulation in patients in whom propanidid or Althesin produce this effect (Watkins et al., 1976a). Anaesthetists with a skin sensitivity to propanidid have been able to use Althesin without trouble (Sneddon and Glew, 1973; Dundee et al., 1974).

However, there appears to be some association between previous exposure to propanidid and a reaction to Althesin. It addition diazepam in its usual formulation has not been reported as causing any anaphylactic reactions, whereas the preparation in Cremophor EL (Stesolid), while producing no pain on injection, has led to a number of anaphylactoid collapses in Scandinavia. Glen et al. (1979) have carried out studies with the miniature pig comparing alphaxalone + alphadolone in Cremophor EL with the same steroids dissolved in ethyl alcohol + propylene glycol. When a dose of Althesin was repeated within seven days there was a reaction resembling the subclinical manifestations of histamine liberation in man, described by Watkins, Clark and their colleagues (1976). These effects were less frequent when the steroids were dissolved in the organic solvents, and did not occur at all with thiopentone. It would seem therefore that the surfactant properties of Cremophor EL may enhance the immunogenicity of propanidid and Althesin, thereby rendering subclinical effects potentially more dangerous.

MECHANISMS

The combination of clinical signs described suggest a variety of mechanisms and only by a set of laboratory measurements carried out at the time of the reaction can we distinguish between them.

Overdosage

This has been recognised as a cause of hypotension since the days of Pearl Harbour but with the understanding that hypotension is closely related to the rate of injection, the dose administered and the circulatory state of the patient, there is rarely a problem with thiopentone in experienced hands. The same is not true for propanidid and although this agent is virtually equipotent (W/W) with thiopentone (Clarke et al., 1968), anaesthetists tend to use doses of 6–8 mg · kg^{-1} to produce a longer duration of action. However the dose/toxicity curve of propanidid appears to be steeper than that of thiopentone for most side effects including hypotension (Clarke and Dundee, 1970). Soon after the first reports of hypersensitivity reactions to propanidid the suggestion was made that overdosage was a possible cause (Clarke and Dundee, 1969; Grimmeisen, 1971). However Doenicke (1975) by analysing the dose versus the frequency of reaction has shown that this is not the whole explanation. Neither the occurrence rate nor the severity of reaction appears to be dose dependent.

Althesin has a higher therapeutic index than the barbiturates both in animal studies (Child et al., 1971) and in man (Clarke et al., 1972). Although 50 μl · kg^{-1} is approximately equipotent with thiopentone 4 mg · kg^{-1} (Carson et al., 1975) there is little hypotension with a dose three times as high. This safety is emphasized even more strongly by the case report from Canada (Boggild-Madsen and Cargnelli, 1978) where 35 ml of pure "Alfathesin" were infused accidentally over 2 min. The mean arterial blood pressure was 70 mm Hg before the episode and remained unchanged. The only apparent effect of the infusion was a fall in body temperature to 31°C in spite of the fact that all infusions were warmed to 37°C. It must be concluded therefore that although side effects are, as with other drugs, dose and rate related (Clarke et al., 1972; Samuel and Dundee, 1973) there is no reason to attribute the "hypersensitivity" reactions to overdosage. In general, it would seem that though overdosage can cause profound hypotension during induction it is unlikely to cause erythema, oedema, wheals and bronchospasm.

Direct release of histamine

This occurs most frequently with drugs such as tubocurarine and pethidine which act on the mast cells without antibody or complement involvement. It can occur with intravenous anaesthetics (Watkins, 1979) and is related to dose and speed of injection. However, it is distinguishable from direct pharmacological action of the drug only by measurement of plasma histamine, an estimation which is possible in very few centres.

Anaphylactic or anaphylactoid reactions

(Type I to Type IB hypersensitivity reactions) are described in detail in another section, but it is necessary here to emphasize that analysis is only possible by studying blood soon after the reaction, for complement and immunoglobulin (Watkins, Thornton et al., 1976). Intradermal testing can give a lead to the causative agent (Fisher, 1979) but does not clarify the mechanism involved.

PREDISPOSING FACTORS

Atopy

Table 1 shows that about 9 per cent of all reactors have a history of atopy (asthma, hay fever or eczema). This however is likely to be a considerable underestimate because only some of the patients had been directly questioned on this point. The earlier survey by Clarke and his colleagues (1975) put the figure at 15 per cent and presumably this more nearly approaches the minimum figure. It is, however, also striking to see both in Table 2.1 and the 1975 study that a history of atopy is about three times as common in barbiturate reactors than in those reacting to propanidid or Althesin.

The incidence of an atopic history in patients reacting to intravenous anaesthetics must be compared with the incidence in the general population to determine whether it is a true predisposing factor. This information was not available and a study was carried out to discover the atopic, allergic and anaesthetic history of 10,000 surgical patients in the UK (Dundee et al., 1978). As a result it was found that 8.5 per cent of patients presenting for anaesthesia reported an atopic history. This figure is not significantly different from that in patients who have had hypersensitive reactions to intravenous anaesthetics or more specifically in those reacting to Althesin. There is however a significant difference between the frequency of atopic history in barbiturate reactors and the general population ($x^2 = 12.36$; P <0.0005). The fact that an atopic history is recorded in only one propanidid reactor is probably due to lack of questioning rather than a genuine difference from those reacting to barbiturates or Althesin.

Allergy

A history of allergy to food or drugs is found in 19 per cent of patients having reactions to intravenous anaesthetics (Table 2. 1) and again this is probably an underestimate. When the figures are broken down into barbiturate reactors and those reacting to other intravenous anaesthetics the frequency of allergic history is again higher in the former group though the difference is less marked than for atopy.

The incidence of a history of allergy in the general surgical population has been found to be 13.5 per cent (Dundee et al.m 1978) and the incidence in reactors in general (Table 2. 1) is significantly higher than this ($x^2 = 8.66$; P <0.005). When reactors are divided into those to barbiturates and the others, it appears that this correlation is all with the former group in whom almost one third give a history of allergy. The difference between barbiturate-reactors and the surgical population regarding allergic history is highly significant ($x = 30.88$; P <0.0005). Again, history of allergy is less common in the propanidid reactors.

It appears therefore that a history of atopy or allergy is a predisposing factor to barbiturate reactions, though the same cannot be demonstrated for reactions to Althesin or propanidid. Watkins (1980) has demonstrated that 7 of the thirtyfive Althesin reaction investigated between 1974 and 1978 are probably pharmacological, whereas none of the reactions after other drugs fell into this category. In addition many of the reactions with this drug occur on first exposure by complement C_3 activation and this would suggest that the immunoglobulins are not involved. Logically it is more appropriate to withhold the barbiturates rather than Althesin from atopic/allergic individuals, but the particularly high frequency of reactions with the steroids outweighs this consideration.

A relationship between allergy and reactions to propanidid is suggested by the retrospective survey of 2209 propanidid anaesthetics by Doenicke (1975). He found that 15.6 per cent of patients reacting to propanidid gave a history of allergy compared with 8.2 per cent of the surgical patients as a whole.

Previous anaesthetics

The figures in Table 2. 1 show that approximately 50 per cent of patients having reactions have been previously exposed to the same drug. Again, these are minimum

TABLE 2.1

Summary of published reports of hypersensitivity reactions to various intravenous anaesthetics up to the end of 1978. Most of those up to 1977 are listed by Clarke (1979) but additional reports are listed below. The numbers of unpublished reports listed were obtained from the Committee on Safety of Medicines or communicated directly to the authors, 1974–1978.

		Site of clinical features				History			Deaths
	No	Skin	CVS	RS	GI	Atopy	Allergy	Same anaesthetic	
Thiopentone									
See Clarke (1979) for detailed list	45	36	34	24	5	9	22	21	6
Chung (1976)	1	1	1	1	–	–	–	1	–
Unpublished	35	23	29	21	2	5	8	13	4
Methohexitone									
Shafto (1969)	1	–	1	–	–	–	–	–	–
Driggs and O'Day (1972)	6	6	6	5	3	3	1	–	–
Reichert and Basset (1972)	1	1	–	–	1	–	–	–	–
Wyatt and Watkins (1975)	1	11	1	–	–	1	–	–	–
Unpublished	6	5	4	2	–	1	1	–	–
Thiamylal									
Thompson, Eason and Flacke (1973)	1	1	1	1	–	–	–	–	–
Dohi, Naito and Takahashi (1975)	1	11	–	1	–	–	–	–	–
Ketamine									
Mathieu, Goudsouzian and Snider (1975)	1	1	–	–	–	–	1	1	–
Propanidid									
See Clarke (1979) for detailed list	52	49	49	9	5	–	6	31	2
Unpublished	19	19	13	3	1	1	1	9	2
Althesin									
See Clarke (1979) for detailed list	91	62	67	63	5	7	16	42	–
Hughes, Inglis and Campbell (1977)	1	1	1	–	–	–	–	1	–
Jago and Restall (1978)	1	1	1	–	1	–	–	1	–
Unpublished	134	103	111	59	3	9	18	67	3

CVS = Cardiovascular system; RS = Respiratory system; GI = Gastrointestinal.

estimates as the anaesthetic history of all patients is not known. In a control group of patients who had not had reactions Fee and his colleagues (1978) found the surprisingly high figure of 67 per cent as having had an anaesthetic at some time in their lives. It was not possible to tell exactly which anaesthetics all had received. However, extrapolation from the replies indicates that approximately 80 per cent of those anaesthetised had received thiopentone and 18 per cent had received Althesin; i.e. 54 per cent of the surgical population had received thiopentone previously and 12 per cent had had Althesin. (This survey was carried out in 1976 and unfortunately, propanidid was not included). These figures show that a history of previous exposure to thiopentone is no more frequent in thiopentone-reactors than in the general population but a history of exposure to Althesin is commoner in those reacting to Althesin. There is therefore no contra-indication to repeat administrations of thiopentone but, on this evidence, Althesin should not be repeated within a short time interval. It is probably undesirable to repeat Althesin before 8 weeks on the evidence of Glen et al. (1979) that the minature pig is particularly sensitive to repeat administrations of Althesin, the critical time being 7 days.

PREVENTION AND INVESTIGATION

It is not possible to prevent adverse reactions completely because almost any drug can cause such a reaction even with a test dose and skin testing of every patient is impracticable and unsafe. However the severity of the reaction can be reduced by slowly administering only moderate doses of the drug. There seems little point in avoiding a particular drug in patients with a general atopic or allergic history though the findings given earlier suggest that thiopentone is no more safe than Althesin. If a patient is known to be sensitive to a particular drug this should obviously be avoided. However, it is not easy positively to incriminate one agent when two are given in close succession. Studies of IgE and complement after a reaction (Watkins, 1979) can usually identify it as being hypersensitivity in type rather than due to overdosage or other causes. They can suggest a likely agent. However, they are not as clear as intradermal testing for establishing the causative agent, in particular for distinguishing between the anaesthetic and the muscle relaxant.

Intradermal testing has been advocated most strongly by Fisher (1976b, 1977a, 1979), whose general technique is as follows: prepare fresh solutions of all drugs and solvents that are relevant, dilute them to 1:1000 and inject 0.1 ml intradermally on the anterior surface of the forearm after cleaning with alcohol. A positive reaction is a flare with a wheal of at least 1.0 cm appearing within 30 min and persisting for 30 min. If there is a reaction with more than one drug, both should be tested in a dilution of 1:10000. Fisher (1975) states that the risks of provoking a generalised reaction by skin testing in this way are small, though he has had one using 1:100. Resuscitation facilities should always be available. When testing with induction agents, a dilution of 1:100 gives more consistent results and 1:10,000 is safer for tubocurarine (Fisher, 1979).

Sources of error include false positives from failure to dilute solutions sufficiently, especially the myoneural blocking drugs. False negatives can occur at extremes of age and in the 3–4 weeks after a reaction. Sympathomimetic drugs, antihistamines and steroids may also inhibit a skin reaction. It is probably more dangerous to be misled by false negatives into giving an allegedly safe drug to a patient who has already had one severe reaction. For this reason many anaesthetists prefer to warn against all drugs which could have been involved in causing a reaction. However, this makes things very difficult for the next anaesthetist involved and it is probably useful to narrow down the field of incriminated drugs provided one remembers that no tests are infallible.

The commonest situation to be faced with is to decide on a sequence of drugs for an individual with an atopic or allergic history. Premedication with an antihistamine has been shown to reduce the frequency and severity of reactions (Lorenz et al., 1972; Doenicke, 1975), promethazine 50 mg being the most suitable drug. If both H_1 and H_2 receptors are to be blocked (and this is doubtful) cimetidine 400 mg should also be given 2 hours before operation. Steroids such as prednisolone or hydrocortisone also reduce the severity of reactions but their potential toxicity makes routine use undesirable in the large numbers of patients involved. Disodium chromoglycate has been shown to block signs of immune recognition in vitro (Watkins et al. 1976a) but its clinical value is still unknown.

A patient who has already had a reaction to one agent can probably be anaesthetised with another but he is still at considerable risk and the anaesthetist should consider the above measures as well as being prepared to resuscitate if necessary. Local anaesthesia is, of course, the least likely to provoke a hypersensitivity reaction but an inhalational induction with or without intravenous diazepam is an alternative. Pancuronium appears to be the safest of the non-depolarising neuromuscular blocking drugs though even it has been incriminated in one of Fisher's cases (Fisher, 1979).

TREATMENT

The commonest manifestation of the hypersensitivity reaction is vasodilatation and extravasation of fluid into the tissue spaces. The logical treatment is therefore administration of fluid, preferably a colloid plasma expander. Fisher (1977b) has calculated that the volume lost is 1–2 litres and this volume should be rapidly infused. Progress can be monitored by the central venous pressure but urgent restoration of the blood volume should not wait for this. The exact nature of the fluid is less critical. A solution of a colloid will remain in the vascular compartment for longer than Ringer-lactate or normal saline, but in a patient having on anaphylactoid reaction it would seem preferable to use human plasma protein rather than a dextran or gelatin, both of which carry considerable risk of their own. Tilting of the table into the head-down position is also a useful first-aid measure to counteract the tendency to venous pooling in the legs. The trachea will also need to be intubated if this has not already taken place, and inhalational anaesthesia should, of course, be replaced by oxygen. This will be valuable whether or not there is bronchospasm or laryngeal oedema.

Since both vasodilation and myocardial failure are involved in these histamine-mediated reactions, a drug of multiple actions such as adrenaline or isoprenaline is most effective, as well as being readily available. However, to be effective in shock they must be given intravenously and this necesitates dilution of the standard 1:1000 solution to 1:10,000 and administration in 1 ml increments. The alpha stimulators such as metaraminol (1–10 mg) may have a place if the heart rate is already rapid, which is a likely consequence of the action of histamine.

Adrenaline has the additional advantage of being a potent bronchodilator but slow intravenous injection of aminophylline 250 mg is probably safer if this is the main problem. Other drugs are of less certain value though hydrocorisone (100–150 mg) is beneficial to counteract more slowly both the bronchospasm and the cardiovascular collapse. Antihistamines (promethazine 25–50 mg or chlorpheniramine 10 mg intravenously) may also be given to help terminate the reaction.

Continued observation and supportive treatment will probably be necessary but reactions, especially those following Althesin, are often surprisingly brief in duration and it may be possible to proceed with the operation. Since most anaesthetists only experience one or two of these reactions in a career, it is surprising that treatment is so effective and complete recovery occurs in about 95 per cent of cases.

REFERENCES

Avery, A.F. and Evans, A. (1973): Reactions to Althesin. *Brit. J. Anaesth.*, *45*, 301-303.

Beck, L. (1965): Erfahrungen mit dem Kurznarkotikum propanidid in der Geburtshilfe. In: *Die intravenose Kurznarkose mit dem neuen Phenoxyessigsaurederivat. Propanidid (Epontol).* Editors: K. Horatz, R. Frey and M. Zindler. Springer-Verlag, Berlin, p. 223.

Boggild-Madsen, H.B. and Gargnelli, T. (1978): Accidental over-dose of Alfathesin under general anaesthesia: case report. *Canad. Anaesth. Soc. J.*, *25*, 245-246.

Carson, I.W., Dundee, J.W. and Clarke, R.S.J. (1975): The speed of onset and potency of Althesin. *Brit. J. Anaesth.*, *47*, 512-515.

44

Child, K.J., Currie, J.P., Davis, B., Dodds, M.G., Pearce, D.R. and Twissell, D.J. (1971): The pharmacological properties in animals of CT 1341 – a new steroid anaesthetic agent. *Brit. J. Anaesth., 43*, 2-13.

Chung, D.C.W. (1976): Anaphylaxis to thiopentone: a case report. *Canad. Anaesth. Soc. J., 23*, 319-322.

Clark, M.M. and Cockburn, H.A. (1971): Anaphylactoid response to thiopentone. *Brit. J. Anaesth., 43*, 185-189.

Clarke, R.S.J. (1979): Hypersensitivity reactions to intravenous anaesthetics. In: *Current Topics in Anaesthesia. Intravenous Anaesthetic Agents.* Editor: J.W. Dundee. Arnold, London, pp. 87-118.

Clarke, R.S.J. and Dundee, J.W. (1969): Hypotensive reaction after propanidid and atropine. *Brit. Med. J., 4*, 369.

Clarke, R.S.J. and Dundee, J.W. (1970): Toxic effects of intravenous anaesthetics: a comparison of propanidid with thiopentone. In: *Progress in Anaesthesiology. Proc. 4th World Congress of Anaesthesiologists, Amsterdam.* Editors: T.B. Boulton, R. Bryce-Smith, M.K. Sykes, G.B. Gillett and A.L. Revell. Excerpta Medica, Amsterdam. pp. 1189-1191.

Clarke, R.S.J., Dundee, J.W., Barron, D.W. and McArdle, L. (1968): Clinical studies of induction agents. XXVI: The relative potencies of thiopentone, methohexitone and propanidid. *Brit. J. Anaesth., 40*, 593-601.

Clarke, R.S.J., Dundee, J.W. and Carson, I.W. (1972): Some aspects of the clinical pharmacology of Althesin. *Postgrad. med. J., 48*, 62-65.

Clarke, R.S.J., Dundee, J.W., Garrett, R.T., McArdle, G.K. and Sutton, J.A. (1975): Adverse reactions to intravenous anaesthetics. A survey of 1000 reports. *Brit. J. Anaesth., 47*, 575-585.

Dannemann, H. and Lubke, P. (1970): Komplikationen wahrend Narkosen mit Epontol. *Z. prakt. Anaesth. Wiederbeleb., 5*, 273.

Davis, J. (1971): Thiopentone anaphylaxis. Case report. *Brit. J. Anaesth. 43*, 1191-1193.

Doenicke, A. (1975): Propanidid. In: *Recent Progress in Anaesthesiology and Resuscitation. Proceedings of the IV European Congress of Anaesthesiology. Madrid.* Editors: A. Arias, R. Llaurado, M.A. Nalda and J.N. Lunn. Excerpta Medica, Amsterdam. pp. 107-113.

Dohi, S., Naito, H. and Takahashi, T. (1975): A case of anaphylactoid reaction to thiamylal. *Jap. J. Anesth., 24*, 743-748.

Driggs, R.L. and O'Day, R.A. (1972): Acute allergic reaction associated with methohexital anesthesia: report of six cases. *J. oral Surg., 30*, 906-909.

Dundee, J.W. (1956): *Thiopentone and Other Thiobarbiturates.* Livingstone, Edinburgh and London.

Dundee, J.W., Assem, E.S.K., Gaston, J.H., Keilty, S.R., Sutton, J.A., Clarke, R.S.J. and Grainger, D. (1974): Sensitivity to intravenous anaesthetics: report of three cases. *Brit. med. J., 1*, 63-65.

Dundee, J.W., Fee, J.P.H., McDonald, J.R. and Clarke, R.S.J. (1978): Frequency of atopy and allergy in an anaesthetic patient populations. *Brit. J. Anaesth., 50*, 793-798.

Evans, F. and Gould, J. (1952): Relation between sensitivity to thiopentone, sulphonamides and sunlight. *Brit. med. J., 1*, 417.

Evans, J.M. and Keogh, J.A.H. (1977): Adverse reactions to intravenous anaesthetic induction agents. *Brit. med. J., 2*, 735-736.

Fee, J.P.H., McDonald, J.R., Dundee, J.W. and Clarke, R.S.J. (1978): Frequency of previous anaesthesia in an anaesthetic patient populations. *Brit. J. Anaesth., 50*, 917-920.

Fisher, M.M. (1975): Severe histamine-mediated reactions to intravenous drugs used in anaesthesia. *Anaesth. intens. Care, 3*, 180-197.

Fisher, M.M. (1976a): Severe histamine-mediated reactions to Althesin. *Anaesth. intens. Care, 4*, 33-35.

Fisher, M.M. (1976b): Intradermal testing after severe histamine reactions to intravenous drugs used in anaesthesia. *Anaesth. intens. Care, 4*, 97-104.

Fisher, M.M. (1977a): Intradermal testing after severe reactions to anaesthetic drugs. *Anaesth. intens. Care, 5*, 272.

Fisher, M.M. (1977b): Blood volume replacement in acute anaphylactic cardiovascular collapse related to anaesthesia. *Brit. J. Anaesth., 49*, 1023-1026.

Fisher, M.M. (1979): Intradermal testing in the diagnosis of acute anaphylaxis during anaesthesia − results of five years experience. *Anaesth. intens. Care, 7*, 58-61.

Galley, A.H. (1963): methohexitone (discussion) *Proc. roy. Soc. Med., 56*, 377-8.

Glen, J.B., Davies, G.E., Thompson, D.S., Scarth, S.C. and Thompson, A.V. (1979): An animal model for the investigation of adverse responses to i.v. anaesthetic agents and their solvents. *Brit. J. Anaesth., 51*, 819-827.

Grimmeisen, H. (1971): Epontol anaesthesia. *Med. Klin., 66*, 1417.

Gunner, B.W., Harrison, G.A. and Walker, W.D. (1965): Propanidid, a new short-acting anaesthetic. *Med. J. Aust., 2*, 327-329.

Haslett, W.H.K. and Dundee, J.W. (1968): Studies of drugs given before anaesthesia. XIV. Two benzo-diazepine derivatives − chlordiazepoxide and diazepam. *Brit. J. Anaesth., 40*, 250-258.

Hughes, R.L., Inglis, M. and Campbell, D. (1977): Althesin reactions. *Anaesthesia, 32*, 910-911.

Hunter, A.R. (1943): Dangers of pentothal sodium anaesthesia. *Lancet, 1*, 46-48.

Kay, B. (1972): Brietal sodium in children's surgery. In: *Das Ultrakurznarkoticum Methohexital.* Editor: C. Lehmann. Springer-Verlag, Berlin. pp. 149-158.

Jago, R.H. and Restall, J. (1978): Sensitivity testing for Althesin. *Anaesthesia, 33*, 644-645.

Lorenz, W., Doenicke, A., Meyer, R., Reinmann, J., Kusche, J., Barth, M., Geesing, H., Hutzel, M. and Weissenbacher, B. (1972): Histamine release in man by propanidid and thiopentone: pharmacological effects and clinical consequences. *Brit. J. Anaesth., 44*, 355-369.

Mathieu, A., Goudsouzian, N. and Snider, M.T. (1975): Reaction to ketamine: anaphylactoid or anaphylactic. *Brit. J. Anaesth., 47*, 624.

Radnay, P. (1965): Allergic and anaphylactic reactions, decrease in blood pressure. In: *Intravenous anaesthesia for outpatients.* Editor: M. Zindler. *Acta anaesth. scand., Suppl. 17*, 79-80.

Reichert, E.F. and Bassett, P.A. (1972): A rare allergic reaction to sodium methohexital. *J. oral Surg., 30*, 910.

Samuel, I.O. and Dundee, J.W. (1973): Clinical studies of induction agents. XLII: Influence of injection rate and dosage on the induction complications with Althesin. *Brit. J. Anaesth., 45*, 1215-1216.

Savege, T.M., Foley, E.I. and Simpson, B.R. (1973): Some cardiorespiratory effects of Cremophor EL in man. *Brit. J. Anaesth., 45*, 515-517.

Shafto, C.E. (1969): Continuous intravenous anaesthesia for paediatric dentistry. *Brit. J. Anaesth., 41*, 407-416.

Shaw, H. (1974): Anaesthetic complications. *N.Z. Soc. Anaesth. Newsletter, 21*, 144.

Sneddon, I.B. and Glew, R.C. (1973): Contact dermatitis due to propanidid in an anaesthetist. *Practitioner, 211*, 321-323.

Soga, D., Beer, R., Bader, B., Andrae, J. and Gotz, E. (1973): Die Beëinflussung der linksventrikularen Myokardkontraktilitat und Haemodynamik durch Propanidid beim Menschen. In: *Intravenose Narkose mit Propanidid.* Editors: M. Zindler, H. Yamamura and W. Wirth. Springer-Verlag, Berlin. pp. 78-87.

Uppington, J. (1973): Epileptiform convulsions with Althesin. *Anaesthesia, 28*, 546-550.

Watkins, J. (1980): Adverse reactions to intravenous induction agents. In: *Adverse responses to anaesthetic drugs.* Editor J.A. Thornton. Elsevier, North-Holland Biomedical Press.

Watkins, J., Clark, A., Appleyard, T.N. and Padfield, A. (1976a): Immune-mediated reactions to Althesin (Alphaxalone). *Brit. J. Anaesth., 48*, 881-886.

Watkins, J., Thornton, J.A. and Clarke, R.S.J. (1976b): Adverse reactions to intravenous anaesthetics. *Brit. J. Anaesth., 48*, 118.

Watkins, J., Udnoon, S., Appleyard, T.N. and Thornton, J.A. (1976c): Identification and quantitation of hypersensitivity reactions to intravenous anaesthetic agents. *Brit. J. Annesth., 48*, 457-461.

Watt, J.M. (1975): Anaphylactic reactions after use of CT 1341 (Althesin). *Brit. med. J., 3*, 205-206.

Whitwam, J.G. (1978): Adverse reactions to i.v. induction agents. *Brit. J. Anaesth., 50*, 677-687.

Wyatt, R. and Watkins, J. (1975): Reaction to methohexitone. *Brit. J. Anaesth., 47*, 1119-1120.

Zindler, M. (1965): Allergic and anaphylactic reactions, decrease in blood pressure. *Acta anaesth. scand., Suppl. 17*, 79-80.

3

Adverse reactions to intravenous agents: side effects

J.G. Whitwam

INTRODUCTION

The induction of anaesthesia by the intravenous route was introduced over forty five years ago. Many of the drugs which have been used for this purpose are now of little more than historial interest and a complete list of all the sequelae which have been associated with their use would be too long for inclusion in this short review.

In recent years, particularly since the introduction of non-barbiturate induction agents, there has been an increasing awareness and emphasis on the occurence of acute reactions involving the immune system, some of which occur on first exposure to the drugs and there is a tendency to equate the term "adverse reaction" with "immune mediated". However, the majority of adverse reactions to the intravenous induction agents are not immune based but are caused by side effects, secondary effects or overdose in either normal subjects or those who are intolerant to the drug and have exaggerated responses. This article is restricted to these types of reactions in otherwise healthy subjects, which may follow single or repeated administration of drugs used to induce anaesthesia by the intravenous route. The drugs and techniques which will be considered are listed in Table 3.1. The problems associated with drug interactions will be considered only where relevant, for example, the effects of premedication. The common aim with all these drugs is to induce loss of awareness and "anaesthesia" rapidly (e.g. within one arm brain circulation time), and pleasantly, without any serious adverse physiological effects. Ideally there should be sufficient reflex depression to allow surgery without the addition of other drugs. Recovery should also occur free from side effects at a time which can be determined accurately by the anaesthetist. The number and variety of drugs currently under investigation implies that as yet no one drug fulfils these requirements. Indeed if such an ideal drug ever becomes available then this type of review would cease to have any relevance except as an historial document.

The following classification provides a basis for a comparison of the effects of the drugs under consideration (Table 3.1).

Induction complications. Probably the best approach to a discussion of the induction characteristics of these drugs is that introduced by Dundee and his colleagues (Dundee, Barron and King, 1960; Dundee and Riding, 1960; Dundee and Moore, 1961a,b). Induction complications are classified as follows: (a) excitatory phenomena, that is tremors and involuntary muscle movements mostly involving the limbs; (b) respiratory upset, that is cough, hiccup and laryngospasm; (c) respiratory depression; (d) cardiovascular changes.

Tissue irritation and damage. (Drug and solvent). For example, pain on injection and venous complications. Effects of accidental arterial injection.

Duration of action

Recovery. (a) Psychic phenomena − dreaming, hallucinations, dissociative phenomena, delirium, anxiety and agitation, emotional reactions, longterm effects of frequent repeated administrations; (b) motor phenomena, for example, increased tone, tremors and convulsions; (c) effects on pain; (d) nausea and vomiting.

TABLE 3.

CLASSIFICATION OF INTRAVENOUS INDUCTION AGENTS

Barbiturates	− Thiopentone
	Methohexitone.
Euglenols	− Propanidid
Steroids	− Althesin
	Minaxolone
Imidazole derivatives	− Etomidate
Phenol derivative	− Di-isopropyl phenol
	(I.C.I. 35868).
Benzodiazepines	− Diazepam
	Midazolam
Phenylcyclohexamines	− Ketamine
Opiates	Morphine
	Papaveretum
	Fentanyl
Neuroleptanalgesia	− Combination of an opiate with a "neuroleptic" agent such as a butyrophenone derivative, e.g. fentanyl and droperidol.

INDUCTION COMPLICATIONS

Excitatory phenomena

The systematic study, documentation and classification of excitatory phenomena started with the introduction of methohexitone. These phenomena had been observed previously with drugs such as hexobarbitone, (Dundee and Wyant, 1974), but it was the interest taken by the Belfast group under Professor Dundee which led to a formal description of these phenomena and subsequently to study of the possibility of reducing their incidence, for example by the use of opiates.

Muscle movements and tremors were not mentioned in the original report on the clinical effects of methohexitone (Stoelting, 1957). Since then their reported incidence has varied from very low, for example 3% (Taylor and Stoelting, 1960) to as high as 35 − 40% depending principally on the dose of the drug and the premidication used (e.g. Redish et al., 1958; Wyant and Chang, 1959; Dundee and Moore, 1961a,b; Moore and Dundee, 1961; Whitwam and Manners, 1962).

Propanidid induces muscle movements and tremor in about 11% of patients (Dundee and Clarke, 1964) and in this respect it is better than methohexitone but worse than thiopentone. Although althesin is a much "smoother" induction agent than methohexitone it also causes these phenomena in up to 20% of patients (Clarke, Dundee and Carson, 1972) and in one report, in paediatric anaesthesia (Keep and Manford, 1974) their frequency and severity were greater than with methohexitone. Etomidate causes the highest incidence of muscle movements during induction of anaesthesia of any of the intravenous agents currently available. For example Holdcroft and her colleagues (1976) reported a 60% incidence of muscle movements in unpremedicated patients while Zacharias, Dundee and Clarke, 1978 suggested that the incidence might be as high as 95%. Holdcroft et al. (1976) also noticed an increase in muscle tone in up to 8% of unpremedicated patients during recovery from etomidate and this has been confirmed in patients during recovery from etomidate anaesthesia for bronchoscopy. (McIntosh et al., 1979). However, unlike ketamine which may cause prolonged changes in muscle tone, the incidence of involuntary muscle movements during recovery is relatively short lived and did not last longer than 10 min in any case.

The incidence of involuntary muscle movements, and increased muscle tone is also high during induction of anaesthesia with minaxolone, varying between 16% and 70% in different reports. (Aveling et al., 1979); McNeill et al., 1979; Punchihewa et al., 1980) depending on the dose and the associated use of other drugs such as fentanyl. Punchihewa et al. (1980) also observed that these movements persisted into the post operative period in 22% of patients who wee premedicated with atropine alone and in 6% of patients who also received fentanyl; in some patients these movements persisted up to 20 min.

Early reports on midazolam and ICI 35868 suggest that both these drugs are associated with smooth induction of anaesthesia, relatively free from adverse reactions of this type (Conner et al., 1978; Reves et al., 1978; Kay and Rolly 1977a,b).

Ketamine causes tremor and involuntary muscle movements fairly frequently, and there is often an incrase in muscle tone to such an extent that the airway can become difficult to manage (Dundee and Wyant, 1974). Foldes and his colleagues (1966) observed that fentanyl could cause muscle rigidity and laryngospasm and Corssen (Corseen, Domino and Sweet, 1966; Corssen, 1966) also commented on the "lead pipe" rigidity which was sometimes associated with the administration of mixtures of droperidol and fentanyl. Schotz and Zeigler (1967) expressed the opinion that muscle rigidity was related to the speed of administration rather than to the total dose of fentanyl. This view has been confirmed by Fox, Fox and Crandell (1967) and Morgan, Lumley and Gillies (1974). In terms of the modern use of high-dose fentanyl (e.g. 50 μg $\cdot$ kg^{-1}) during induction of anaesthesia, the tendency to muscle rigidity will be abolished by the use of muscle relaxants which are administered ot provide conditions suitable for intubation and artificial respiration.

Respiratory upset

There is a low frequency of cough, hiccup and laryngospasm with thiopentone (Dundee and Moore, 1961a), Althesin (Clarke Dundee and Carson, 1972) and propanidid (Dundee and Clarke, 1964). The frequency with etomidate is also low and does not appear to be dependent on the dose (Holdcroft et al., 1976). With methohexitone, a frequency as high as 40–45% has been reported (Moore and Dundee, 1961; Young and Whitwam, 1964a).

Laryngospasm, when it occurs while the patient is mainly under the influence of methohexitone, is usually mild and passes off rapidly (Taylor and Stoelting, 1960; Young and Whitwam, 1964a). In preliminary reports with minaxolone the incidence has varied between 3% and 20% (Aveling et al., 1979; McNeill et al., 1979; Punchihewa et al., 1980). The incidence of these complications with midazolam and ICI 35868 appears to be very low (e.g. Dundee, 1979).

Factors influencing excitatory phenomena and respiratory upset

Dose of the drug. As mentioned above, with fentanyl the frequency and severity of muscle rigidity are related to the dose. Greater frequency and severity of these reactions occur when the induction doses of thiopentone, methohexitone, Althesin and propanidid are increased, but this is not true of etomidate (Holdcroft et al., 1976). McNeill et al. (1979) have suggested that with minaxolone the incidence of excitatory effects was less when the dose was increased from 0.5 mg · kg^{-1} to 1.0 mg · kg^{-1}. Were this observation to be confirmed then in this respect minaxolone would be different to the other drugs in this group.

Speed of administration. This is an important factor with fentanyl (Morgan, Lumley and Gillies, 1974) and methohexitone (Barron, 1968).

Influence of other drugs. Dundee and his associates (1961) made a detailed study of the effect of premedication on these complications with methohexitone. Hyoscine causes a higher frequency than atropine. Promethazine should be avoided because of the frequency and severity of the reactions during subsequent administration of methohexitone. Drugs with analgesic properties decrease the frequency, and this is also true for thiopentone, propanidid and Althesin (Dundee, Carson and Clarke, 1972) and etomidate (Holdcroft et al., 1976). Goroszeniuk and colleagues observed that a small dose of fentanyl (for example 0.1 mg) administered i.v. would abolish the muscle movements associated with methohexitone (Goroszeniuk, Whitwam and Morgan, 1977). Diazepam also reduces their frequency with etomidate, but is not as effective as the opiates (Doenicke et al., 1973; Holdcroft et al., 1976). Fentanyl reduces the incidence of excitatory phenomena following minaxolone (Punchihewa et al., 1980). The position can be summarized by saying that, in order to minimize these complications and ensure "smooth" induction of anaesthesia, the patient should be premedicated with opiates, the dose of the drug should be kept to the minimum and it should be injected slowly. However, this last remark may not be true for etomidate and minaxolone.

Respiratory depression

All the opiates and their derivatives can produce respiratory arrest and the subject has been reviewed by Swerdlow (1967). The barbiturates cause respiratory depression and, in equipotent doses, thiopentone and methohexitone cause similar effects with a high frequency of apnoea, for example as great as 70% (Whitwam, 1962). Opiates enhance the adverse effects of both thiopentone and methohexitone on respiration (Eckenhoff and Helrich, 1958; Dundee et al., 1961). The frequency of apnoea is also markedly increased by pre-oxygenation as a result of the reduction of activity of the peripheral chemoreceptors (Fry, Whitwam and Chakrabarti, 1973). One of the striking features of the administration of propanidid is an initial period of respiratory stimulation. However, this is followed very often by a period of apnoea which may be as long as that seen following the administration of the barbiturates (Zindler, 1965). A brief period of hyperventilation also occurs in the majority of patients following the induction of anaesthesia with etomidate and Althesin, but this is less marked than with propanidid. A brief period of hyperventilation sometimes occurs towards the end of the injection of minaxolone and this is similar to that seen following etomidate and althesin (Punchihewa et al., 1980). Hall, Whitwam and Morgan (1973) and Morgan, Lumley and Whitwam (1977) reported a frequency of apnoea of 41% and 30% following Althesin and etomidate respectively. The incidence of apnoea following the administration of minaxolone is less than that observed with either althesin or etomidate. It was observed in 20–35% of patients by Punchihewa et al. (1980) and in 4 out of 66 patients by Aveling et al. (1979). McNeill et al. (1979) noticed no pronounced respiratory depression in patients receiving $0.5 \text{ mg} \cdot \text{kg}^{-1}$ or less of minaxolone, and there was only a 10% incidence of pronounced respiratory depression when a dose of $1.0 \text{ mg} \cdot ^{-1}$ was used. Punchihewa et al. (1980) found that premedication with papaveretum did not increase the incidence of apnoea following minaxolone, but that the minute volume, 3 min after injection was significantly less than patients who had not received opiates. The very limited early experience with ICI 35868 suggests that it does cause a transient dose related period of respiratory depression but that this is less than that seen following methohexitone (Dundee, 1979). Midazolam can cause short periods of apnoea but the respiratory depression caused by hypnotic doses of this drug appears to be of little clinical significance (Dundee, 1979). The depression of minute volume caused by etomidate is relatively transient (Morgan, Lumley and Whitwam, 1977), and its effects on respiration are less than with Althesin and the barbiturates. However, one advantage of Althesin is that although Hall, Whitwam and Morgan (1973) observed that the frequency of apnoea using a dose of $100 \mu l \cdot \text{kg}^{-1}$ was 50% compared with 32.5% using a dose of $50 \mu l \cdot \text{kg}^{-}$, 3 min after injection there was no significant difference in the degree of respiratory depression between the high and low doses and it was suggested that this may be of value in obstetric anaesthesia. Ketamine causes a very low frequency of apnoea, for example under 1% (Morgan et al., 1971). Droperidol does not have any significant effect on respiratory function (Prys-Roberts and Kelman, 1967). Usually the effects of diazepam on the respiratory system are minimal (Healy, 1969). However, some workers have observed marked hypoventilation with diazepam, for example a reduction in minute volume of 20–30% (Stovner and Endressen, 1965, 1966) and respiratory arrest have been reported (Buskop, Price and Molmar, 1967). Both opiates (Dundee et al., 1970) and barbitures (Prensky et al., 1967) markedly increase the depressant effects of diazepam on respiration.

Cardiovascular effects

Lyons and Clarke (1972) observed that thiopentone, methohexitone and Althesin in relatively equipotent doses caused similar decreases in arterial pressure in heavily pre-medicated cardiac patients. Dundee and Clarke (1964) found that the frequency of hypotension was similar with thiopentone, methohexitone and propanidid when given in equipotent low doses; however, when the dose was increased propanidid consistently produced considerably more cardiovascular depression. Conway, Ellis and King (1968) showed that propanidid was capable of causing profound cardiovascular depression. I.C.I 35868 causes similar haemodynamic changes to those produced by thiopentone althesin (Dundee 1979). Clinical doses of midazolam have only minimal effects on the circulation (Dundee 1979). Ketamine, given as a single dose of 2 mg · kg^{-1} i.v., has been observed to cause a large increase in systemic and pulmonary arterial pressure, heart rate, and central venous and wedge pressures and cardiac index (Savege et all., 1976). However, when a second dose of ketamine was administered after the first dose, they observed a decrease in cardiac output and heart rate and very little change in arterial pressure. It would appear that the previous administration of diazepam prevents the stimulatory effects of ketamine on the circulation (Jackson et al., 1978). In general, opiates will cause cardiovascular depression when administered i.v. in large doses, and again the subject has been reviewed by Swerdlow (1967).

In animals fentanyl causes a decrease in arterial pressure and heart rate and it has been suggested that the bradycardia is caused by sensitization of the baroreceptor reflex (Laubie et al., 1974). Stanley (1978) has shown that fentanyl, when administered to patients in a dose of 20 μg · kg^{-1}, causes a significant reduction in heart rate and arterial pressure. However, he found that additional fentanyl up to 50 μg · kg^{-1} did not increase this effect.

The i.v. injection of droperidol in man causes a relatively small reduction in arterial pressure and it antagonizes the peripheral vasoconstriction caused by cate-cholamines, but these effects are transient (Whitwam and Russell, 1971. The combined effects of fentanyl and droperidol on the circulation are depressant (Prys-Roberts and Kelman, 1967). In normal, healthy subjects the effects of diazepam in moderate clinical doses on the circulation are minimal (Healy, Robinson and Vickers, 1970). However, cardiovascular collapse has been reported following the use of this drug (Rollason, 1968).

TISSUE IRRITATION

Pain on injection

Any combination of a drug and a solvent, either of which is irritant to the tissues, is likely to cause pain on injection. When administered in water, etomidate causes a pain in between 15% (Morgan, Lumley and Whitwam, 1975) and 50% (Zacharias, Dundee and Clarke, 1978) of patients. However, this is reduced when the drug is presented in either cremophor or propylene glycol. Taylor and Stoelting (1960) reported a high frequency of pain on injection of methohexitone, but subsequent papers failed to confirm this finding (Coleman and Green, 1960). Rowlands (1969) estimated that the frequency for methohexitone was between 1% and 5%. Diazepam causes either pain or an unpleasant sensation during injection in a high percentage of patients. Minazolam is a water soluble benzodiazepine, it causes no pain on injection and does not cause venous thrombosis. The injection of I.C.I. 35868 is associated with pain in a high percentage of patients.

Venous complications

Any i.v. injection may be followed by tenderness, thrombosis or thrombophlebitis (Riding, 1975). Venous complications occur in about 2–3% of patients who receive thiopentone, methohexitone and Althesin, but with propanidid the frequency may increase to approximately 10% (Carson et al., 1972). These figures can be made worse by increasing the concentration of the drugs. Holdcroft and colleagues (1976) reported that only one of 400 patients who received etomidate developed thrombophlebitis. Hegarty and Dundee (1977) observed a frequency of venous thrombosis of 23%, 2–3 days after the i.v. injection of diazepam 10 mg and this increased to 39% after 7–10 days.

Intra arterial injection

The i.v. agents arrive at the tissues through the arterial system, and hence all injections eventually become intra-arterial. However, by the time the drugs have passed from a peripheral vein into the pulmonary circulation, they are sufficiently diluted various physiochemical changes will have occurred so that the pulmonary arteries are not routinely damaged. When a barbiturate is injected into an artery, crystal formation is caused by the decrease in pH; in addition red cell haemolysis and platelet aggregation occur and the result is intravacular thrombosis (Dundee and Wyant, 1974).

Since the descriptions of the sequelae of the intra-arterial injection of thiopentone (macintosh and Heyworth, 1943; Cohen, 1948), this has been an important consideration when administering any drug intravenously. Francis (1964) and Mather and Goodhead (1966) found that thiopentone and methohexitone in equal amounts caused similar damage when injected intra-arterially into the ears of rabbits. Since methohexitone is normally administered in only one-third the dose of thiopentone, they considered methohexitone, as used in clinical practice, to be safer in this respect. What evidence there is, suggests that the intra-arterial injection of propanidid in man does not necessarily cause vascular damage (Dundee and Wyant, 1974). However, it would be most unwise to say that the intra-arterial injection of any of these drugs wil be without risk under all circumstances.

The case reported by Schneider and Mace (1974) should be a reminder of the need for extreme care when injecting these drugs. A 4-yr-old epileptic male child was admitted with uncontrolled seizures. Diazepam 10 mg (in 2 ml) was injected i.v. on the volar surface of the left wrist. Four hours later the hand and forearm were observed to be swollen and dusky, and in spite of all treatment an above-elbow amputation was required 6 days later. Pathology showed extensive thrombosis of the ulnar, radial and brachial arteries, and a prominent feature was extensive platelet thrombi. Platelet antibodies of diazepam have been described (Baume, 1971), but were not tested in this patient. They concluded that it is possible that at least part of the injection may have been intra-arterial the wrist, but that the mechanism for the extensive arterial damage and thrombosis was not clear. The author has been informed of another patient who had necrosis of relevant tissue after the accidental administration of diazepam into the radial artery.

Perhaps the ventral aspect of the wrist, where the veins are located adjacent to either radial or ulnar arteries, should be avoided for intravenous injections, just as one avoids the veins on the medial side of the antecubital fossa close to the brachial artery.

DURATION OF ACTION

This is not really an adverse reaction but, since it is a property of these drugs which may complicate their application and use, a few observations are relevant.

Propanidid, which is rapidly metabolized, has a very short duration of action (Doenicke et al., 1968).

Etomidate has a short duration of action when administered in single doses. However McIntosh et al. (1979) compared methohexitone and etomidate for bronchoscopy and found that recovery in the patients who had received methohexitone was quicker than those who received etomidate.

In terms of immediate recovery, methohexitone has a shorter duration of action than Althesin and thiopentone (Clarke et al., 1971). The reasons for this are not very clear, but recently Briemer (1976) has shown that the terminal elimination half-life of methohexitone is relatively short (70–125 min) and he concluded that, after initial redistribution, the relatively rapid recovery was a result of rapid metabolism. Minaxolone is associated with a much longer period of recovery than the other drugs of similar purpose (Aveling et al., 1979; Punchihewa et al., 1980). Recovery from midazolam is also relatively slow, compared for example with thiopentone and althesin (Dundee, 1979). Potentially one of the major advantages of I.C.I. 35868 is its short duration of action and apparent lack of cumulative effects (Dundee, 1979).

Ketamine, the butyrophenones and the benzodiazepines all have a long duration of action, particularly the latter group (Dundee and Wyant, 1974). Occasionally ketamine may fail to produce anaesthesia and this is thought to be a result of the absence of appropriate cerebral development (Wyant, 1971; Janis and Wright, 1972).

RECOVERY

Psychic phenomena

It is not uncommon for patients recovering from anaesthesia to be restless and occasionally to show emotional reactions; however, the problem of psychic reactions during recovery from anaesthesia became the subject of intense research following the introduction of ketamine. Domino, Chodoff and Corssen (1965), in the first detailed report of the use of ketamine in man, described the sequelae as followed: "During the recovery period the subjects showed considerable variation in psychic reaction. Some were completely orientated in time and space, and showed no significant changes. Others showed marked alteration in mood and affect, some becoming apprehensive and aggressive, and other markedly withdrawn. Almost all subjects felt entirely numb, and in extreme instances stated that they had no arms or legs or that they were dead". Other reactions noted included feelings of estrangement or isolation, negativism, hostility, apathy, drowsiness inebriation, hypogenic states and repetitive motor behaviour. Diplopia and other visual disturbances sometimes occurred on return to consciousness, and some patients thought they were blind. The patient may have difficulty in speaking and severe emergence delirium may occur. Reactions of this type following ketamine in hypnotic doses occur in a high percentage of patients.

Much effort has been spent in seeking ways of eliminating these reactions, either by avoiding stimulation of the patient (Corssen, Miyasaka and Domino, 1968) or by the use of other drugs such as diazepam. Reports on the ability of diazepam to modify these emergence reactions are conflicting. For example, Loh and colleagues (1972) failed to find any effect of the benzodiazepine on emergence reactions. However, Coppell, Bovill and Dundee (1973), using much larger doses of diazepam, found that they were able to reduce the frequency of unpleasant dreams and delirium to acceptable values. Johnstone (1972) completely abolished the emergence reactions by the use of oral nitrazepam and droperidol. The frequency of reactions following ketamine anaesthesia in children appears to be less than in adults (Wilson, Nichols and McCoy, 1967; Page Morgan and Loh, 1972). A very small frequency of emergence reactions has been reported in obstetrics (moore, McNabb and Dundee, 1971). Peltzand Sinclair (1973) found that the frequency of awareness during Caesarean section was lower using ketamine as an induction agent than using thiopentone. They also observed no significant difference in the frequency of unpleasant dreams and post-partum psychosis between these two drugs.

The butyrophenones can cause feelings of anxiety and agitation when they are administered alone (Hider, 1964; Clark, 1969). The patients may appear placid and are easily rousable, but their subjective experience is one of being agitated and ill at ease. However, this should not be a problem when droperidol is used as part of a neuroleptic technique, as it will always be administered with other drugs, such as fentanyl, in relatively large amounts which will suppress these reactions. One of the features of minaxolone is the high level of patient acceptability (Aveling et al., 1979).

Motor phenomena

Increased muscle tone is a common feature of ketamine anaesthesia and often persists into the period after operation. When excessive doses of the butyrophenones are used the patient may remain in an agitated state and also exhibit increased motor activity for a considerable period of time. Other drugs may be effective in controlling these phenomena. For example, Johnstone (1972) observed that a combination of nitrazepam and droperidol given before ketamine anaesthesia suppressed the musclar catatonia which would otherwise have been observed.

As mentioned above motor phenomena have been observed during the recovery period following both etomidate and minaxolone.

Effects on pain

Although induction agents are "short-acting" drugs, in sub-hypnotic doses they may alter pain thresholds and, therefore, following a relatively short procedure their effects may persist into the time following surgery. Pain is a very complex issue and the majority of the studies on the effects of theintravenous induction agents on pain have been performed using sub-hypnotic doses and some form of algesimetry.

Although these studies are open to criticism, the general conclusions are as follows. The barbiturates general conclusions are as follows. The barbiturates depress pain thresholds, that is they are "anti-analgesic" (Dundee, 1960; Clutton-Brock, 1961). Morgan, Whitwam and Page (1973) showed that, in its effects on pain, Althesin was very similar to the barbiturates.

Ketamine has very powerful analgesic properties (Domino Chodoff and Corssen, 1965), and, as with the barbiturates, its effects persist into the posthypnotic phase (Bjarnsen and Corssen, 1967). As a result, it has been suggested (Sadove et al., 1971) that small doses of ketamine can produce an analgesic effect in sub-dissociative doses (for example, $0.4 \text{ mg} \cdot \text{kg}^{-1}$), and it is being used in small doses for minor, potentially painful procedures such as the removal of chest drains.

Diazepam, when used for sedation, has the advantage that, unlike the barbiturates, it has little effect on experimentally-induced pain (Hall, Whitwam and Morgan, 1974). Droperidol has no analgesic effects itself. However, it may prolong the effectiveness of fentanyl and, like diazepam, does not appear to be contraindicated in the management of the patients after operation, inspite of its potentially adverse effect on pain sensibility (Morrison, Loan and Dundee, 1971).

Nausea and vomiting

Droperidol is a powerful anti-emetic agent and therefore a low frequency of nausea and vomiting would be anticipated following its use. Of the other agents, propanidid causes the greatest frequency of nausea and vomiting (up to 40% of patients) ketamine is a little better, with a frequency of nausea and vomiting of something under 40%. Of the remaining "short-acting" induction agents, that is althesin, thiopentone and methohexitone, althesin produces the smallest frequency of nausea and vomiting and methohexitone the greatest (Dundee and Wyant, 1974). However, these figures will depend on many factors, for example the type of surgery, the use of other drugs etc. For example, Young and Whitwam (1974b) observed an extremely small frequency of nausea and vomiting following dental anaesthesia induced with methohexitone and continued with nitrous oxide with or without the addition of halothane. Etomidate is associated with a relatively high incidence of postoperative nausea e.g. up to 30% (Holdcroft et al., 1976). When fentanyl is used together with etomidate the incidence of nausea and vomiting sufficiently high to limit its potential use in out patients (Dundee, 1979). Minaxolone is associated with a very low incidence of post anaesthetic nausea and vomiting

(Aveling et al., 1979; Punchihewa et al., 1979) It seems likely that Midazolam and I.C.I. 35868 will also be relatively trouble free in this respect (Dundee, 1979).

CONCLUSION

After over forty five years thiopentone remains the most commonly used induction agent and provides a standard by which other drugs of similar purpose can be compared. Methohexitone is still the induction agent of choice where rapid recovery is important, and in over twenty years of use it has proved safe and reliable. Of the newer agents, etomidate causes minimal cardiorespiratory depression and although it has only been in use a few years it also is proving to be a safe drug. ketamine has a place for the induction of anaesthesia in patients who are hypotensive due to haemorrhage, and also in whom ready and continuous access to the airway may not be available, (e.g. radiotherapy). It also has the advantage that it can be used intramuscularly when access to veins is difficult. If midazolam proves to have minimal effects on the cardiorespiratory system and is free from excitatory effects, then providing a dose which will consistently induce sleep can be established, it may have a significant role for the induction of anaesthesia in patients undergoing relatively long procedures and may provide a serious challenge to thiopentone. The new phenol derivative I.C.I. 35868 appears to be extremely promising for a trial as an intravenous agent where an absence of excitatory effects and cumulation are important e.g. for the induction of anaesthesia for short procedures and for the maintenance of anaesthesia by the intravenous route.

REFERENCES

Aveling, W., Sear, J.W., Fitch., Ahang, H., Waters A., Cooper, G.M., Simpson, P., Savege, T.M., Prys-Roberts, C. and Campbell, D. (1979): Early clinical evaluation of minaxolone: new intravenous steroid anaesthetic agent. *Lancet, 2,* 71-73.

Barron, D.W. (1968): Clinical studies of induction agents. XXII: Effect of rate of injection on incidence of side-effects with thiopentone and methohexital. *Anesth. Analg. (Cleve.), 47,* 171.

Baume, R. (1971): Cytopnies medicamenteuses: Purpura thrombopeenique origine et anticorps anti-plaquetaires actifs en presence de Valium. *Maroc. Med., 546,* 321.

Bjarnsen, W. and Corssen, G. (1967): CI 581: a new nonbarbiturate short acting anaesthetic for surgery in burns.

Brimer, D.D. (1976): Pharmacokinetics of methohexitone following intravenous infusion in humans. *Brit. J. Anaesth., 48,* 743.

Buskop, J.J., Price, M. and Malmar, I. (1967): Untoward effect of diaxepam. *New Engl. J. Med., 277,* 316.

Carson, I.W., Alexander, J.P., Hewitt, J.C. and Dundee, J.W. (1972): Clinical studies of induction agents. XLI: Venous sequelae following the use of steroid anaesthetic agent Althesin. *Brit. J. Anaesth., 44*, 1311.

Clark, M.M. (1969): Droperidol in preoperative anxiety. *Anaesthesia, 24*, 36.

Clarke, R.S.J., Dundee, J.W. and Carson, I.W. (1972): Some aspects of the clinical pharmacology of Althesin. *Postgrad. med. J. (Suppl. 2), 48*, 62.

Clarke, R.S.J., Dundee, J.W., Garrett, A.T., McArdle, G.K. and Sutton J.A. (1975): Adverse reactions to intravenous anaesthetics: a survey of 100 reports. *Brit. J. Anaesth., 47*, 575.

Clarke, R.S.J., Montgomery, S.J., Dundee J.W. and Bovill J.G. (1971): Clinical studies of induction agents. XXXIX: CT 1341 a new steroid anaesthetic. *Brit. J. Anaesth., 43*, 847.

Clutton-Brock, J. (1961): Pain and the barbiturates. *Anaesthesia, 16*, 80.

Cohen, S.M. (1948): Accidental intra-arterial injection of drugs. *Lancet, 2*, 361.

Coleman, J. and Green, R.A. (1960): Methohexital, a short acting barbiturate. *Anaesthesia, 15*, 411.

Conner, J.T., Katz, R.L., Pagano, R.R. and Graham, C.W. (1978): RO 21-3981 for intravenous surgical premedication and induction of anaesthezia. *Anesth. Analg. (Cleve.)., 51*, 1.

Conway, C.M., Ellis, D.B. and King, N.W. (1968): A comparison of the acute haemodynamic effects of thiopentone, methohexitone and propanidid in the dog. *Brit. J. Anaesth, 40*, 736.

Coppell, D.L., Bovill, J.G. and Dundee, J.W. (1973): The taming of ketamine. *Anaesthesia, 28*, 293.

Corssen, G. (1966): Neuroleptanalgesia and anaesthesia: its usefulness in poor-risk surgical cases. *South. Med. J., 59*, 801.

Corssen, G., Domino, E.F. and Sweet, R.B. (1964): Neuroleptanalgesia and anaesthesia. *Anesth. Analg. (Cleve.), 43*, 748.

Corssen, G., Miyasaka, M. and Domino, E.F. (1968): Changing concepts in pain control during surgery. Dissociative anesthesia with CI-581. A progress report. *Anesth. Analg. (Cleve.), 47*, 746.

Doenicke, A., Krumby, I., Kugler, J. and Klempa, J. (1968): Experimental studies of the breakdown of epontol: determination of propanidid in human serum. *Brit. J. Anaesth., 40*, 415.

Doenicke, A., Kugler, J., Penzel, G., Laub., Kalmer, L., Killian, I., and Bezecny. (1973): Hirnfunktion und Toleranzbreite nach Etomidate einem neuer barbituratfreien i.v. applizierbaren Hypnoticum. *Anaesthesist, 22*, 357.

Domino, E.F., Chodoff, P. and Corssen, G., (1965): Pharmacological effects of CI 581 a new dissociative anesthetic in man *Clin. pharmacol. Ther., 6*, 279.

Dundee, J.W. (1960): Alterations in response to somatic pain. *Brit. J. Anaesth., 32*, 407.

Dundee, J.W. (1979): New i.v. anaesthetics. *Brit. J. Anaesth., 51*, 641-648.

Dundee, J.W., Barron, D.W. and King, R. (1960): The effect of methylation on the anaesthetic action of ethyl-methyl-propyl-thiobarbiturate. *Brit. J. Anaesth., 32*, 566.

Dundee, J.W., Carson, I.W. and Clarke, A.S.J. (1972): kA comparison of Althesin (CT 1341) with methohexitone and propanidid as induction agents. In: *Proc. 5th World Congr. Anaesthesiologists, Kyoto*. Excerpta Medica, Amsterdam. p. 124.

Dundee, J.W. and Clarke, R.S.J. (1964): Clinical studies of induction agents IX: A comparative study of a new euglenol derivative FBA 1420 with G 29,505 and standard barbitutates. *Brit. J. Anaesth., 36*, 100.

Dundee, J.W., Haslett, W.H.K., Keilty, S.R. and Pandit S.K. (1970): Studies of drugs given before anaesthesia. XX: Diaxepam-containing mixtures. *Brit. J. Anaesth., 42*, 143.

Dundee, J.W. and Moore, J. (1961a): Thiopentone and methohexital. A comparison as main anaesthetic agents for a standard operation. *Anaesthesia, 16*, 50.

Dundee, J.W. and Moore, J. (1961b): The effect of Scopolamine on methohexital anaesthesia. *Anaesthesia, 16*, 194.

Dundee, J.W. and Riding, J.E. (1960): A Comparison of inactin and thiopentone as intravenous anaesthetics. *Brit. J. Anaesth., 32*, 206.

Dundee, J.W., Riding, J.E., Barron, D.W. and Nicholl, R.M. (1961): Some factors influencing the
induction characteristics of methohexitone anaesthesia. *Brit. J. Anaesth. 33*, 296.

Dundee, J.W., and Wyant, G.M. (1974): *Intravenous Anaesthesia, 1st edn.* Churchill Livingstone,
Edinburgh and Londen.

Eckenhoff, J.E. and Helrich, M. (1958): The effect of narcotics, thiopental and nitrous oxide upon respiration and respiratory responses to hypercapnia. *Anesthesiology, 19*, 240.

Foldes, F.F., Kepes, E.R., Kronfield, P.P. and Siffman, H.P. (1966): A rational approach to neuro-
leptanesthesia. *Anesth. Analg. (Cleve.), 45*, 642.

Fox. J.W.C., Fox, E.J. and Crandel L. (1967): Neuroleptanalgesia for heart and major surgery. *Arch.
Surg., 94*, 102.

Francis, J.G. (1964): Intra-arterial methohexitone. *Anaesthesia, 19*, 501.

Fry, D.E., Whitwam, J.G. and Chakrabarti M.K. (1973): Induction apnoea and the peripheral chemoreceptors. *Brit. J. Anaesth., 45*, 1054.

Goroszeniuk, T., Whitwam, J.G. and Morgan, M. (1977): Use of methohexitone, nitrous oxide and
fentanyl for short surgical procedures. *Anaesthesia, 32*, 209.

Goroszeniuk, T., Morgan, M. and Whitwam, J.G. (1977): An evaluation of etomidate-fentanyl-
nitrous oxide for short surgical procedures. *Anesth. rean. intens. Ther., IX*, 147.

Hall, G.M., Whitwam, J.G. and Morgan, M. (1973): Some respiratory effects of Althesin. *Brit. J.
Anaesth., 45*, 629.

Hall, G.M., Whitwam, J.G. and Morgan, M. (1974): Effect of diazepam on experimentally induced
pain. *Brit. J. Anaesth., 46*, 50.

Healy, T.E.J. (1969): Intravenous diazepam for cardiac catheterisation. *Anaesthesia, 24*, 537.

Healy, T.E.J., Robinson, J.S. and Vickers, M.D. (1979): Physiological responses to intravenous diazepam as a sedative for conservative dentistry. *Brit. med. J., 3*, 10.

Hegarty, J.E. and Dundee, J.W. (1977): Sequelae after the intravenous injection of three benzodiazepines – diazepam, lorazepam and flunitrazepam. *Brit. med. J., 2*, 1384.

Hider, C.F. (1964): In the application of neuroleptanalgesia. In: *Anaesthesia and Other Practice.*
Editors. N.W. Shephard. Pergamon Press, London.

Holdcroft, A., Morgan, M., Whitwam, J.G., and Lumley, J. (1976): Effect of dose and premedication
on induction complications with etomidate. *Brit. J. Anaesth., 48*, 199.

Jackson, A.P.F., Dhadphale, P.R., Callaghan, P.L. and Alseri, S. (1978): Haemodynamic studies
during induction of anaesthesia for open heart surgery using diazepam and ketamine. *Brit. J.
Anaesth., 50*, 375.

Janis, K.M. and Wright, W. (1972): Failure to produce analgesia with ketamine in two patients with
cortical disease. *Anesthesiology, 36*, 405.

Johnstone, M. (1972): The prevention of ketamine dreams. *Anesth. intens. Care, 1*, 70.

Kay, B. and Rolly, G. (1977a): I.C.I. 35868, a new intravenous induction agent. *Acta anaesthesiol. belg.,
28*, 303.

Kay, B. and Rolly, G. (1977b): I.C.I. 35868 – The effect of a change of formulation on pain after intravenous injeciton. *Acta anaesthesiol. belg., 28*, 317.

Keep, P.J. and Manford, M.L.M. (1974): A comparison of Althesin and methohexitone in paediatric
anaesthesia. *Brit. J. Anaesth., 46*, 685.

Laubiem L., Schmitt, H., Canellas, J., Roquebert, J. and Demichel, P. (1974): Centrally mediated
bradycardia and hypotension induced by narcotic analgesics: dextromoramide and fentanyl. *Europ. J.
Pharmacol., 28*, 66.

Loh, L., Singer, L., Morgan, M. and Moore, P.H. (1972): Influence of diazepam on the emergence reactions following ketamine anaesthesia. *Canad. Anaesth. Soc. J., 19*, 421.

Lyons, S.M. and Clarke, R.S.J. (1972): A comparison of different drugs for anaesthesia in cardiac surgical patients. *Brit. J. Anaesth., 44*, 575.

Macintosh, R.R. and Heyworth, P.S.A. (1943): Intra-arterial injection of pentothal. *Lancet, 2*, 571.

McIntosh, B.M.M., Lumley, J., Morgan, M. and Stradling, P. (1979): Methohexitone and etomidate for bronchoscopy, *34*, 239-244.

McNeill, M.G., Clarke, R.S.J. and Dundee, J.W. (1979): Minaxolone: a new water soluble steroid anaesthetic. *Lancet, 2*, 73-74.

Mather, J.S. and Goodhead, B. (1966): Intra-arterial methohexitone and thiopentone. *Anaesthesia, 21*, 81.

Moore, J. and Dundee, J.W. (1961): Promethazine, Its influence on the course of thiopentone and methohexital anaesthesia. *Anaesthesia, 16*, 61.

Moore, J., McNabb, T.G. and Dundee, J.W. (1971): Preliminary report on ketamine in obstetrics. *Brit. J. Anaesth., 43*, 779.

Morgan, M., Loh, L., Singer, L. and Moore, P.H. (1977): Ketamine as the sole anaesthetic agent for minor surgical procedures. *Anaesthesia, 26*, 158.

Morgan, M., Lumley, J. and Gillies, I.D.S. (1974): Neuroleptanaesthesia for major surgery. Experience with 500 cases. *Brit. J. Anaesth., 46*, 288.

Morgan, M., Lumley, J. and Whitwam, J.G. (1975): Etomidate – a new water-soluble, non-barbiturate intravenous induction agent. *Lancet, 1*, 955.

Morgan, M., Lumley, J. and Whitwam, J.G. (1977): Respiratory effects of etomidate. *Brit. J. Anaesth., 49*, 233.

Morgan, M., Whitwam, J.G. and Page, P. (1973): Influence of subnarcotic doses of Althesin (CT 1341) on pain induced by two types of pain stimuli. *Brit. J. Anaesth., k45*, 481.

Morrison, J.D., Loan, W.B. and Dundee, J.W. (1971): Controlled comparison of the efficacy of fourteen preparations in the relief of postoperative pain. *Brit. med. J., 3*, 287.

Page, P., Morgan, M. and Loh, L. (1972): Ketamine anaesthesia in paediatric procedures. *Acta anaesthesiol. Scand., 16*, 155.

Peltz, B. and Sinclair, D.M. (1973): Induction agents for Caesarean sections: a comparison of thiopentone and ketamine. *Anaesthesia, 28*, 37.

Prensky, A.L., Raff, M.C., Moore, M.J. and Schwab, R.S. (1967): Intravenous diazepam in the treatment of prolonged seizure activity. *New Engl. J. Med., 276*, 779.

Prys-Roberts, C. and Kelman, G.R. (1967): The influence of drugs used in neuroleptanalgesia on cardiovascular and ventilatory function. *Brit. J. Anaesth., 39*, 134.

Punchihewa, V.G., Morgan, M., Lumley, J. and Whitwam, J.G. (1980): Initial experience with minaxolone: a water soluble steroid intravenous anaesthetic agent. *Anaesthesia, 35*, in press.

Punchihewa, V.G., Whitwam, J.G., Morgan, M., and Lumley, J. Respiratory effects of minaxolone. In preparation.

Redish, C.H., Vore R.E., Chernish, S.M. and Gruber, C.M. (1958): A comparison of thiopental sodium, methitural sodium and methohexital sodium in oral surgery patients. *J. oral Surg., 11*, 603.

Reves, J.G., Corssen, G. and Holcomb, C. (1978): Comparison of two benzodiazepines for anaesthesia induction: midazolam and diazepam. *Canad. Anaesth. Soc. J., 25*, 211.

Riding, J.E. (1975): Minor complications of general anaesthesia. *Brit. J. Anaesth., 49*, 91.

Rollason, W.N. (1968): Diazepam as an intravenous induction agent for general anaesthesia. In: *Diazepam in Anaesthesia*. Editors: P.F. Knight and C.G. Burgess. Wright. Bristol. p. 70.

Rowlands, D.E. (1969): Comments on injection pain. In: *Symposium on Methohexitone.* Eli Lilly and Co.

Sadove, M.S., Shulman, M., Hatano, S. and Fevold, N. (1971): Anesthetic effect of ketamine administered in subdissociative doses. *Anesth. Analg. (Cleve.), 50,* 452.

Savege, T.M., Colvin, M.P., Weaver, E.J.M., Bond, C., Drake, J. and Inniss, R. (1976): A comparison of some cardiorespiratory effects of Althesin and ketamine when used for induction of anaesthesia in patients with cardiac disease. *Brit. J. Anaesth., 48,* 1071.

Schneider, S., Mace, J.W. (1974): Loss of Limb following intravenous diazepam. *Paediatrics, 53,* 112.

Schotz, S. and Zeigler, M.L. (1967): Neuroleptanalgesia with Innovar. *Anesth. Analg. (Cleve.), 46,* 69.

Stanley, T.H. (1978): Anaesthetic requirements and cardiovascular effects of fentanyl-oxygen and fentanyldiazepam-oxygen anaesthesia in man. *Proc. roy Soc. Med.*

Stoelting, V.K. (1957): The use of a new intravenous oxygen barbiturate 25398 for intravenous anaesthesia (a preliminary report). *Anesth. Analg. (Cleve.), 36,* 49.

Stovner, J. and Endressen, R. (1965): Diazepam in intravenous anaesthesia. *Lancet, 2,* 1298.

Stovner, J. and Endressen, R. (1966): Intravenous anaesthesia with diazepam. Proceedings, of the 2nd European Congress of Anaesthesiology, *Acta anaesthesiol. scand., (Suppl.) 24,* 223.

Swerdlow, M. (1967): (General analgesics used in pain relief: Pharmacology. *Brit. J. Anaesth., 39,* 669.

Taylor, C. and Stoelting, V.K. (1960): Methohexital sodium − a new ultrashot acting barbiturate. *Anesthesiology, 21,* 29.

Whitwam, J.G. (1962): A clinical comparison of the incidence and duration of apnoea following methohexitone and thiopentone. *Brit. J. Anaesth., 24,* 729.

Whitwam, J.G. and Manners, J.M. (1962): Clinical comparison of thiopentone and methohexitone. *Brit. Med. J., 1,* 1663.

Whitwam, J.G. and Russell, W.T. (1971): The acute cardiovascular changes and adrenergic blockade by droperidol in man. *Brit. J. Anaesth., 43,* 581.

Wilson, R.D., Nichols, R.J. and McCoy, N.R. (1967): Dissociative anesthesia with CI-581 in burned children. *Anesth. Analg. (Cleve.), 46,* 719.

Wyant, G.M. (1971): Intramuscular Ketalar (CI-581) in paediatric anaesthesia. *Canad. Anaesth. Soc. J., 18,* 72.

Wyant, G.M. and Chang, C.A. (1959): Sodium methohexitone: a clinical study. *Canad. Anaesth. Soc. J., 6,* 40.

Young, D.S. and Whitwam, J.G. (1964a): Observations on dental anaesthesia introduced with methohexitone. I: Induction of anaesthesia. *Brit. J. Anaesth., 36,* 31.

Young, D.S. and Whitwam, J.G. (1964b): Observations on dental anaesthesia introduced with methohexitone. II: Maintenance and recovery. *Brit. J. Anaesth., 36,* 94.

Zacharias, M., Dundee, J.W. and Clarke, R.S.L. (1978): Eavaluation of Etomidate. *Brit. J. Anaesth., 50,* 634.

Zindler, M. (1965): Changes of respiration and blood gases after propanidid. *Acta anaesthesiol. scand. (Suppl.) XVII,* 67.

Thornton (ed.) Adverse Reactions of Anaesthetic Drugs
© Elsevier/North-Holland Biomedical Press, 1981

4

Adverse effects of neuromuscular blocking drugs

M. Lim and H.C. Churchill-Davidson

INTRODUCTION

In attempting to discuss adverse effects, the literature has been scanned for case reports implicating a particular muscle relaxant. It is necessary to remind the reader that in this field "the last drug given" is often blamed for any untoward effect yet conceivably it played no part. For example, in the past, muscle relaxants were often held to be responsible for the occurrence of prolonged post-operative apnoea; but the regular use of the peripheral nerve stimulator has shown that many such cases are the result of central respiratory depression rather than failure of peripheral mechanisms. Alternatively, a diagnosis of bronchospasm was easily made yet the true cause of increased airway resistance lay in some mechanical obstruction of the airway.

Another important element is the reluctance on the part of many anaesthetists to publicise cases with a fatal result. Partly from a feeling of self-embarrassment and partly from a fear of future legal proceeding, these case reports may never appear in the Journals. It is not possible, therefore, to be entirely comprehensive but we present here some of the adverse effecs that have been attributed to the muscle relaxants.

ANAPHYLACTOID REACTIONS

The intravenous administration of muscle relaxants can occasionally lead to the liberation of histamine (and possibly other chemical mediators e.g. serotonin, slow reacting substance (anaphylaxis, bradykinin and prostaglandins) resulting in clinical manifestations ranging from localised erythema and whealing, to generalised flushing, urticaria, abdominal pains, bronchospasm and potentially fatal circulatory collapse. Because of the similarity of the clinical syndrome to that of classical anaphylaxis, this reaction has often been referred to as "allergic", "hypersensitivity-type", "anaphylactic-type" or even "anaphylactic", without proper regard for the precise meaning of the term used. However, it is now apparent that although the end result may be the same, several distinct mechanisms may be involved in the actual histamine-releasing process.

The first involves a direct pharmacological action of the drug on mast cells without participation of immune mechanisms (Paton, 1959). The exact releasing mechanism is uncertain (Goodman and Gillman, 1975), but the extent to which this occurs is thought to be related to the dosage and the speed at which the drug is injected into the circulation (Paton, 1959). D-tubocurarine is believed to be particularly active in this respect.

A second group of aetiological mechanisms consist of those in which immune mechanisms participate in the events leading to histamine release (Watkins, 1979). The most obvious of these is the acute allergic reaction of Type I variety (Coombs and Gel classification) initiated by interaction of specific antigen and cell bound (Immunoglobulin E) antibody, i.e. the typical anaphylactic reaction. A further mechanism may involve the direct activation of the alternate complement pathway (via complement C3) but this has yet to be established as being of significance in the reactions produced by muscle relaxants.

The term "anaphylactoid" is used here (in accordance with recent recommendations – Watkins and Clarke, 1978) in the purely descriptive sense for all such reactions. Differentiation between the different mechanisms is difficult and can only, but not always, be established on the basis of detailed laboratory testing. Prior sensitisation is required for an anaphylactic reaction, but the majority of cases identified as such by immunological testing do not give a history of previous exposure to the drug concerned. A possible explanation is that sensitisation may have occurred with a cross-reacting antigen in the past, but this has yet to be proven.

A survey of the anaphylactoid reactions in which neuromuscular blocking agents have been implicated is given in the following section. It should be noted that in all probability, the number of cases reported in the literature is not a true reflection of the actual incidence of such reactions because of under-reporting and the difficulties associated with retrospective analysis. In the majority of situations, multiple drugs have been used and the incrimination of a particular muscle relaxant is based on circumstantial evidence and the results of skin testing. The latter is not always reliable, and can yield both false positive and false negative results (Fisher, 1976). Inadequate testing also makes it difficult to distinguish between the different underlying mechanisms in most cases.

Summaries of the individual case histories are given in the Appendix. It will be seen that the evidence is somewhat tenuous for some, but for the sake of completeness, these have been included in this review.

d-Tubocurarine

This is generally regarded as the most potent histamine liberator among the muscle relaxants in current use. Mild cutaneous reactions consisting of erythema and whealing at the site of injection can occur in up to 60 per cent of cases (Bush, 1965), and are presumed to be the result of localized histamine release. It is also a commonly held view that histamine release has a central role to play in causing the transient hypotension which often follows the administration of d-tubocurarine (See section on Cardiovascular Effects). The occurrence of bronchospasm, again presumed to be histamine induced, was first reported by West (1936) and several other cases are to be found in the early literature (Whiteacre and Fisher, 1945; Griffith, 1946; Holaday, 1946 and Smith and Volpitto, 1960). More detailed studies aimed at evaluating this effect indicate that although d-tubocurarine generally produces insignificant and variable changes in airways resistance (Landmesser et al., 1952); Gerbeshagen and Bergman, 1967), marked increases can occasionally occur in some individuals, particularly if there is pre-existing obstructive airway disease (Westgate et al., 1962; Crago et al., 1972).

The case reports of eight severe anaphylactoid reactions involving the use of d-tubocurarine are summarised in the Appendix. The clinical manifestations of these were of the following nature:

  (a) Circulatory collapse with or without cutaneous manifestations: 3 cases: Salem et al., 1968; Hainsworth and Bingham, 1970; Fisher, 1976; Baldwin and Churcher, 1979.
  (b) Bronchospasm followed by circulatory collapse:
      1 case: Harrison, 1966.
  (c) Bronchospasm and facial erythema:
      1 case: Brandus et al., 1970.
  (d) Urticarial reactions:
      2 cases: Westgate et al., 1961; and Brandus et al., 1973.

It should be stressed once again that the evidence for incrimination of d-tubocurarine as the causative agent is poor in many of these reports. Four patients had histories of allergies, and of the two who reacted with bronchospasm, one had a past history of asthma. No patient had been exposed previously to d-tubocurarine and, furthermore, none were confirmed as being true anaphylactic reactions. There were no fatalities, the most severe reaction being that documented by Fisher (1976) in which the patient required application of external cardiac massage and had to be subsequently maintained on intermittent positive pressure ventilation over the next 13 days. Residual mental confusion was still evident six weeks after the event.

Gallamine

Histamine release following the administration of gallamine was demonstrated by Mushin and his colleagues (1949), but the available evidence suggests that this occurs to a much lesser extent than with d-tubocurarine (Sniper, 1952). The literature contains reports of 14 anaphylactoid reactions which may have been precipitated by gallamine (See Appendix for case summaries). The clinical features of these consisted of the following:
  (a) Circulatory collapse, bronchospasm and generalised erythema:
    1 case: Okazaki et al., 1969.
  (b) Circulatory collapse with or without cutaneous manifestations:
    6 cases: Hainsworth and Bingham, 1970; Fisher, 1976, 1978; Evans and McKinnon, 1977; and McKie, 1978.
  (c) Bronchospasm and circulatory collapse:
    3 cases: Sniper, 1971; Holmes et al., 1971; and Watt, 1973.
  (d) Bronchospasm and facial oedema:
    1 case: Fisher, 1978.
  (e) Generalised erythema and urticaria:
    3 cases: Lopert, 1955; and Walmsley, 1959.
It will be seen that the majority of these cases were females (12 out of 14 cases). Four patients had histories of allergies, and of the 4 who reacted with bronchospasm, 1 had a history of asthma. Immunological testing identified 3 cases as being anaphylactic in nature (Fisher, 1976 and 1978) although none of these 3 patients had had previous exposure to gallamine. The patient described by Watt (1973) had a history of previous exposure to gallamine, suggesting the possibility of sensitisation, but no confirmatory immunological tests were performed. There was one fatality following severe circulatory collapse (Holmes et al., 1971). However, thiopentone and penicillin had also been given and either of these agents could have been responsible for the reaction. Six other cases of circulatory collapse occurred of which only one (Fisher, 1976) required external cardiac massage. This same patient was thought to have sustained permanent myocardial damage from hypoxia, but all the other cases made uneventful recoveries.

Suxamethonium

Om the basis of intradermal tests, Bourne and his colleagues (1952) concluded that suxamethonium had one per cent of the activity of d-tubocurarine in liberating histamine and it was initially thought that this was of little practical importance (Davies, 1956). However, Smith (1957) reported marked localised wheal and flare reactions at the sites of suxamethonium injections in 3 patients, and there are now at least 14 reports of more systemic anaphylactoid reactions involving the use of suxamethonium in the literature (See Appendix). The clinical manifestations of these reactions were as follows:

   (a) Bronchospasm, circulatory collapse and cutaneous manifestations: 6 cases:
      Jerums et al., 1967; Sitarz, 1974; Mandappa et al., 1975; Fisher, 1975;
      Matthews et al., 1977; and Royston and Wilkes, 1978.
   (b) Bronchospasm and circulatory collapse without cutaneous manifestations:
      1 case: Fisher, 1975.
   (c) Circulatory collapse and cutaneous manifestations:
      4 cases: Kepes and Haimovici, 1959; Mandappa et al., 1975;
      Fisher, 1975; St. Maurice et al., 1976.
   (d) Bronchospasm with no other features:
      6 cases: Smith, 1957; Fellini et al., 1963; Eustace, 1967;
      Katz and Mulligan, 1972; Bele-Binda and Valeri, 1971.

There is again a preponderance of females in these cases (12 out of 17). Six cases had histories of allergies, and of the 13 cases who reacted with bronchospasm, 2 had asthma while 2 others were chronic bronchitics. There is good evidence to suggest that anaphylactic reactions occurred in the 4 cases described by Jerums and his associates (1967), Fisher (1975) and Royston and Wilkes (1978). There were no deaths although circulatory collapse occurred in 7 cases and external cardiac massage had to be administered to 3 patients (Jerums et al., 1967; Fisher, 1975 and Royston and Wilkes, 1978). One patient (Jerums et al., 1967) has some residual neurological deficit for several weeks after the reaction, while recovery was apparently uneventful in all the other instances.

Pancuronium

Studies of pancuronium in animals showed no evidence of histamine release (Buckett et al., 1968), and initial clinical studies, reporting a lack of cutaneous manifestations with accompanying cardiovascular stability, suggested that this was also the case in man (Baird and Reid, 1967; McDowall and Clarke, 1969; Crul, 1970; Dobkin et al., 1973). Nana et al. (1972) studied its use in 9 patients with obstructive airways disease who had marked bronchial sensitivity to acetylcholine, and reported no clinical signs of bronchospasm. However, Bodman (1978) recently demonstrated that the intradermal injection of pancuronium can produce wheal and flare reactions in man (although to a significantly lesser extent than d-tubocurarine), and the following adverse reaction implicating pancuronium have been reported (See Appendix for case summaries):

   (a) Bronchospasm with no other features:
      2 cases: Heath, 1973; Clark, 1973.
   (b) Bronchospasm and facial flushing:
      1 case: Buckland and Avery, 1973.
   (c) Bronchospasm and moderate hypotension:
      1 case: Tweedie and Urdish, 1974.

Two of the patients had histories of asthma, while another had had a previous reaction to aspirin. Bronchospasm was the main problem in all 4 cases. There were no fatalities. Immunological testing was incomplete in all cases and no conclusions can be drawn regarding the aetiological mechanisms involved.

Alcuronium

Alcuronium has been suggested as the cause of the following anaphylactoid reactions (case summaries in the Appendix).

   (a) Circulatory collapse, bronchospasm and cutaneous manifestations:
      2 cases: Fisher et al., 1978.
   (b) Circulatory collapse and cutaneous manifestations:
      3 cases: Fisher et al., 1978; Chan and Yeung, 1972.
   (c) Circulatory collapse:
      1 case: Fisher et al., 1978.

Four of these cases had no history of previous allergies. One was allergic to codeine, and the case described by Chan and Yeung (1972) appeared to have multiple sensitivities having apparent reactions to Biligraffin, alcuronium and ampicillin over a 2-month period. There were no fatalities although 2 cases experienced hypotension severe enough to warrant external cardiac massage. Immunological testing suggested that 3 cases were anaphylactic reactions (Fisher et al., 1978).

The aetiology of the remaining cases remain obscure. Direct release of histamine may possibly have occurred, but the available evidence suggests that alcuronium is relatively free of histamine-releasing properties (Lund and Stovner, 1962; Bush, 1965; Waser and Harbeck, 1962).

Fazadinium

It has been suggested that fazadinium does not usually cause significant histamine release (Brittain and Tyers, 1973) and there is, to date, only one report of a possible anaphylactoid reaction to this agent (Rowlands and Fidler, 1978; See Appendix for case summary).

Decamethonium

Decamethonium has been shown to have only very weak histamine-releasing properties (Sniper, 1952), and clinical use of the drug is not usually accompanied by any signs of histamine release (Enderby, 1959). There have been no recorded cases of severe anaphylactoid reactions following its administration.

ADVERSE CARDIOVASCULAR EFFECTS

When considering the effects of the various relaxants on the cardiovascular system, it is important to remember that they are usually given to patients who are already receiving various other pharmacological agents, and that their administration is invariably accompanied by a number of procedures which can alter cardiovascular haemodynamics of their own accord (e.g. artificial ventilation, endotracheal intubation). The general condition of the patient, and the time relationship of any observed changes to the onset of the surgical stimulus are other important variables. It is, therefore, hardly surprising that there are a vast number of conflicting reports on the cardiovascular responses to these agents. Having said this, certain trends can generally be identified from the multitude of studies which have been performed. It is the aim of the following section to indicate these where relevant, and to review the current theories on the underlying mechanisms involved. The reader should also bear in mind that although these changes are discussed as "adverse effects", they are not necessarily always undesirable. For example, while the hypotension associated with d-tubocurrarine may be detrimental in an elderly arteriosclerotic patient anaesthetised with halothane, this same effect may constitute a useful adjunct in achieving hypotensive anaesthesia in a suitable patient.

d-tubocurarine

One of the main reservations regarding the use of d-tubocurarine is the hypotension which may occur following its intravenous administration. This was reported soon after its introduction to clinical anaesthesia, and it is now well recognised that this effect is more pronounced with increasing age, halothane anaesthesia, and situations where the anaesthetised patient is incapable of responding with adequate compensation e.g. hypovolaemic states or patients with fixed cardiac outputs (Cullen, 1943; Johnstone, 1956; Thomas, 1957; Chatas et al., 1963; Stoelting and Longnecker, 1972a; Smith and Whitcher, 1967; and Miller and Munger, 1972). The mechanisms which have been suggested to account for this hypotensive effect have centered round its well known histamine-releasing and ganglion-blocking activities (both resulting in a reduction of total peripheral resistance – as observed by Smith and Whitcher, 1967; Longnecker et al., 1970; and Coleman et al., 1972), and a possible direct negative inotropic effect on the myocardium.

Histamine release was first demonstrated by Alam and his co-workers (1939) and subsequently suggested as a cause for the hypotensive effect (Comroe and Dripps, 1946). Supportive evidence was presented by Lee and Johnson (1970), who showed that D-tubocurarine produced only minor changes in histamine-depleted dogs; but pre-treatment with anti-histamines does not completely abolish the hypotension following d-tubocurarine (Stoelting and Longnecker, 1972b Tashiro and Jordan, 1976), and there is no correlation between other clinical signs of histamine release and the hypotension (McDowall and Clarke, 1969; and Feldman, 1973).

Although D-tubocurarine has been conclusively shown to have autonomic ganglion-blocking activity in numerous animal experiments (Guyton and Reeder, 1950; Alper and Flacke, 1969; Hughes and Chapple, 1976a; and McCullough et al., 1970), this is a dose-related phenomenon and doubt remains as to whether or not, at neuromuscular blocking doses, a sufficient degree of ganglionic blockade occurs which would account solely for the hypotensive effect of this agent. Certainly, it has been shown that vasomotor responses (to endotracheal intubation) are relatively well preserved following the administration of doses of d-tubocurarien which produced hypotension (Johnstone et al., 1978).

Finally, it has been suggested that d-tubocurarine may have a negative inotropic effect on the myocardium. Evidence for this was first presented by Iwatsuki, Yusa and Kataoka (1965) and Dowdy and her co-workers (1965). The Japanese workers attributed their findings to the effects of histamine on the myocardium, while Dowdy and Sullivan in a subsequent publication (1968) concluded that their findings were related to decreased calcium exchange in the myocardium. Further studies have indicated that these observations may have been due to the preservatives added to some commercial preparations, and not to the pure form of the drug itself (Carrier and Murphy, 1970; Dowdy et al., 1971). However, more recently, Johnstone and his colleagues (1978) have again presented evidence suggesting that D-tubocurarine in simple aqueous solution (without any added preservatives) can produce myocardial depression and that this is exerted via calcium ion antagonism. It remains to be seen if this finding will be substantiated by further studies.

Pancuronium

Reports indicate that the administration of pancuronium results in either insignificant changes in heart rate and blood pressure (Baird and Reid, 1967; McDowall and Clarke, 1969; Dobkin et al., 1971; Levin and Dillon, 1971; Harrison, 1972; Lyons and Clarke, 1972; and Brown et al., 1973) or transient tachycardia and hypertension (Loh; 1970; Kelman and Kennedy, 1971; Coleman et al., 1972; Gertel et al., 1972; Stoelting, 1972; Miller et al., 1975a; and Parmentier and Dagnelie, 1979). While these latter effects may be desirable in preventing catastrophic hypotension in the poor-risk patient, the combination of the resultant increase in myocardial oxygen demand and decreased coronary perfusion has obvious disadvantages in ischaemic hearts. Very severe hypertension has also been observed (Fraley et al., 1978). Other cases have been described in which there were strong reasons for suspecting that pancuronium had precipitated the occurrence of ventricular tachycardia (Anderson and Rosenthal, 1975; Roizen and Feeley, 1978). However, these patients were on concurrent therapy with potentially dysrhythmogenic agents (aminophylline and tricyclic antidepressants) and it is probable that it was the interaction of pancuronium with these drugs which precipitated the adverse reactions.

The mechanisms underlying these responses have been extensively investigated. Bonta, Goorissen and Derkx (1968) first reported that pancuronium could prevent the bradycardia produced by the electrical stimulation of the vagus nerve in cats; since then a considerable amount of evidence has been accumulated suggesting that the administration of neuromuscular-paralyzing doses will result in significant blockade of cardiac muscarinic receptors, thereby causing a tachycardia (Saxena and Bonta, 1971; Goat and Feldman, 1972; Hughes and Chapple, 1976a; and Lee, Son and Waud, 1977). This has received some support from the finding that the prior administration of atropine will modify the cardiovascular response to pancuronium in man (Kelman and Kennedy, 1971; Coleman et al., 1972; and Miller et al., 1975a).

The possibility of an indirect sympathomimetic action was raised by Nana, Cardan and Domokos (1973) who reported a rise in plasma catecholamine levels following the administration of pancuronium during halothane anaesthesia. Further evidence has been presented by Ivankovich and his co-workers (1975) who showed that pancuronium blocks the in-vitro re-uptake of catecholamines in noradrenergic nerve terminals; and Domench and his colleagues (1976), who reported that pre-treatment of dogs with peripheral adrenergic depletors blocked the pressor effect of pancuronium. In the same experiment, repeated doses of pancuronium produced a diminishing pressor response which could be restored by noradrenaline infusion. It should be noted however, that other workers have been unable to demonstrate rises in catecholamine levels following the administration of pancuronium (Takki and Tammisto, 1973; and Zsigmond et al., 1974).

A third possibility is that pancuronium may have a direct positive inotropic effect. This was investigated by Duke and his associates (1975) who found no change in isometric contraction of rabbit atrial or cat papillary muscle following perfusion with pancuronium. However, their findings have been disputed by Seed and Chamberlain (1977), who found an increase in myocardial contractility in the denervated, paced heart, and concluded that pancuronium has a significant positive inotropic effect which is independent of an increase in heart rate.

Gallamine

It is well recognised that the use of gallamine in man is associated with a consistent increase in heart rate (Lamoureux and Bourgeois-Gavardin, 1949; Doughty and Wylie, 1951; Marbury et al., 1951; Riker and Wescoe, 1951; Smith and Whitcher, 1967; Eisele et al., 1971; and Kennedy and Farman, 1968). The tachycardia occurs within 1–1.5 min of the administration of gallamine, is apparent with sub-paralysing doses, and outlasts the paralysis produced by larger doses (Doughty and Wylie, 1951; Marbury et al., 1951). Eisele, Marta and Davis (1971) found a dose-related response to 20 mg increment doses up to a total dosage of 100 mg following which no further increase in heart rate occurred. Large bolus doses (up to 400 mg) failed to elicit a greater response than that achieved with 100 mg gallamine. In both instances, the administration of atropine following the maximum response to gallamine, produced further increases in heart rate.

There is less unanimity of opinion on the effect of gallamine on other cardiovascular parameters (Thomas, 1963) but increases in blood pressure, cardiac output, and left ventricular stroke work may accompany the tachycardia (Smith and Whitcher, 1967 and Kennedy and Farman, 1968). As has been pointed out earlier, this may impose an undesirable strain on the heart in certain circumstances and also possibly contribute towards increased intra-operative bleeding (Casale and Farman, 1970). An increased incidence of dysrhythmias following the use of gallamine during cyclopropane anaesthesia was noted by Walts and Prescott (1965).

The chronotropic effect of gallamine has long been assumed to be the result of an atropine-like blockade of cardiac muscarinic receptors (Riker and Wescoe, 1951; Rathbun and Hamilton, 1970; Goat and Feldman, 1972; and Lee Son and Waud,

1977). However, gallamine has a much less potent effect than atropine, and the vagolysis produced is incomplete in that a further increase in heart rate can be elicited by atropine following a maximal response to gallamine (Eisele et al., 1971). It also differs from atropine in being remarkably specific in its actions on cardiac muscarinic receptors, being devoid of other atropine-like effects (Riker and Wescoe, 1951).

It is possible that gallamine may have an indirect sympathomimetic effect, bringing about the release of noradrenaline from adrenergic nerve endings in the heart by an unidentified mechanism. This was postulated by Brown and Crout (1970) on the basis of their experimental studies showing that gallamine produced positive chronotropic and inotropic effects which could be blocked by propanolol and pretreatment with reserpine. However, attempts to demonstrate this effect in man have so far been unsuccessful (Longnecker et al., 1973. Reitan et al., 1973).

Alcuronium (diallyl-nor-toxiferine)

Studies on the cardiovascular effects of alcuronium have produced conflicting results, with some investigators reporting the occurrence of hypotension and tachycardia and others finding cardiovascular stability. Early studies by Hugin and Kissling (1961), Waser and Harbeck (1962), Foldes and his associates (1963) and Wordsworth (1964) all showed no significant changes in heart rate or blood pressure. Lund and Stovner (1962) similarly found no change in blood pressure, but observed a mild degree of tachycardia in some patients, and later reports by Kennedy and Kelman (1970) and Tammisto and Welling (1969) agreed with this. However, hypotension following the use of this agent has been shown by other studies. Hunter (1964) found a marked fall in blood pressure accentuated by high dosage and the concomitant administration of halothane; hypotension comparable with that produced by d-tubocurarine has been reported by Baraka (1967), Pandit et al. (1971), Lyons and Clarke (1972) and Coleman et al. (1972).

No satisfactory mechanism has been proposed to account for the hypotensive effect of alcuronium. Unlike d-tubocurarine, it is thought to be relatively free of histamine-releasing properties (Lund and Stovner, 1962; Bush, 1964a and 1965; Waser and Harbeck, 1962), and Hughes and Chapple (1976a) could find no significant effects on sympathetic mechanisms with neuromuscular blocking doses in cats. To date, there has been no suggestion of a negative inotropic effect on the myocardium.

Metocurine (Dimethyl tubocurarine)

Metocurine was first synthesised as the trimethylated derivative of d-tubocurarine by King in 1935 and subsequently intorduced into clinical practice by Stoelting, Graf and Vieira (1948) and Wilson, Gordon and Raffan (1950). However, despite initial favourable reports suggesting greater potency than d-tubocurarine with no significant hypotensive effect and less tendency to release histamine, it did not gain widespread clinical use – possibly because of difficulties with synthesis and preparing batches of regular consistency (Mogey and Trevan, 1950).

More recently, interest has been revived in metocurine and reports are again emphasising its relative lack of adverse cardiovascular effects. Thus, using doses not greater than 0.3 mg/kg on patients undergoing elective surgical procedures, no significant changes in heart rate or blood pressure were found during both nitrous oxide-narcotic and nitrous oxide-halothane anaesthesia (Stoelting, 1974; Hughes et al., 1976a; Savarese et al., 1977; and Vitez, 1978). In a study on patients with severe heart disease undergoing coronary artery surgery, Basta and Lichtiger (1977) found smaller rises in heart rate, blood pressure and myocardial tension-time index following intubation with 0.3 mg/kg metocurine (as compared to pancuronium) during nitrous oxide-halothane anaesthesia and concluded that the use of metocurine in these patients is associated with a smaller myocardial oxygen demand. It should be noted, however, that cardiovascular changes do occur when doses higher than 0.3 mg/kg are used (Savarese et al., 1977; and Zaidan et al., 1977).

Animal experiments indicate that the cardiovascular stability associated with the use of metocurine is the result of its highly specific action at the neuromuscular junction, so that, at paralysing doses, there is minimal or no effect on autonomic ganglia and cardiac muscarinic receptors (Hughes and Chapple, 1976 a and b; McCullough et al., 1972, Lee Son and Waud, 1977; and Savarese, 1979); and less tendency to cause histamine release (McCullough et al., 1972; and Savarese, 1979). If these reports are substantiated following more widespread use of the drug, it would appear that metocurine may have much to recommend itself as the relaxant of choice in situations where minimal disturbance to the cardiovascular system is desired.

Fazadinium

Fazadinium was first introduced into clinical practice by Simpson and his colleagues (1972) as a rapidly acting non-depolarising agent with minimal cardio-vascular effects. However, further experience has shown that it often produces a consistent and considerable tachycardia (Arora et al., 1973; Savege et al., 1973; Blogg et al., 1973; Coleman et al., 1973; Lyons et al., 1975; Hughes et al., 1976b;

and Rowlands and Fidler, 1978). This may be accompanied by a fall in stroke volume (in contrast to gallamine and pancuronium), and decreased total peripheral resistance (Coleman et al., 1973; Savege et al., 1973). Stability of blood pressure, hypotension and hypertension have all been reported following its administration Arora et al., 1973; Coleman et al., 1973; Savege et al., 1973; Lyons et al., 1975; Blogg et al, 1973; and Hughes et al., 1976b), illustrating once again the difficulties of assessing cardiovascular changes in patients subjected to different anaesthetic regimes.

Animal experiments have demonstrated that fazadinium has marked vagolytic properties at sub-paralysing doses, and it is probable that this has a major role to play in the production of the tachycardia in man (Brittain and Tyers, 1973; Marshall, 1973; and Hughes and Chapple, 1976a). Although ganglionic blockade has been shown to occur only with supramaximal doses in animals (Hughes and Chapple, 1976a) it is conceivable that this may account for the observed fall in total peripheral resistance, and also contribute in part towards the increase in heart rate. At the present time, there is no evidence to suggest that histamine release is involved in the cardiovascular responses associated with this agent (Blogg et al., 1973).

Suxamethonium

The effects of suxamethonium on the cardiovascular system are complicated and a multitude of reports claiming both rises and falls in heart rate and blood pressure abound in the literature (Graf et al., 1963; and Goat, 1972). However, from the clinical point of view, interest has centred mainly on its effects on heart rate and rhythm, and it is towards these features that the following discussion will be directed.

A slowing of the heart rate (consisting of either a simple sinus bradycardia or more complicated bradydysrhythmias) following the first dose of suxamethonium is commonly observed in infants and children (Leigh et al., 1957; Telford and Keats, 1957; Craythorne et al., 1960b; and Mazze and Dunbar, 1968) but in adults, it would appear that some sensitisation mechanism is involved because this is observed only with the second and subsequent doses (Bullough, 1959; Lupprian and Churchill-Davidson, 1960; Williams et al., 1961; Williams and Gain, 1962; Schoenstadt and Whitcher, 1963; Mathias and Evans-Prosser, 1970; and Viby-Mogensen et al., 1976). The intensity of the response is dose-dependent (Lupprian and Churchill-Davidson, 1960); if the initial dose is high (1.6 mg/kg) then a subsequent large dose will be followed by a bradydysrhythmia and, in extreme cases, ventricular standstill. The smaller the initial and subsequent doses, the less the cardiac disturbance. There is also a critical period following the initial injection during which the response is most likely to occur; estimates of this vary between 20–10 min (Williams et al., 1961; and Mathias and Evans-Prosser, 1970), with a peak incidence at around 5 min. After an interval of 20 min, further doses do not produce any dramatic change in rhythm. There are isolated case reports of episodes of cardiac standstill occurring after a first dose of suxamethonium, but these are rare and are certainly the exceptions to the rule (Wong and Brodsky, 1978; and Loennecken et al., 1970).

Thiopentone has been reported to protect against the occurrence of this phenomenon (Williams et al., 1961, McIntyre, 1962; and Schoenstadt and Whitcher, 1963) but other reports involving the use of thiopentone would suggest that the protection is incomplete (Johnstone, 1955; Bullough, 1959; and Lupprian and Churchill-Davidson, 1960). Most authors are agreed that while intramuscular atropine given as a premedicant is ineffective, intravenous atropine, in sufficient dosage, can both block and correct this response (Leigh et al., 1957; Verner and Comty, 1959; Lupprian and Churchill-Davidson, 1960; and Williams et al., 1961). It has been pointed out that the minimum dosage required for adequate protection carries with it the risk of marked and potentially dangerous tachycardia in some patients (Viby-Mogensen et al., 1976). Brandt and Viby-Mogensen (1978) have suggested that for optimal protection, atropine (in a dose not exceeding 0.01 mg/kg) should be given 30 sec before the repeat administration of suxamethonium. Other measures reported to prevent the development of this response include the use of trimetaphan (Williams et al., 1961), hexafluorenium (Schoenstadt and Whitcher, 1963) and small doses of the nondepolarising blocking agents, d-tubocurarine, pancuronium, alcuronium, c-toxiferine and gallamine (Mathias et al., 1970; Karhunen et al., 1972; and Stoelting, 1977). The effectiveness of this latter measure has been questioned recently by Wisborg, Christensen and Viby-Mogensen (1977).

Because of the structural similarity between acetylcholine and suxamethonium, attempts to explain this particular action of suxamethonium have centred on the stimulation of cholinergic receptors in the heart, either directly (Goat, 1972) or via reflex vagal activity following stimulation of peripheral sensory receptors in the carotid body (Mathias and Evans-Prosser, 1970). However, these theories do not offer an adequate explanation as to why repeated doses over a critical period of time are usually required to elicit the response. Biochemical changes initiated by the first dose, particularly in potassium levels or the potassium/calcium ratio, are attractive possibilities as sensitising factors (List, 1971; Smith, 1976), but there is as yet little evidence to support this. Attempts to correlate its occurrence with changes in either the plasma potassium or potassium/calcium ratio have failed (Williams et al., 1961; and List, 1971). Even so, this does not necessarily rule out a possible role for these factors since plasma values may not reflect physiologically significant changes at cellular level. An alternative possibility suggested by Schoenstadt and Whitcher (1963) is that choline, produced from the hydrolysis of suxamethonium may sensitise the myocardium to further doses.

Ventricular dysrhythmias have also been reported following the administration of suxamethonium. Of these, the potentially lethal episodes of ventricular fibrillation resulting from the severe hyperkalaemic response in certain conditions (e.g. para-plegics and burns victims) have been well documented and defined (see section on Hyperkalaemia). Isolated reports in the literature have suggested that ventricular dysrhythmias may also occur following intralingual injection of suxamethonium to children (Mazze and Dunbar, 1968), administration of suxamethonium to a patient with a phaeochromocytoma (Stoner and Urbach, 1968), and in patients with heart disease undergoing elective cardiac surgery (List, 1971). This last claim (incidence of 33 per cent) is difficult to evaluate because control studies were not performed. Dowdy and Fabian (1963) reported that suxamethonium appeared to potentiate the effects of cardiac glycosides leading to an increased incidence of ventricular dysrhythmias in digitalised patients, but Perez (1970) and List (1971) were unable to confirm this.

Galindo and Davis (1962) have postulated that a combination of post-ganglionic sympathetic stimulation, direct myocardial effect, potassium changes and possibly stimulation of the adrenergic glands may all contribute towards an increase in cardiac excitability and the devlopment of dysrhythmias "given the proper circum-stances". Experimental studies on the effects of suxamethonium on adrenaline induced dysrhythmias in dogs have produced conflicting claims, with Wong et al. (1971) suggesting that suxamethonium has antidysrhythmic properties and Tucker and Munson (1975) finding the opposite effect.

To summarise, the main adverse effects of suxamethonium on the cardiovascular system are the possible occurrence of a marked reduction in heart rate, and ventricular dysrhythmias. The former is probably the result of direct or indirect stimulation of cholinergic receptors in the heart (following an, as yet, undefined sensitising mechanism), while the latter has been shown to be related to an abnormal hyperkalaemic response occurring in certain circumstances.

Decamethonium

In general, there are no significant haemodynamic changes following single injections of decamethonium (Enderby, 1959; and Lawson, 1958). However, a slowing of the heart rate can occur following repeated injections (Guernier and Mason, 1952) and the administration of a dose of suxamethonium following an injection of decamethonium can also elicit this response (Williams and Gain, 1962;

Williams et al., 1961). It would thus appear that the mechanisms by which these two depolarising agents exert their effects on cardiac rate and rhythm are essentially similar in nature.

PROLONGED PARALYSIS

Although the introduction of muscle relaxants has revolutionized the practice of anaesthesia, it should be stressed that the single most important consequence of their use is that adequate ventilatory support must be provided during the period of paralysis. Failure to ensure this — either inadvertently (for example, disconnected ventilator tubing) or as the result of inadequate reversal of paralysis — will lead inevitably to respiratory failure with its attendant morbidity and mortality (Stoddart, 1978; Editorial, Brit. med. J, 1979). In most cases, reversal of competitive neuromuscular blockade is satisfactorily achieved following the administration of a maximum of 5.0 mg of neostigmine (Bridenbaugh and Churchill-Davidson, 1968), but this may prove to be inadequate in the face of overdosage or significant potentiation of neuromuscular blockade.

Some of the factors which may influence the intensity and duration of action of the muscle relaxants are discussed below. An awareness of these, and the appropriate use of the peripheral nerve-stimulator (Churchill-Davidson and Wise, 1960; and Ali et al., 1975) should help to identify and prevent cases of inadequate reversal from developing respiratory failure post-operatively.

Non-depolarising muscle relaxants

(a) Acid-base disturbances. The effects of alterations in acid-base balance on the actions of the muscle relaxants are complex, and several conflicting observations on this matter have been reported. Thus, while there appears to be general agreement that respiratory acidosis augments the neuromuscular blockade induced by D-tubo-curarine and pancuronium (Baraka, 1964; Katz and Wolf, 1964; Norman et al., 1970; Miller et al., 1975b; and Miller and Roderick, 1978a); the effect of metabolic acidosis are, unfortunately, less clear. It has often been suggested that this latter condition results in a similar potentiation of the effects of these agents (Bush and Baraka, 1964; Gamstorp and Vinnars, 1961; Crul-Sluijter and Crul, 1974), but recent studies by Miller and co-workers (1975b and 1978a) have indicated that this may not be the case. The results from these latter studies also suggest that metabolic

alkalosis following prolonged vomiting (e.g. in pyloric stenosis) may enhance the actions of d-tubocurarine and pancuronium, and oppose antagonism of the resultant neuromuscular blockade by neostigmine. Several studies have suggested that hypercapnia antagonizes and hypocapnia augments the neuromuscular block induced by gallamine (Bridenbaugh et al., 1966; Walts et al., 1967, Foldes, 1959; Hughes, 1970), while Coleman and his colleagues (1975) have claimed that the activity of fazadinium is unaffected by changes in acid-base balance.

(b) Electrolyte disturbances. (See also page 84) The normal resting membrane potential is primarily dependent on the distribution of potassium ions between the intracellular and extracellular compartments. Thus, a fall in extracellular potassium concentration (relative to intracellular potassium concentration) will result in hyperpolarization of the cell membrane and potentiation of competitive neuromuscular blockade; whereas comparable falls in potassium occurring in both compartments will have no discernible effects. The basic problem encountered in attempting to apply these theoretical considerations to the clinical situation is that the serum potassium per se does not give any indication regarding the changes in transmembrane potential. Feldman (1963) has suggested that in the majority of cases where a low serum potassium is found (e.g. following defective intake or excessive diuretic therapy), comparable falls will have occurred in both compartments with no resultant effect on neuromuscular blockade; but on the other hand, Miller and Roderick (1978b) has been able to demonstrate potentiation of pancuronium-induced paralysis and increased resistance to neostigmine antagonism following diuretic induced potassium depletion in cats. The significance of the finding of a low serum potassium in relation to neuromuscular blockade is therefore still very much open to debate, but it would seem prudent in the circumstances to titrate the dose of muscle relaxant very carefully in those patients with hypokalaemia.

Acetylcholine release from the nerve ending is inhibited by a rise in magnesium ion concentration, and a fall in calcium ion concentration (Del Castillo and Engbaek, 1954; Katz and Miledi, 1965) and, as would be expected, experimental studies have demonstrated potentiation of non-depolarising blockade by magnesium and hypocalcaemia (Ghoniem and Long, 1970; Giescke et al., 1968 and Waud and Waud, 1978). Cases of prolonged paralysis following the use of muscle relaxants in pre-eclamptic patients treated with magnesium sulphate have been described (Ghoniem and Long, 1970; and De Silva, 1973). There are, as yet, no clinical reports of a similar problem arising in hypocalcaemic states.

(c) Renal failure. Gallamine is mainly dependent on the kidneys for its excretion (Agoston et al., 1978), and numerous reports of prolonged paralysis and recurarisation following its use in patients with renal failure support the view of

most anaesthetists that it is contraindicated in these circumstances (Churchill-Davidson et al., 1967; Singer et al., 1971; McLaughlin, 1972 and Anand et al., 1972). It has also been shown that although d-tubocurarine and pancuronium have alternative routes of excretion (Cohen et al., 1967; and Agoston et al., 1973), there is delayed clearance of both drugs in the presence of renal failure (Gibaldi et al., 1972; Miller et al., 1973; McLeod et al., 1976; D'Hollander et al., 1978) and prolonged paralysis may occur following the use of large or repeated doses of these agents (Riordan and Gilbertson, 1971; Miller and Cullen, 1976; Rouse et al., 1977; and Geha et al., 1976). Alcuronium has also been shown to be excreted more slowly in the presence of renal disease (Raaflaub and Frey, 1972). The use of fazadinium was recently investigated by Camu and D'Hollander (1978) who concluded that single doses in the therapeutic range did not result in prolonged or enhanced blockade, but additional incremental doses did produce a prolonged duration of action.

(d) Liver disease. Patients in liver failure do not exhibit increased sensitivity to the non-depolarising agents, rather the reverse, i.e. decreased sensitivity being the case with d-tubocurarine (Dundee and Gray, 1953). However, occasional cases of prolonged paralysis have been observed following the administration of pancuronium to patients with obstructive biliary disease (Ward et al., 1975). Decreased plasma clearance of pancuronium has been demonstrated in this group of patients (Somogyi et al., 1977). It has also been suggested (Duvaldestin et al., 1978) that a prolonged duration of action of pancuronium may occur in patients with cirrhosis because of a large distribution volume of the drug (necessitating high initial dosage, while simultaneously decreasing the rate of clearance).

(e) Neuromuscular disease. It is well recognised that increased sensitivity to the action of the non-depolarising agents is exhibited by patients with myasthenia gravis, the myasthenic syndrome, and ocular myopathy (Bennett and Cash, 1943; Dundee, 1951; Wise, 1962; Jacob and Varkey, 1966; Ross, 1963; Blitt et al., 1975, Lake, 1978). Prolonged responses to non-depolarising agents have also been reported in some cases of von Recklinghausen's disease (Manser, 1970; Magbagbeola, 1970; Baraka, 1974; and Yamashita and Matsuki, 1975).

(f) Administration to neonates. As a result of the clinical observations of Stead (1955), Bush and Stead (1962) and Bennett et al. (1975), it is widely believed that neonates are more sensitive to the effects of non-depolarising agents than subjects from other age groups. However, further studies using electromyographic and twitch response techniques have produced conflicting results, with Churchill-Davidson and Wise (1964) and Goudsouzian (1975) reporting no demonstrable sensitivity using dosages calculated on the basis of body surface area. For practical purposes, there is general agreement that neonates have a much smaller margin of

safety, and Goudsouzian (1975) has stressed the importance of careful titration against requirements to avoid overdosage. Feldman (1978a) has further stated that adequate dilution of the agents used is the single most important factor in the administration of relaxant drugs to the newborn and that provided an excessive dose is not used, adequate reversal will be achieved.

(g) Hypothermia. The effects of non-depolarising agents have long been thought to be antagonised by hypothermia (Zaimis et al., 1958). This led to speculation that relative overdosage and recurarisation following rewarming might occur after hypothermic surgery, but there is in fact, little evidence that this occurs (McKlveen et al., 1973). Indeed, more recent studies by Foldes et al. (1974), Miller and his colleagues (1975c and 1978), Thornton and his co-workers (1976), Park et al. (1977) and Park and Macnamara (1979) have all shown that hypothermia augments rather than antagonises non-depolarising blockade.

(h) Drug interactions. (See also page 85) Enhancement of competitive neuromuscular blockade may occur following the administration of the following drugs: *antibiotics* (Miller, 1975; Becker and Miller, 1976, Lee et al., 1977a; Waterman and Smith, 1977; and Rawlins, 1978); *quinidine* (Miller et al., 1967); *lithium* (Borden et al., 1974; and Hill et al., 1977); *propanolol* (Wislicki and Rosenblum, 1967); *trimetaphan* (Wilson et al., 1976); *frusemide* (Miller et al., 1976) and *local anaesthetics* (Telivuo and Katz, 1970). It is also well known that the volatile anaesthetic agents (e.g. ether, halothane, enflurane) can potentiate the actions of the competitive blocking agents (Feldman, 1978a).

(i) Dehydration, hypovolaemia and alterations in regional blood flow. All these are factors which may possibly alter the distribution and elimination kinetics of the individual muscle relaxants. Their significance has been discussed by Feldman (1963 and 1978a).

(j) Protein binding. Studies by Baraka and Gabali (1968) and Stovner et al. (1971a,b and 1972) have shown a correlation between d-tubocurarine requirements and the gamma-globulin protein fraction, while alcuronium and gallamine requirements were related to the albumin fraction. It is thus conceivable that marked variations in plasma protein fractions may influence the activity of the neuromuscular blocking agents concerned. However, while this has been suggested as the explanation for the observed resistance to d-tubocurarine in liver disease (where albumin/globulin ratios are often reversed – Dundee and Gray, 1953), there is little evidence of clinically excessive blockade arising from changes in the opposite direction.

Depolarising muscle relaxations

Suxamethonium

A single injection of suxamethonium (50–75 mg) on average produces respiratory paralysis for 2 to 4 min (Feldman, 1978b) this short duration of action being primarily due to the fact that suxamethonium is rapidly hydrolysed by the enzyme cholinesterase. Prolongation of paralysis for more than 10 min is abnormal and may occur either because hydrolysis is impaired (as a result of genetic or acquired factors) or overdosage has occurred (with or without the development of Phase II block).

(A) Genetic factors

The serum cholinesterase enzyme system is considered to be a polymorphic one involving several co-dominant allelic genes and isoenzymes. Phenotyping of these isoenzymes is based on the differential inhibition of their activity by several substances (e.g. dibucaine, fluoride, chloride, succinylcholine) and four cholinesterase genes have been identified to date. These are the usual (E_1^u), atypical (E_1^a, Kalow and Genest, 1957), fluoride-resistant (E_1^f, Harris and Whittaker, 1961), and silent (E_1^s, Liddell et al., 1962) genes. The enzymes determined by the variants E_1^a and E_1^f have a qualitative difference in a reduced ability to hydrolyse suxamethonium, while the E_1^s variant is associated with a complete lack of cholinesterase activity. The estimated frequency of occurrence of the 10 possible genotypes is shown in Table 4.1. The silent gene is usually thought of as being particularly rare, but a recent survey by Viby-Mogensen and Hanel (1978) has suggested that it may occur with a greater frequency than previously assumed. Homozygotes and heterozygotes containing the variant genes ($E_1^aE_1^a$, $E_1^fE_1^f$, $E_1^sE_1^s$, $E_1^aE_1^s$, $E_1^aE_1^f$, $E_1^fE_1^s$) exhibit abnormal sensitivity of varying degrees to suxamethonium (Viby-Mogensen and Hanel, 1978), the most severely affected being those homozygous for the silent gene ($E_1^sE_1^s$). Heterozygotes with one normal gene ($E_1^uE_1^f$, $E_1^uE_1^a$, $E_1^uE_1^s$) would theoretically be expected to have adequate quantities of the normal enzyme, but for reasons which are as yet unclear, it would appear that 1 in 480 (or more) of these individuals do display abnormal sensitivity (Lehman and Liddell, 1969; Viby-Mogensen and Hanel, 1978).

(B) Acquired factors

(i) Physiological. It is well established that low levels of serumcholinesterase occur during pregnancy and the early puerperium (Shnider, 1965; Robertson, 1966; Hazel and Monier, 1971; Blitt et al., 1977; and Oropollo, 1978), and several cases of

TABLE 1

ESTIMATED INCIDENCE OF THE CHOLINESTERASE GENOTYPES

Genotype	Incidence
$E_1{}^uE_1{}^u$	0.94
$E_1{}^uE_1{}^a$	0.04
$E_1{}^uE_1{}^f$	0.004
$E_1{}^uE_1{}^s$	0.006
$E_1{}^aE_1{}^a$	0.0004
$E_1{}^aE_1{}^f$	0.00003
$E_1{}^aE_1{}^s$	0.0001
$E_1{}^fE_1{}^f$	0.000003
$E_1{}^fE_1{}^s$	0.000005
$E_1{}^sE_1{}^s$	0.00001

(After Smith, 1976, published by Springer Verlag).

prolonged apnoea following the administration of suxamethonium have been reported (Shnider, 1965; Robertson, 1966; MacDonald and Graham, 1968; and Wildsmith, 1972). No adequate explanation for this decrease in enzymatic activity has yet been advanced, but it is possible that increased oestrogens may play a central role since women on oral contraceptives (see below) are also known to have low serumcholinesterase levels.

Low enzyme levels have been found in neonates and infants under 6 months of age (Zsigmond and Downs, 1971), but would appear to be of little significance in view of the reported resistance of neonates to suxamethonium (Stead, 1955; Telford and Keats, 1957; Nightingale et al., 1966; and Cook and Fischer, 1975).

(ii) Diseased states. Reduced serumcholinesterase activity has been reported in the following conditions: chronic liver disease (McArdle, 1940; Foldes et al., 1956) malnutrition (McCance et al., 1948; and Waterlow, 1950); malignancy (McComb et al., 1964; and Kaniaris et al., 1979); blood dyscrasias (Scudamore et al., 1951); chronic renal failure (Thomas and Holmes, 1970; and Ryan, 1977); hypothyroidism (Thompson and Whittaker, 1965); burns (Bush, 1964b; and Viby-Mogensen et al. 1975a); some connective tissue disorders (Potts and Thornton, 1961; Eielsen and Stovner, 1978); tetanus (Porath et al., 1977). Low levels have also been reported following therapeutic radiation (Hodges and Harkness, 1954); albumin transfusion (Vorhaus et al., 1950); and plasmapheresis (Wood and Hall, 1978).

(iii) Drug interactions. (See also page 83) Several drugs are known to interfere with the activity of serumcholinesterase. These include the well recognised anticholinesterases ecothiopate iodide (McGavin, 1965; deRoetth et al., 1965;

Pantuck, 1966, Gestzes, 1966; and Cavallaro et al., 1968), tacrine and hexafluo-renium — both of which are used to produce deliberate prolongation of the action of suxamethonium in clinical practice (Gordh and Wahlin, 1961; Barrow and Smethurst, 1963; and Katz et al., 1965). Inhibition of serumcholinesterase activity may also occur following therapy with the phenothiazines promethazine, diphenhy-dramine and chlorpromazine (Todrick, 1954; Erdos et al., 1956; and Hofstee, 1960); phenelzine (Bodley et al., 1969); certain cytotoxic agents (Wang and Ross, 1963; Mone and Mathie, 1967; Zsigmond and Robins, 1972; and Gurman, 1972); procaine (Foldes et al., 1953). ketamine (Schuh, 1975), oral contraceptives (Robertson, 1967), trasylol (Chasapakis et al., 1968 and Doenicke et al., 1970); propanidid (Doenicke et al., 1968; Torda et al., 1972; and Taussig et al., 1979); trimetaphan (Tewfik, 1957; Sklar and Lanks, 1977; and Poulton et al., 1979); and some of the competitive muscle relaxants, particularly pancuronium (Stovner et al., 1975; and King, 1976).

In addition to the above, several other drugs been shown to potentiate the neuro-muscular blockade produced by suxamethonium, although not necessarily by inhibition of serumcholinesterase activity. These are lignocaine (Usubiaga et al., 1967a); quinidine (Grogono, 1963; Cuthbert, 1966); various antibiotics (Miller, 1975, and Lithium (Hill et al., 1976). Hodges (1958) suggested a possible interaction between oxytocin and suxamethonium, but subsequent workers (Keil, 1962; and Ichiyanagi et al., 1963) have been unable to substantiate this.

In conclusion it will thus be seen that there are a wide variety of situations which can produce a reduction in serumcholinesterase activity. Studies by Borders and his coworkers (1955). and Oropollo (1978) indicate that the incidence of this occurring in a general surgical population is approximately five per cent. The actual incidence of prolonged paralysis sufficient to cause concern clinically is much smaller than this — in the region of 1 in 1800 anaesthetics (Bauld et al., 1974). This is probably a reflection of the fact that most of the acquired factors mentioned above cause only a relatively minor fall in enzymatic activity, and gross reductions are required before clinically significant impairment occurs.

The results of several surveys of reported cases of suxamethonium apnoea have shown that while 40–60 per cent of such cases possessed abnormal genotypes which would be expected to result in a severe reduction of serumcholinesterase activity, of the remainder, 30–50 per cent were homozygous, and 10–20 per cent heterozygous for the normal gene (Kalow, 1965; Thompson and Whittaker, 1966; Lehmann and Liddell, 1969; Whittaker and Vickers, 1970, Bauld et al., 1974 and Viby-Mogensen and Hanel, 1978). The significance of these figures is that apart from the occasional heterozygote with abnormal sensitivity, between 40–60 per cent of cases of presumed suxamethonium apnoea could not be accounted for by inherited pseudocholinesterase abnormalities. Acquired factors (e.g. liver diseases, malignancy, concurrent drug therapy) were held to be responsible for 17 per cent and 6 per cent respectively in the series described by Bauld et al., 1974 and Viby-Mogensen and Hanel, 1978. Hyperventilation and respiratory depression, either of central or peripheral origin (from non-depolarising agents or overdosage of suxamethonium) probably accounted for the majority of the remaining cases, although the possibility remains that hitherto undetected variants may have played a role in some of these.

(C) Overdosage

This is essentially a problem of the past when the use of intermittent injections or continuous infusions of large doses of suxamethonium were prevalent, and monitoring with the peripheral nerve stimulator not generally practised. In such situations, it is easy to see how an overdose of suxamethonium sufficient to swamp the body's capacity for hydrolysis could have occurred. Prolonged exposure to suxamethonium may also result in the development of full phase II block, with delayed recovery of normal neuromuscular transmission (Feldman, 1978b).

Decamethonium

The following points should be noted in considering recovery of normal neuro-muscular transmission following the administration of decamethonium. Firstly, there is no satisfactory clinical antidote which is available for reversing the block induced following a normal dose of this agent. Secondly, phase II block readily occurs following repeated doses, making the use of the drug hazardous for prolonged operations (Feldman, 1973). It should also be remembered that the drug is excreted largely unchanged in the urine, and potentiation of its effects will occur in the presence of renal failure.

MUSCLE PAINS

Suxamethonium

The syndrome of muscle aches and pains which may occur following the administration of suxamethonium is well recognised. Churchill-Davidson (1954) reported an incidence of 66 per cent in out-patients and 14 per cent in inpatients, and various estimates since then have ranged between the extremes of 1.7 per cent (Edmunds-Seal and Eve, 1962) and 89 per cent (Mayrhofer, 1959). This range is undoubtedly a reflection of the variety of factors which may influence its occurrence and severity, and the occasional difficulty in differentiating it from other aches and pains incurred as a result of the surgical procedure. A higher incidence is reported following early ambulation (Churchill-Davidson, 1954) and the pain may occur at any time up to the fourth post-operative day (Burtles and Tunstall, 1961). Women and patients unaccustomed to exercise are more susceptible (Hegarty, 1956; and Newnam and Loudon, 1966) while children, the aged and pregnant mothers are reported to be relatively free from this complication (Bush and Roth, 1961; Burtles and Tunstall; 1961 and Crawford, 1971). The use of thiopentone for induction prior to the administration of suxamethonium is also claimed to result in a lower incidence of pain (Craig, 1964). There is no simple correlation between the development of muscle pains and the severity of visible muscle fasciculations (Morris and Dunn, 1957; Lamoreaux and Urbach, 1960; and Brodsky and Brock-Utne, 1979). The mechanism whereby the aches and pains are produced is still unresolved. Most suggestions have, in the past, favoured structural damage sustained during the fasciculations as the cause of the pains (Paton, 1959; Waters and Mapleson, 1971).

Raised creatine phosphokinase (CPK) levels and the occasional finding of myoglobin in the blood and urine following the administration of suxamethonium (Tammisto and Airaksinen, 1966; Innes and Stromme, 1973; and Ryan et al., 1971) have been interpreted as supportive evidence for this. However, no microscopic evidence of damage has been shown (Mayrhofer, 1959 and Hegab et al., 1974) and there is no significant correlation between the incidence of pain and CPK levels. Moreover myoglobinaemia and elevated CPK levels tend to occur most frequently in children, an age group with a relatively low incidence of muscle pains. Interest has also been focused on the muscle spindle fibres as a source of the pains. Rack and Westbury (1966) reported irreversible changes in the function of cat spindle fibres following administration of suxamethonium, and Collier (1975 and 1978) has suggested that spindle damage resulting from tetanic contraction (possibly enhanced by increased influx of calcium into the cell) may occur in man. The resultant loss of fine control of the muscle groups they subserve would result in excessive use and overstretching following the commencement of physical activity − thus giving rise to the pains and stiffness described.

The most convenient method of reducing theincidence of the pains appears to be pre-treatment with small doses of non-depolarising agents (Churchill-Davidson, 1954; Foster, 1960; White, 1962; Glauber, 1966 and Lamoreaux and Urbach, 1960), although there is the possibility of the development of antagonism between the two types of relaxants if an excessive dose of non-depolariser is used (Cullen, 1971). Other measures which have been claimed to be successful include the administration of procaine (Morris and Dunn, 1957); lignocaine (Usubiaga et al., 1967b);

diazepam (Verma et al., 1978; and Maryellen et al., 1978); oral vitamin C (Gupte and Savant, 1971); a combination of propanidid induction followed by lignocaine mixed with suxamethonium (Fry, 1975) and more recently, dantrolene given orally 2 hours pre-operatively (Collier, 1979). Baraka (1977) noted that pre-treatment with a small dose of suxamethonium resulted in a reduction of fasciculations when the full dose was subsequently given, but Brodsky and Brock-Utne (1979) have suggested that this is not accompanied by a reduction in the incidence and severity of the muscle pains.

Decamethonium

Muscle pains may also occur with this agent, but are reported to be of lesser frequency and intensity as compared to the pains produced by suxamethonium (Feldman, 1973). It has also been suggested that the pains, when they occur, tend to be largely confined to the jaw and calf muscles, and in contrast to suxamethonium are observed in conscious volunteers immediately following administration.

HYPERKALAEMIA

Suxamethonium

It is well recognised that the depolarisation induced by suxamethonium is associated with a release of potassium ions from inside muscle cell. In normal circumstances, this shift results in a small rise of serum potassium of the order of 0.5 mmol/L, with no significant clinical sequelae (Paton, 1959). An abnormal massive efflux of potassium ions can, however, occur in certain clinical situations, resulting in hyperkalaemia which has, on occasions, been severe enough to cause fatal cardiac dysrhythmias.

The danger of cardiac arrest following the administration of suxamethonium to patients with burns was established following reports by various authors (Forrest, 1959; Finer and Nylen, 1959; Fleming et al., 1960; Allan, 1961; McCaughey, 1962; Bush, 1964b; and Belin and Karleen, 1966). However, it was not until 1967 that Tolmie, Joyce and Mitchell, working with burns casualties in Vietnam, presented unequivocal evidence that hyperkalaemic ventricular fibrillation following suxamethonium was the mechanism by which circulatory arrest occurred. This hyperkalaemic response to suxamethonium in burns victims has since been confirmed by several other investigators (Schaner et al., 1969; Gronert et al., 1969; and Viby-Mogensen et al., 1975b).

Suxamethonium-induced hyperkalaemic circulatory arrests have also been reported in patients with massive tissue trauma (Mazze et al., 1969; Birch et al., 1969; Weintraub et al., 1969), tetanus (Roth and Wuthrich, 1969) and a variety of neurological disorders involving either focal or general motor abnormalities e.g. the stroke syndrome, cerebral palsy, multiple sclerosis, encephalitis, spinal cord transections and peripheral neuropathy (Cooperman 1970; Cooperman et al., 1970; Smith and Grenvik, 1970; Tobey, 1970; Tobey et al., 1972; Stone et al., 1970a; Thomas, 1969; Cowgill et al., 1974 and case history no. 62, 1971). It will be noted that both upper and lower motor neurone-type lesions are susceptible to the dangers of the hyperkalaemic response. The period of risk may begin as early as four days after injury and persist for 2 to 3 months in patients with burns or trauma, and perhaps 3 to 6 months (or more) in patients with neurological disorders (Tobey et al., 1972; Gronert and Theye, 1975; Viby-Mogensen et al., 1975b; and John et al., 1976). Pre-treatment with non-depolarising agents before the administration of suxamethonium can attenuate the rise in serum potassium (Konchigeri and Tay, 1976), but dangerously high levels can still occur in individual patients who are at risk, in spite of this (Weintraub et al., 1969; Tobey et al., 1972).

It is now universally accepted that this hyperkalaemic response is the result of an excessive loss of potassium from the abnormal muscles involved in all the above lesions. The reason for this excessive loss has been fairly well defined for patients with chronic denervation of their muscles. Thus, changes are thought to occur in the muscle cell which effectively enlarges the area of suxamethonium-sensitive membrane, thereby resulting in a greater surface from which potassium leakage occurs on exposure to suxamethonium (Axelson and Thesleff, 1959; Stone et al., 1970b and Kendig et al., 1972). The situation regarding upper motor neurone lesions and burn injuries is, however, rather more complex since the lower motor neurone is intact in the former and, similarly, denervation does not necessarily occur following burns. Furthermore, simple immobilisation cannot be invoked as a possible cause, since this has been shown to be free of an abnormal hyperkalaemic response (Gronert and Theye, 1974). A review of other possible mechanisms which may be involved has been presented by Gronert and Theye (1975).

Circulatory arrests following the administration of suxamethonium to patients in renal failure were described by Roth and Wuthrich (1969) and Powell (1970). These authors went on to suggest that the use of suxamethonium is contraindicated in the presence of renal failure. However, studies by Miller and his associates (1972), Koide and Waud (1972), Powell and Miller (1975), Day (1976) and Walton and Farman (1973) have demonstrated conclusively that an exaggerated hyperkalaemic response does not usually occur, and that only those patients with pre-operative hyperkalaemia or uremic neuropathy are at risk.

Decamethonium

A small rise in serum potassium has also been documented following the use of decamethonium in normal patients (Weintraub et al., 1969, Fahmy et al., 1975). Although there are non recorded cases of a severe hyperkalaemic response, it is reasonable to assume that subjects known to be at risk from this phenomenon (following the administration of suxamethonium) will react in a similar fashion if exposed to decamethonium.

MALIGNANT HYPERTHERMIA

Suxamethonium

Suxamethonium shares with halothane the unenviable record of being the anaesthetic agents whichf are most often implicated as "trigger agents" in precipitating the rare, but potentially fatal syndrome of malignant hyperthermia (Relton et al., 1973). The syndrome characteristically manifests itself as a fulminant, rapidly progressive rise in body temperature usually, but not always, accompanied by muscle rigidity, and the subsequent development of a hypermetabolic state resulting in acidosis, hyperventilation and hyperkalaemia. In cases precipitated by suxamethonium, failure of the jaw muscles to relax after its administration is often an early warning sign (Denborough, 1977). Tachydysrhythmias, myoglobinuria and renal failure may develop and, unchecked, the disease progresses to haemolysis, consumption, coagulopathy, acute heart failure, neurological deficit and often, death (Britt, 1972). It occurs most frequently in children and young adults, males being more commonly affected than females; the incidence has been estimated as 1 in 14,000 anaesthetics administered to children (Britt and Kalow, 1970). The mortality is high, of the order of 60–70 per cent (Britt and Kalow, 1970; Denborough, 1977), and the chances of survival are related to the speed with which the diagnosis is made and treatment instituted.

There is a familial incidence with early genetic studies indicating that the condition is inherited as a simple autosomal dominant trait with variable expression and incomplete penetrance (Denborough et al., 1962; Britt et al., 1969) Subsequently, abnormally high serum levels of muscle enzymes with or without clinical evidence of myopathy were found in many asymptomatic relatives of affected patients, suggesting that the condition exists as a subclinical myopathy which can progress to malignant hyperthermia when exposed to the appropriate triggering agent (Isaacs and Barlow, 1970a,b; Denborough et al., 1970). More recent studies have suggested that the inheritance of the trait may be more complex and multifactorial (Ellis et al., 1978), and there is evidence that there may be a second distinct predisposing myopathy occurring in young boys with a number of striking physical abnormalities (Denborough, 1977). It is thought that this second myopathy is inherited as a recessive characteristic. Serum creatinine phosphokinase levels are unreliable as a diagnostic indicator of the malignant hyperthermia trait and more definitive screening depends on the results of light and electron microscopy, and in vitro pharmacological testing of muscle biopsy specimens, although these are not infallible (Isaacs, 1978).

The primary abnormality in this condition is thought to reside within the muscle cell, exposure to an appropriate stimulus resulting in an excessive accumulation of calcium in the myoplasm (Kalow et al., 1970), which then triggers off a variety of complex exothermic reactions. The exact nature of this abnormality has not been fully elucidated, current interest being focused on a primary lesion in the mechanism linking depolarisation of the muscle end plate to contraction of the myofibrils (via release of calcium from the sarcoplasmic reticulum) − the so called "excitation-contraction coupling (ECC) mechanism" (Nelson, 1978; Denborough, 1977). The concept has also been advanced that malignant hyperthermia is the result of an exaggerated endocrine-metabolic response to stress, with the sympathetic nervous system playing a central role in its genesis (Wingard, 1974; Lister et al., 1975; Moulds, 1975 and Williams, 1976). However, Gronert and his colleagues (1977) have suggested that the increased sympathetic activity, while contributing to the overall syndrome, is a secondary and expected response to the generalised stress of the primary muscle abnormality.

The likelihood of a favourable response to treatment is related to the speed with which the diagnosis is made, anaesthesia aborted and vigorous therapy instituted. The latter consists firstly of correcting or preventing hyperthermia, acidosis, hyperkalaemia and any other fluid or electrolyte disturbances. More specific measures which have been suggested include the use of procaine (Harrison, 1971), steroids (Ellis et al., 1974; Raitt and Merrifield, 1974; and Cain and Ellis, 1977) and, more recently, dantrolene sodium − a drug which is believed to block the ECC mechanism, possibly by suppressing release of calcium from the sarcoplasmic reticulum, and/or attenuating transmission of the excitation signal from the T-tubule to the sarcoplasmic reticulum (Anderson et al., 1978). The value of procaine has been questioned (Clarke and Ellis, 1975; Hall et al., 1975; and Gronert et al., 1976a), but the results from animal experiments and in-vitro studies on human muscle specimens, using dantrolene, have been most promising (Harrison, 1975 and 1977; Anderson and Jones, 1976; Gronert et al., 1976b; Hall et al., 1977; Austin and Denborough, 1977; and Nelson and Flewellen, 1979). There are reports on the use of oral dantrolene as part of a successful prophylactic regime for managing patients known to be susceptible to malignant hyperthermia (Kerr et al., 1978; and Pandit et al., 1979), but its clinical effectiveness in treating an established case of malignant hyperthermia has yet to be fully assessed in man.

It has been suggested that the non-depolarising agents may also act as triggering agents for the syndrome (Britt and Kalow, 1970; Chalstrey and Edwards, 1972; and Britt et al., 1974), but this is by no means proven and Cain and Ellis (1977) were in fact able to demonstrate that pancuronium can inhibit halothane-induced muscle contracture in human malignant hyperthermia-susceptible muscle.

RHABDOMYOLYSIS AND MYOGLOBINURIA

Suxamethonium

Acute rhabdomyolysis and myoglobinuria without an accompanying fulminant rise in temperature can sometimes occur following exposure to suxamethonium. This was first reported by Bennike and Jarnum (1964) in a 29-year-old female who developed myoglobinuria and renal failure following anaesthesia with nitrous oxide-oxygen-halothane and suxamethonium. Serum levels of creatine phosphokinase (CPK), lactic dehydrogenase and transaminase were all elevated, and subsequent muscle biopsy revealed changes consistent with rhabdomyolysis. The author concluded that the patient had paroxysmal idiopathic myoglobinuria, provoked in this instance by suxamethonium.

Since then, there have been further reports of myoglobinuria and elevated serum CPK levels occurring following exposure to halothane and suxamethonium anaesthesia. Some of these were asymptomatic, occurring as an isolated phenomenon (Airaksinen and Tammisto, 1965; Moore et al., 1976), while others were associated with inadequate relaxation (Jensen et al., 1968 and Bernhardt and Hoerder, 1978), generalised myotonia (McLaren, 1968), myotonia and cardiac arrest, with hyperkalaemia, hypocalcaemia and hyperphosphatemia (Schaer et al., 1977), acidosis, tachycardia and ventricular dysrhythmias (Miller, E.D. et al., 1978).

The case described by Miller, E.D. and his colleagues (1978) was subsequently shown to have Duchenne's muscular dystrophy, while Moore, Watson and Summary (1976) and Schaer and his associates (1977) considered that their patients suffered from subclinical myopathies. The foregoing cases would, therefore, suggest that a rare, but potentially dangerous interaction resulting in acute rhabdomyolysis and myoglobinuria (without hyperthermia) can occur when suxamethonium and halothane are used in patients with underlying muscle disease (which may or may not be clinically apparent). Whether or not this represents one end of the spectrum of the malignant hyperthermia syndrome, remains a matter for speculation at the present time.

MYOTONIC RESPONSE

Suxamethonium

An abnormally prolonged contracture of muscles can occur following the administration of suxamethonium to patients with certain muscle diseases. The conditions which have been most identified with this response are the myotonic syndromes, consisting of Dystrophia myotonica, Myotonnia congenita, and Paramyotonia congenita (Mitchell et al., 1978). Several reports have been published describing severe generalised spasm in these patients (Paterson, 1962; Thiel, 1967; Kaufman, 1960; and Orndahl, 1962), with the resultant difficulties in maintaining an adequate airway, intubation and controlling ventilation.

The response of myotonic patients to suxamethonium is, however, unpredictable and not all respond with severe generalised spasms. Some have shown no abnormal response at all (Kaufman, 1960; and Haley, 1962), while others experience only localised spasms (Kaufman, 1960). Suxamethonium has also been reported to achieve relaxation of myotonic contractures which were precipitated during anaesthesia, either by other agents, or the drug itself (Cobham and Davis, 1964; Talmadge and McKechnie, 1959; and Haley, 1962).

Other conditions in which a myotonic response has occurred following the administration of suxamethonium include amyotrophic lateral sclerosis, unilateral brachial plexus palsy resulting from a Pancoast's tumour, carpal tunnel syndrome and traumatic nerve injuries (Orndahl and Sternberg, 1962, Brim, 1973, Lee et al., 1977b; and Baraka, 1978). In all of these cases the response consisted of a localised contracture of the affected limbs and was interpreted as a manifestation of denervation hypersensitivity. Myotonia was also reported in a patient with suspected polymyositis (Davies, 1970) although, in this instance, the response could possibly have been part of a malignant hyperthermic syndrome, whilst in 3 other patients, no subsequent definitive diagnosis was made (Relton et al., 1967; Cody, 1968; and Baraka et al., 1970).

Decamethonium

This agent has been shown to provoke a similar myotonic response in susceptible patients (Kaufman, 1960, Orndahl, 1962).

Non-depolarising relaxants do not appear to lead to a myotonic response

(Orndahl, 1962; Mitchell, 1978). In fact, Baraka et al. (1970) was able to reverse suxamethonium-induced myotonia with d-tubocurarine, and has suggested that pre-treatment with a small dose may prevent such a response from occurring.

INTRAOCULAR PRESSURE

Suxamethonium

Following the initial report by Hoffman and Holzer (1953), it has now been fully established that suxamethonium can produce a rise in intracular pressure (Lincoff et al., 1955; Dillon et al., 1957a,b; Schwartz and de Roetth, 1958; Craythorne et al., 1960a; Wynands and Crowell, 1960; Goldsmith, 1967; Taylor et al., 1968; and Robertson and Gibson, 1968). This starts within 30 sec of the administration of suxamethonium and is of a transient nature, the intraocular pressure generally returning to basal levels or less within 5 to 6 min (Schwartz and de Roetth, 1958; Carballo, 1965; Robertson and Gibson, 1968; and Pandey et al., 1972). However, not all patients respond with an elevation of intraocular pressure, the incidence in most studies ranging from 50 to 70 per cent, with a wide variation in the actual degree of the observed rise. The dangers of vitreous expulsion resulting from this pressure elevation is well recognised, and it is generally agreed that the use of suxamethonium is contraindicated in penetrating eye injuries and during the course of intraocular surgery when the eye is open.

It is often stated that the main mechanism responsible for the rise in intraocular pressure is the mechanical pressure exerted as the result of suxamethonium-induced tonic contracture of the extraocular muscles (Lincoff et al., 1955; Macri and Grimes, 1957; Dillon et al., 1957a; and Smith, 1976). However, in experiemntal work on animals, suxamethonium has been shown to produce a rise in intraocular pressure in spite of prior curarisation (Wretlind and Wåhlin, 1959) and division of all extraocular muscles (Adams kand Barnett, 1966; and Katz and Eakins, 1969). Adams and Barnett (1966) were able to mimic the suxamethonium-induced rise in intraocular pressure with an injection of bradykinin into the carotid artery and suggested from their findings that the pressure rise after suxamethonium is, in part, due to a vascular effect, possibly a transient dilatation of the choroidal vessels. A further piece of evidence to support this is the demonstration by Wahlin (1960) that suxamethonium causes a transient dilatation of the conjunctival vessels in man. Katz and Eakins (1969) suggested that contraction of intra-orbital smooth muscle might contribute towards the rise in intraocular pressure, but Smith (1976) has pointed out that this would also result in opening of the irido-corneal angle, thereby increasing drainage of aqueous humor and bringing about a lowering of intraocular pressure instead.

Pre-treatment with small doses of non-depolarising agents has been claimed to attenuate the suxamethonium induced rise in intraocular pressure (Miller et al., 1968; Dickman et al., 1969), but subsequent reports have disputed this (Bowen et al., 1976 and 1978 and Meyers et al., 1978). Other measures which have been advocated include pre-treatment with hexafluorenium (Sobel, 1962; and Katz et al., 1968) and acetazolamide − a carbonic anhydrase inhibitor which reduces the secretion of aqueous humor (Carballo, 1965).

Decamethonium

In a study on 30 patients, Maier and Clark (1965) found that decamethonium caused no statistically significant change in intra-ocular pressure although three patients did show a transient rise. No other studies are available for comparison but, if valid, these results would suggest that the depolarisation process on its own does not usually produce a significant rise in intraocular pressure.

RAISED INTRAGASTRIC PRESSURE

Suxamethonium

Significant rises in intragastric pressure occurring at the time of suxamethonium-induced fasciculations have been observed by several workers (Andersen, 1962; La Cour, 1969; and Miller and Way, 1971) and it has been suggested that this may predispose to regurgitation of stomach contents. However, it is important to realise that a rise in intragastric pressure per se, need not necessarily lead to regurgitation. For one thing, the intragastric pressure necessary to open the gastro-oesophageal sphincter has been shown to vary with the angle of entry of the oesophagus into the stomach, higher pressures being required the more acute the gastro-oesophageal angle (Marchand, 1955; and Greenan, 1961). Furthermore, it is believed that there is a "Physiological sphincter" consisting of a high pressure zone in the lower oesophagus (Fyke et al., 1956; Atkinson et al. 1957; and Botha et al., 1957). Smith and his colleagues (1978) have pointed out that it is more relevant to evaluate the effects of suxamethonium on the pressure gradient between the stomach and this region, rather than on intragastric pressure alone. These latter workers were able to demonstrate that suxamethonium produced concurrent pressure rises in both regions, with no resultant change in the pressure gradient, thus suggesting that there is, in fact, no increased tendency to regurgitation. They were careful to point out, however, that this study was performed on patients with clinically normal cardio-oesophageal junctions and, therefore, not necessarily applicable to patients with hiatus herniae or other abnormalities of the cardio-oesophageal junction.

CENTRAL NERVOUS SYSTEM EFFECTS

General considerations

(a) Passage across the blood–cerebro-spinal fluid barrier: It has been demonstrated that the passage of small amounts of D-*tubocurarine* and *gallamine* across the blood–cerebro-spinal fluid barrier does occur (Haranath et al., 1973; Devasankaraiah et al., 1973; Matteo et al., 1977). There is some dispute on the significance of this finding (Haranath, 1978; and Matteo and Khambatta, 1978) but most anaesthetists would agree with Matteo and his associates in their conclusion that the quantities passing into the cerebrospinal fluid after intravenous administration are insufficient to cause any significant pharmacological effects in man.

(b) Accidental intrathecal injection: There are two documented cases of the occurrence (Mesry and Baradaran, 1974; and Goonewardene et al., 1975). In both instances, *gallamine* was accidentally injected instead of a local anaesthetic for spinal anaesthesia and this was followed by the development of convulsions which persisted for more than 24 hours.

(c) Increase in cerebro-spinal fluid pressure: The administration of D-*tubocurarine* may be followed by a rise in cerebro-spinal fluid pressure (Tarkannen et al., 1974). This effect is probably related to an increase in cerebral blood flow arising either as the result of histamine release, or a direct action of d-tubocurarine on cerebral haemodynamics (Tarkannen et al., 1974; and Savarese, 1975). *Suxamethonium* may also cause an increase in cerebro-spinal fluid pressure (Wåhlin, 1960) via a direct vasodilatory effect on cerebral blood vessels. These rises are generally considered to be mild and probably of no great significance in normal patients but they may be potentially harmful when used in patients with pre-existing raised intracranial pressure.

PLACENTAL TRANSFER

General considerations

Although placental transfer of d-tubocurarine (Elert and Cohen, 1962), alcuronium (Thomas et al., 1969), gallamine (Crawford, 1956), pancuronium (Booth et al., 1977), fazadinium (Blogg et al., 1975), dimethyl-tubocurarine (Kivalo and Saarikoski, 1976) and suxamethonium (Drabkova et al., 1973) have been demonstrated, administration in normal dosages do not usually result in significant neuromuscular blockade in the newborn. A potential danger does, however, exist, as illustrated by the following cases:

(1) Older and Harris (1968) reported curarisation in a 28 weeks old neonate born to an epileptic mother who had received a total of 285 mg of d-tubocurarine for control of status epilepticus in the preceeding 16 hours prior to delivery. The authors also mentioned another case where it was thought likely that *arthrogryphosis multiplex congenita* in a newborn infant was the result of assumed curarisation sustained during the 8th to 12th weeks of pregnancy, when the mother had been curarised and ventilated following infection with tetanus.

(2) Baraka et al. (1975) reported that administration of *suxamethonium* to an atypical homozygous mother resulted in prolonged paralysis of the newborn child who was subsequently shown also to be an atypical homozygote. In a second case, the heterozygotic child of a homozygous mother appeared to be spared from this effect.

CONCLUSIONS

This chapter reviews in detail the adverse effects of the muscle relaxants. The bulk of the evidence for a specific side-effect centres around the depolarising relaxants — particularly, suxamethonium. Quite reasonably this has led some anaesthetists to suggest that there is no longer any place for suxamethonium in clinical practice. This is too extreme a view and it is necessary to re-iterate some of the advantages of this drug which go some way to off-setting the disadvantages.

First, after some thirty years of intensive search, a short-acting, *non-depolarising* drug, with minimal side-effects, still eludes the pharmacologist. The outstanding advantage of suxamethonium has lain in its rapid metabolism by plasma cholinesterase enzyme, thereby enabling some 5–10 times the paralysing dose (in absence of enzyme) to be administered to give a very short duration of activity. It seems hardly surprising, therefore, that such large doses should stimulate other cholinergic receptors and lead to multiple side actions. Conversely, if a non-depolarising relaxant was discovered (which also was capable of rapid breakdown by plasma cholinesterase) it would not seem surprising if this drug led, in turn, to a *blockade* of cholinergic receptors — again with numerous side actions. To minimise these effects, the relaxant would have to be highly specific for the neuromuscular junction, yet interestingly enough the non-depolarising relaxant which has been found to possess these qualities best i.e. C-Toxiferine, was abandoned early in its clinical trials because it was considered too long-acting.

Secondly, many of the adverse effects of suxamethonium can be modified or prevented by pre-treatment with a small dose of a non-depolarising relaxant. However, the selection of this dose is critically balanced because the two types of neuromuscular block are antagonistic. In the emergency situation where a rapid establishment of the airway is vital, then suxamethonium *alone* still reigns supreme. Newer drugs like fazadinium have been claimed to have a rapid onset of paralysis but this necessitates giving a high dose with its own problems of temporary irreversibility and tachycardia. In situations like burns, trauma or any condition involving recent denervation of the motor nerve, then the use of suxamethonium (even with pre-treatment) is clearly contra-indicated.

As regards the non-depolarising drugs, the presence of some side-actions such as a tachycardia or reduction in blood pressure can often be put to advantage in the clinical situation. If a relaxant such as D-tubocurarine is used in conjunction with halothane anaesthesia, then often a moderate controlled hypotension can be achieved. Conversely, if a raised cardiac output is required, then the cardiovascular effects of gallamine (and to a lesser extent pancuronium) will be found useful.

APPENDIX

(1) Circulatory collapse with or without cutaneous manifestations

d-Tubocurarine

(a) Salem et al. (1968)

51-year-old male. Allergic to penicillin. Premedicated with pethidine, hydroxyzine and atropine. Induced with thiopentone, followed by suxamethonium and intubation. Maintained on nitrous oxide-oxygen-halothane, and then given d-tubocurarine. Profound hypotension occurred 1 minute after the injection of d-tubocurarine, and this was followed by generalised marked flushing of the skin. Treatment was instituted with methoxamine, phynylephrine, hydrocortisone, and fluids, and the blood pressure eventually returned to normal. Skin tests performed the following day, using undiluted solutions of d-tubocurarine. Results unhelpful as positive reactions occurred in the patient and the majority of controls. The patient was re-anaesthetised 3 days later, using the same regime as before, with the substitution of a suxamethonium drip for d-tubocurarine. No abnormal reactions occurred on this occasion.

Comment. Evidence for incriminating d-tubocurarine lies in the timing of the reaction and the uneventful re-exposure to all the other drugs which had been used in the first anaesthetic. There is insufficient data for further definition of the nature of the reaction.

(b) Hainsworth and Bingham (1970)

39-year-old female. History of sensitivity to apples, primula and metallic spectacle earpieces. Anaesthetised 4 months previously without exposure to muscle relaxants. Premedicated with pethidine, promethazine and atropine. Induced with methohexitone, followed by injection of d-tubocurarine and gallamine, subsequently intubated. Circulatory collapse (pulseless, but heart sounds heard) and a generalised rash developed soon after induction. Spontaneous improvement occurred without specific drug therapy. Fluids and steroids subsequently administered for persistent mild hypotension. Strongly positive skin tests obtained for gallamine and d-tubocurarine; negative reaction with methohexitone. Diluted solutions used for testing.

Comment. Reaction could have occurred in response to only one, or both of these drugs. There is insufficient data for more positive identification of the causative agent.

(c) Fisher (1976)

42-year-old female. No history of allergies, no previous anaesthetics. On concurrent therapy with clonidine and propanolol for hypertension. Premedicated with pethidine, promethazine and atropine. Induced with thiopentone and intubated following suxamethonium. Several minutes later, d-tubocurarine administered. Reaction occurred within 2–3 min, consisting of circulatory arrest and obvious cyanosis. (c) continued. Resuscitated over the next 45 minutes with external cardiac massage, intracardiac adrenaline, sodium bicarbonate, steroids and fluids. Further care was required in an intensive care unit over the next 2 weeks, and there was still mental confusion 6 weeks after the reaction, although full recovery was anticipated by the author. Intradermal tests, using dilute solutions, at 4 days were unhelpful, but a positive reaction to D-tubocurarine occurred at 3 weeks. Negative responses were obtained with all the other drugs which had been used. *Comment.* The results of the intradermal tests suggest that d-tubocurarine was the agent responsible. There is insufficient data for further definition of the nature of the reaction.

(d) Baldwin and Churcher (1979)

42-year-old female. No allergies. No previous exposure. Premedicated with papaveratum and atropine. Induced with thiopentone followed by suxamethonium and intubation. Tubocurarine administered after recovery from suxamethonium-induced paralysis; this was followed almost immediately by cardio-vascular collapse and gross generalised oedema. Treated with fluids, methoxamine and steroids. Blood pressure recovered to 40 mm Hg systolic after 7 min and continued to rise steadily over the following half hour. Promethazine administered after successful reversal of neuromuscular paralysis. Oedema gradually subsided and patient went on to make an uneventful recovery. Intradermal tests performed for thiopentone and d-tubocurarine 2 days later. Negative response to thiopentone but minimal dose of tubocurarine produced wheal and flare reaction and a dramatic subjective response which resolved following treatment with steroids. Re-anaesthetised successfully 4 days later using thiopentone, gallamine, nitrous oxide-oxygen-halothane.

Comment. The results of the skin tests suggest that d-tubocurarine was indeed the agent responsible for the reaction but it should be noted that suxamethonium was not subjected to similar testing.

(2) Bronchospasm followed by circulatory collapse

(a) Harrison (1966)

58-year-old female. Episode of allergic asthma 20 years previously. No mention of previous exposure to d-tubocurarine. Premedicated with pethidine and atropine. Induced with thiopentone and intubated, following suxamethonium. Maintained uneventfully on nitrous oxide-oxygen-halothane for 45 min, after which d-tubocurarine injected. Severe bronchospasm occurred almost immediately, and this was soon followed by circulatory collapse. Recovery following therapy with fluids, isoprenaline and aminophylline. No tests performed.

Comment. While the timing of the reaction strongly suggests that d-tubocurarine was the causative agent, the possibility that the other drugs used could have been responsible cannot be excluded.

(3) Bronchospasm and facial erythema

Brandus et al. (1970)

64-year-old female. No history of allergies, no mention of previous exposure to d-tubocurarine. Premedicated with secobarbital. Induced with thiopentone, following which, d-tubocurarine injected intravenously. Bronchospasm and facial erythema appeared almost immediately after this. Reaction apparently resolved following injection of lignocaine. No tests performed.

Comment. Reaction could have occurred to either thiopentone or D-tubocurarine; there is no evidence to favour one or the other of these agents.

(4) Urticarial reactions

(a) Westgate et al. (1961)

25-year-old male. History of urticarial reaction to onions and strawberries. 10 previous uneventful anaesthetics — no previous exposure to d-tubocurarine. Premedication not specified. Induced with thiopentone and d-tubocurarine, and subsequently intubated. Immediately after this, swelling of eyelids noted, and patient rapidly developed facial, pharyngeal and epiglottic œdema. Severe urticarial reactions were also noted at the sites of the wounds from his previous operations. Following treatment with steroids and diphenhydramine, the reaction gradually subsided without further problems. Skin tests, using diluted solutions, showed a positive response to d-tubocurarine and a negative response to thiopentone. Prausnitz-Kuster testing yielded a negative result to d-tubocurarine. Histamine levels were also measured and found to be elevated at the time of the reaction. The significance of this is unclear as no control levels were available, and rises, falls and unchanged levels have all been noted following the uneventful administration of D-tubocurarine (Westgate and Van Bergen, 1962).

Comment. The results of the skin tests suggest that d-tubocurarine was the causative agent. The negative Prausnitz-Kustner reaction does not necessarily rule out the possibility of an anaphylactic reaction, as false negative results can occur.

(b) Brandus et al. (1973)

18-year-old male. Pyrexial. History of sensitivity to laundry detergent. No previous anaesthetics. No premedication. Small test dose of d-tubocurarine administered before induction with no ill-effects. Induced with thiopentone, followed by full dose of d-tubocurarine over 10-sec period. Urticarial rash and tachycardia occurred within seconds of this. No specific treatment instituted; reaction gradually resolved spontaneously. Towards end of operation, further small dose of d-tubocurarine given with no adverse effects. Skin tests performed several weeks later using diluted solutions. Positive reaction obtained with d-tubocurarine at normal temperature; this was more marked when the temperature of the arm was raised. No tests performed for thiopentone.

Comment. The results of skin testing suggest the d-tubocurarine may have caused the reaction. However, thiopentone was not subjected to similar skin testing, and furthermore, no adverse effects were observed following both the initial test dose of d-tubocurarine and the further dose administered after the reaction had occurred.

Gallamine

(1) Circulatory collapse, bronchospasm and generalised erythema

Okazaki et al. (1969)

49-year-old female. No history of allergies or asthma. Previous anaphylactoid reaction (bronchospasm, circulatory collapse and generalised erythema) following induction with thiopentone and hexafluorenium, 12 days before anaesthetic involving gallamine. Following recovery from above, re-anaesthetised with following regime: same premedication as first anaesthetic (atropine and pethidine) with addition of hydrocortisone. Gaseous induction with halothane and nitrous oxide. Intubation following suxamethonium was uneventful: 12 min later, gallamine administered. Immediately following this, patient developed bronchospasm, followed by circulatory collapse and generalised erythema. Treated with aminophylline and "Effortil". Uneventful recovery with no major complications. No tests performed.

Comment. Evidence incriminating gallamine is purely circumstantial and the diagnosis must remain doubtful in view of the lack of any sensitivity tests.

(2) Circulatory collapse with or without cutaneous manifestations

(a) Hainsworth and Bingham (1970) (See under "d-tubocurarine").

(b) Fisher (1976)
   56-year-old female. History of angioneurotic oedema. 4 previous unevertful exposures to thiopentone and one to suxamethonium. Premedicated with pethidine, promethazine and atropine. Induced with thiopentone, gallamine and suxamethonium. Following intubation, noted to be profoundly hypotensive. External cardiac massage performed, and treated with fluids and sodium bicarbonate. Blood pressure gradually returned to normal, but recovery complicated by heart failure, thought to have been the result of myocardial damage sustained during period of anoxia. Skin tests performed 3 months later, using diluted solutions of thiopentone, suxamethonium and gallamine. Positive reaction occurred only with gallamine. Prausnitz-Kustner testing initially reported as negative, but in a later publication (Fisher, 1978), a positive reaction was said to have occurred.

   Comment. In spite of lack of previous exposure, the positive skin test and Prausnitz-Kustner reaction strongly suggest that this was a true anaphylactic reaction to gallamine.

(c) Fisher (1978)
34-year-old female. No history of allergies, no previous anaesthetics. No information regarding premedication. Induced with thiopentone and gallamine. Immediate reaction consisting of generalised erythema and severe hypotension. Prompt recovery following treatment with adrenaline and Haemacel. Residual complaints of abdominal cramps and nausea. Positive reaction to gallamine on intradermal testing. Positive Prausnitz-Kustner reaction with gallamine.

   Comment. Above results suggest that gallamine was a causative agent, and that the reaction was the result of an anaphylactic mechanism.

(d) Fisher (1978)
   42-year-old female. No history of allergies. 3 previous uneventful anaesthetics without exposure to gallamine. No information regarding premedication. Induced with thiopentone and gallamine. Immediate development of erythema and severe hypotension. Recovered following fluid infusion. Positive intradermal reaction for gallamine. Positive Prausnitz-Kustner reaction with gallamine.

   Comment. As in the previous case, the results of sensitivity testing are highly suggestive of an anpahylactic reaction to gallamine.

(e) Evans and McKinnon (1977)
   24-year-old male. No history of allergies. One previous uneventful exposure to thiopentone. Premedicated with papaveratum and scopolamine. Induction with thiopentone and gallamine was followed by coughing, then generalised flushing and circulatory collapse. Treated with hydrocortisone

and fluids with eventual recovery. Intradermal testing revealed strongly positive reaction with gallamine and a negative reaction with thiopentone. Prausnitz-Kustner testing not performed.

Comment. Results of intradermal tests suggest that gallamine was the causative agent. The authors suggest that this reaction was not an anaphylactic one in view of the lack of previous exposure, but as has been emphasised, this is not necessarily the case, and the nature of this particular reaction remains undefined.

(f) McKie (1978)

45-year-old female undergoing laparoscopic sterilisation. Previous uneventful anaesthetic without exposure to gallamine. No history of allergies. Premedicated with morphine and scopolamine. Induction with thiopentone and gallamine, followed by inflation with oxygen and nitrous oxide. Generalised erythema and circulatory collapse noted within 1 minute of induction. Successful resuscitation following intubation, administration of oxygen, fluids, hydrocortisone and chlorpheniramine. Residual complaints of abdominal soreness ("more intense than normal discomfort following laparoscopic procedures"). Skin testing performed 3 months later using diluted solutions of all intravenous agents used, together with pancuronium, alcuronium and suxamethonium. Positive reaction only with gallamine.

Comment. The results of the skin tests suggest that gallamine was the agent responsible. There is insufficient evidence to substantiate the author's claim that this was an anaphylactic reaction.

(3) Bronchospasm and circulatory collapse

(a) Sniper (1971)

19-year-old female. Allergic to penicillin, citrus fruits and IVP contrast medium. No mention of previous exposure to anaesthesia. Premedicated with papaveratum and scopolamine. Induced with thiopentone and gallamine, following which, patient found to be in severe bronchospasm. Profound hypotension and possible cardiac arrest followed. External cardiac massage performed, and treatment instituted with hydrocortisone, dextran, methedrine, mannitol and sodium bicarbonate. Eventually recovered without any ill-effects. Skin-tests performed following day. Negative response with thiopentone, and a reaction with gallamine that was "probably more intense and longer-acting than in controls".

Comment. Skin tests performed too soon after event for reliable interpretation. The reaction could possibly have resulted from the administration of gallamine, but there is insufficient evidence to state this with certainty, or to pronounce on the nature of the reaction.

(b) Holmes et al. (1971)

27-year-old female. One previous uneventful operation — not exposed to gallamine. Allergic to citrus fruits. Premedicated with papaveratum and scopolamine. Penicillin administered with the premedication intramuscularly. Induced with thiopentone and gallamine. Following intubation, patient noted to have severe bronchospasm. Circulatory collapse soon followed. Although resuscitation was initially successful, death occurred 4 days later. The cause of death was recorded as "pulmonary oedema and broncho-pneumonia due to cerebral oedema consequent upon cardiac arrest". Skin tests were performed before death, but results were said to be equivocal.

Comment. It is impossible to attribute this fatal reaction to any particular one of the agents used. It is impossible to attribute this fatal reaction to any particulate one of the agents used, nor is it possible to define the nature of the reaction itself.

(c) Watt (1973)

43-year-old female. Previous uneventful exposure to gallamine. Administration of gallamine was followed by a reaction consisting of bronchospasm and cardiovascular collapse. Intradermal testing for gallmine positive, but other drugs used were not similarly tested.

Comment. Previous uneventful exposure could have sensitised the patient to gallamine, thus resulting in an anaphylactic reaction on this occasion. However, no other confirmatory tests were performed and the diagnosis must therefore remain speculative.

(4) Bronchospasm and facial oedema

(a) Fisher (1978)

31-year-old female. 4 previous uneventful anaesthetics without exposure to gallamine. History of asthma. No information regarding premedication. Induced with thiopentone, gallamine and suxamethonium, following which intubation performed. Immediately after this, found to be in severe bronchospasm which eventually responded to aminophylline and hydrocortisone. Also noted to have facial oedema during the reaction. Intravenous challenge with gallamine, performed the next day, provoked another episode of bronchospasm. No other tests performed.

Comment. The result of intravenous challenge with gallamine confirms that this agent had a part to play in the initial reaction. However, neither thiopentone nor suxamethonium were similarly tested. There is insufficient data for further comment on the nature of the mechanisms involved.

(5) Generalised erythema and urticaria

(a) Lopert (1955)

17-year-old female. No history of allergies and no previous anaesthetics. Induced with thiopentone and gallamine. Generalised urticarial wheals and facial flushing noted approximately 5 min after induction. Spontaneous resolution. Direct intravenous challenge with small dose of gallamine produced generalised erythema which again resolved spontaneously. Repeat challenge with gallamine from a different batch resulted in a similar generalised skin reaction. No tests performed for thiopentone.

Comment. Positive responses to 2 direct intravenous challenges provide unequivocal evidence that gallamine was involved in the original reaction. However, thiopentone was not subjected to similar tests and again, cannot be totally excluded as another possible cause.

(b) Lopert (1955)

3.5-month-old child. No mention of allergies or previous exposures to anaesthetics. Premedicated with pentobarbitone and atropine. Gaseous induction with nitrous oxide, oxygen and trilene followed by ether. Gallamine then injected, and soon after this, generalised erythema occurred. Spontaneous resolution after 1 hour. No tests performed.

Comment. As gallamine was the only intravenous agent administered, it is highly likely that this was a reaction to it. Even so, the other drugs used cannot be totally excluded.

(c) Walmsley (1959)

42-year-old female. Operation 8 years previously but no records available. History of urticarial rash after eating lobster. No premedication. Induced with thiopentone and gallamine. Generalised erythema and urticaria occurred within minutes of induction. Spontaneous resolution without specific therapy. Skin tests performed 2 weeks later using undiluted solution of gallamine, provoked erythema around injection site and on the face and neck. This persisted for 2 days before disappearing.

Comment. In view of the intense and generalised reaction to the skin test, there can be little doubt that gallamine was involved in the initial reaction. However, thiopentone was not subjected to similar testing and cannot therefore be totally excluded as another possible cause. There is insufficient data for further definition of the nature of the reaction.

Suxamethonium

(1) Bronchospasm, circulatory collapse, and cutaneous manifestations

(a) Jerums et al. (1967)
28-year-old female. History of urticarial reaction to penicillin. No previous exposure to suxamethonium. First operation – premedicated with atropine. Induced with halothane, oxygen and nitrous oxide following aborted injection of methohexitone (because of pain). Suxamethonium then administered, and 1 min later, developed tachycardia, hypotension and cyanosis. Recovered following treatment with metaraminol and digoxin (for supraventricular tachycardia which had supervened). Second operation, one month later – premedicated with papaveratum and hyoscine. Induced with thiopentone followed by suxamethonium and intubation. Severe reaction then occurred consisting of bronchospasm, profound hypotension and tachycardia, generalised erythema, facial and glottic oedema. Cardiac massage administered; resuscitation was successful, but the patient had residual neurological deficits for several weeks after the incident. Patch-testing yielded a positive result only with suxamethonium; intradermal testing with thiopentone was negative (suxamethonium not subjected to this test because of fear of precipitation of a severe reaction); Prausnitz-Kustner testing yielded a positive result for suxamethonium.

Comment. The circumstances of the reactions and the positive Prausnitz-Kustner test suggest that this was an anaphylactic reaction to suxamethonium.

(b) Sitarz (1974)
30-year-old female. No history of allergies. Previous uneventful ether anaesthetic. Anaphylactoid reaction (circulatory collapse and erythema) following induction of general anaesthesia for proposed Caesarean Section – no details of agents used. Re-anaesthetised following unspecified interval. Premedicated with atropine. Given vitamin C and hydrocortisone immediately prior to induction with Brevinarcorn, and subsequently intubated under suxamethonium. Florid anaphylactoid reaction occurred 2 min after intubation, consisting of marked hypotension, bronchospasm, generalised flushing and urticaria. Treated with steroids, ephedrine, antihistamines, calcium chloride and fluids, with eventual recovery. Skin tests performed 2 weeks after the event, using undiluted solutions of Brevinarcorn and suxamethonium. Localised wheal and flare reaction occurred at the site of administration of suxamethonium, and this was followed 20 min later by a systemic reaction with restlessness and dyspnoea.

Comment. The results of the skin tests suggest that suxamethonium was the agent responsible for the reaction. However, there is insufficient data to support the author's conclusion that this was an anaphylactic reaction.

(c) Mandappa et al. (1975)
35-year-old male. No history of asthma or allergies. No previous anaesthetics. Premedicated with pethidine and atropine. Induced with thiopentone, followed by suxamethonium. Within 1 minute of intubation, patient developed tachycardia and severe hypotension. A generalised erythematous rash

followed, and mild bronchospasm was also noted. Successful resuscitation achieved with methoxamine, promethazine and dexamethasone. Re-exposed to thiopentone and suxamethonium under steroid cover 9 days later. Several minutes after the uneventful administration of thiopentone, suxamethonium was slowly given in small incremental doses. Within minutes, signs of histamine release were again evident. Skin sensitivity tests using diluted solutions of suxamethonium, were performed some time after the reaction, and reported to show a marked wheal and flare response. No tests were performed for thiopentone.

Comment. Although evidence is more in favour of incriminating suxamethonium, thiopentone was not fully excluded as a causative agent. The author suggested that this was an anaphylactic reaction, but there is insufficient evidence to support this.

(d) Fisher (1975)

28-year-old female. No previous anaesthetics. Wheezing reaction to anti-diarrhoeal tablets in the past. Premedicated with pethidine and atropine. Intubated easily following induction with methohexitone and suxamethonium. Then found to be difficult to inflate, became cyanosed, and rapidly developed cardiac arrest necessitating external cardiac massage. Generalised flushing appeared following resuscitation, and persisted for 2 hours. Subsequently, 2 uneventful anaesthetics were administered under steroid and anti-histamine cover, using propanidid, and halothane-oxygen-nitrous oxide. On skin testing 4 months later, the patient reacted with mild bronchospasm and palpitations following the intradermal injection of a diluted solution of suxamethonium. Negative responses were obtained with methohexitone and several other agents. Prausnitz-Kustner testing performed 16 months later (Fisher, 1976) was positive only for suxamethonium and negative for several other drugs which were also tested.

Comment. The skin tests identified suxamethonium as the causative agent, and the result of Prausnitz-Kustner testing indicate that this was an anaphylactic reaction.

(e) Matthews et al. (1977)

24-year-old female undergoing emergency Caesarean Section. Anaphylactoid reaction (hypotension and erythema) following a general anaesthetic with thiopentone, suxamethonium and alcuronium 3 years previously. No tests performed, but patient informed that she was allergic to alcuronium. In this instance, epidural catheter inserted and bupivacaine administered 50 min before induction with thiopentone, atropine and suxamethonium. Intubation was followed immediately by the onset of bronchospasm, circulatory collapse and the slower developmnt of generalised erythema and urticaria. Treated with steroids, aminophylline, metaraminol, fluids and anti-histamines with eventual recovery. Intradermal skin tests, using diluted solutions, revealed negative results for all the agents used except suxamethonium (wheal and flare reaction).

Comment. The skin tests suggested that suxamethonium was the agent responsible. There is insufficient evidence to support the author's conclusion that this was an anaphylactic reaction.

(f) Royston and Wilkes (1978)

19-year-old male. No history of allergies. Underwent multiple anaesthetics over a 10-month period following a pelvic crush injury. Suxamethonium was administered uneventfully on 4 separate occasions. 18 months later, patient underwent a further anaesthetic. Premedicated with diazepam. Induced with atropine, thiopentone and suxamethonium. Immediately after this, the patient developed severe bronchospasm, cyanosis, and profound hypotension necessitating external cardiac massage. Generalised oedema, most marked on the face, was also apparent. Resuscitation with fluids, sodium bicarbonate, aminophylline and methyl prednisolone was successful, and the patient made a complete recovery within

24 hours. Blood samples taken after the reaction showed a decrease in IgE levels and a mild degree of C3 conversion. The low IgE levels were presumed to be indicative of IgE consumption during the reaction, and it was thought that the mild degree of C3 conversion was of insufficient degree to implicate a direct complement mediated mechanism as the cause of the reaction. 6 months later, prick testing yielded a positive reaction only with suxamethonium, and intradermal injection of the same drug resulted in a strongly positive reaction and the development of early signs of an anaphylactoid reaction. The patient was subsequently subjected to 4 further anaesthetics using thiopentone, alcuronium and nitrous oxide — no reaction occurred during these procedures.

Comment. The occurrence of a reaction following 4 uneventful previous exposures, and the results of the immunological tests strongly suggest that this was an anaphylactic reaction to suxamethonium.

(2) Bronchospasm and circulatory collapse without cutaneous manifestations

Fisher (1975)

15-year-old female. History of asthma and several allergies. No previous exposure to suxamethonium. Induced with methohexitone, gallamine, atropine and suxamethonium. Following nasal intubation, developed severe bronchospasm, cyanosis and hypotension. Treatment instituted with hydrocortisone, aminophylline, and methoxamine. The reaction gradually subsided, but the patient was left with residual complaints of stomach cramp, nausea and vomiting. Intradermal testing testing performed 12 months later gave a positive reaction with suxamethonium (up to 1:10,000 dilution). Negative results were obtained for the other intravenous drugs which had also been administered. Prausnitz-Kustner testing yielded a positive result for suxamethonium (Fisher, 1976).

Comment. In spite of the absence of a history of previous exposure, the intradermal and Prausnitz-Kustner tests indicate that this was an anaphylactic reaction to suxamethonium.

(3) Circulatory collapse and cutaneous manifestations

(a) Kepes and Haimovici (1959)

61-year-old male. Underwent an operation 10 years previously without exposure to suxamethonium. Past history of facial rash of indeterminate origin. Premedicated with secobarbital, meperidine and atropine. Induced with Thiamylal, followed by continuous infusion of suxamethonium. 8 min after induction, a generalised urticarial rash appeared, and this was followed by profound hypotension. Treated with hydrocortisone and diphenhydramine. Blood pressure returned to pre-anaesthetic levels after 19 min. Intradermal tests performed soon after the event revealed negative responses to suxamethonium and Thiamylal. Second anaesthetic operation one week after this, during which thiamylal was omitted from the anaesthetic regime. A similar reaction developed following the administration of suxamethonium for intubation. Intravenous challenge was then performed three days later, using all the drugs that had been previously administered. No reactions occurred with meperidine, atropine or Thiamylal, but suxamethonium produced a generalised urticarial reaction.

Comment. The results from intravenous challenge provide conclusive evidence that suxamethonium was the cause of the reaction. There is insufficient data for further definition of the nature of the reaction.

(b) Mandappa et al (1975)

16-year-old female. No history of allergies or asthma. No previous exposure to suxamethonium. Premedicated with atropine. Anaesthesia induced with nitrous oxide, oxygen, trilene and ether. Suxamethonium then administered and intubation performed. Soon after this, the patient developed hypotension, tachycardia, generalised erythema and facial oedema. Treatment instituted with dexamethasone, chlorpheniramine and calcium gluconate. Skin tests, performed soon after the event, were negative for atropine and weakly positive for suxamethonium. Repeat testing 12 days after stopping steroids yielded a strongly positive response with suxamethonium.

Comment. The skin tests suggest that suxamethonium was the causative agent involved. There is insufficient data to support the author's conclusion that this was an anaphylactic reaction.

(c) Fisher (1975)

29-year-old female. 2 uneventful ethyl chloride/ether anaesthetics as a child. No previous exposure to suxamethonium. Premedicated with pethidine, promethazine and atropine. Induced with thiopentone, gallamine and suxamethonium. Shortly after uneventful intubation, developed generalised flushing, hypotension and tachycardia. The flushing faded over 20 min, and the hypotension responded to fluid infusion. The patient complained of cramp-like abdominal pains and nausea for 4 hours postoperatively. Intradermal testing performed 12 months later yielded positive results only with suxamethonium. Prausnitz-Kustner testing was negative for suxamethonium (Fisher, 1976).

Comment. The intradermal tests suggest that suxamethonium was the agent responsible. The negative Prausnitz-Kustner test does not necessarily rule out the possibility of an anaphylactic reaction, as false negative results can occur.

(d) St. Maurice et al. (1976)

27-year-old female undergoing Caesarean section. 1 previous anaesthetic—no details available. No history of allergies. Premedicated with atropine. Induced with gamma hydroxybutyrate and thiopentone. 5 min later, suxamethonium administered; this was followed immediately by the appearance of widespread urticaria. Pancuronium then given and 10 min after induction, it was noted that the patient was profoundly hypotensive. Treatment with steroids and fluids was given with eventual recovery. Lymphocyte transformation tests performed, giving positive reactions to both suxamethonium and thiopentone.

Comment. The reaction could have been due to either one or both of these agents. There is insufficient evidence for more specific identification of the causative agent.

(4) Bronchospasm

(a) Smith (1957)

72-year-old man. Known asthmatic who was in bronchospasm at time of operation. No information regarding prior exposure to suxamethonium. Premedicated with atropine and ephedrine. Induced with thiopentone and suxamethonium. Following intubation, bronchospasm worsened for a few minutes before spontaneously improving, but then worsened again following a second dose of suxamethonium. Adequate control of ventilation achieved following administration of gallamine, and no further difficulties encountered. Positive results were obtained from skin tests using undiluted solutions of suxamethonium and gallamine (more marked with suxamethonium).

Comment. The results from the skin tests are not necessarily significant in view of the use of undiluted solutions. The evidence for incriminating suxamethonium is purely circumstantial, and the issue is further confused by the fact that the patient was already in bronchospasm before induction.

(b) Fellini et al. (1963)

11-year-old female. No history of allergies and no previous exposure to suxamethonium. Premedicated with pentobarbitone and atropine. Gaseous induction with cyclopropane and oxygen passed uneventfully, but bronchospasm and tachycardia occurred following the start of a suxamethonium infusion. This improved when the suxamethonium infusion was stopped, but recurred on 4 further occasions when suxamethonium was administered during the course of the operation. Intradermal skin testing using undiluted solution of suxamethonium yielded a positive reaction on the 3rd post-operative day.

Comment. No definite conclusions can be drawn from the results of the skin tests because of the use of undiluted solution. However, there are good clinical grounds for incriminating suxamethonium as the causative agent. Insufficient tests were performed to enable further definition of the mechanisms involved.

(c) Eustace (1967)

(i) 57-year-old man. Chronic bronchitic, and more recently, periodic attacks of severe bronchospasm. No history of previous exposure to suxamethonium. Premedicated with pethidine and phenergan. Uneventful gaseous induction using halothane and oxygen (preceeded by intravenous atropine). Suxamethonium infusion started after a short interval, and this was soon followed by transient bronchospasm which persisted for 2 to 3 min before spontaneous improvement. No further suxamethonium administered until the end of the operation when a further small dose provoked bronchospasm again. Negative result obtained from skin testing using undiluted solution of suxamethonium one week after event.

(ii) 54-year-old female. Chronic bronchitic. Two previous exposure to suxamethonim following which, apparent bronchospasm had occurred. Premedicated with papaveratum and atropine. Uneventful anaesthetic using thiopentone, nitrous oxide-oxygen-halothane. At the end of the operation, a test dose of suxamethonium produced an attack of bronchospasm which passed off in 2-3 min. Skin tests performed soon after the operation yielded negative results.

Comment. The skin tests were performed too soon after the operation to provide any helpful information. However, in both cases, intravenous challenge at the end of the operation appeared to produce immediate bronchospasm; it is very likely, therefore, that suxamethonium was the causative agent.

(d) Katz and Mulligan (1972)

53-year-old female. Suffered from hay fever, and had developed allergic skin rash following sulphur medication in the past. No information regarding previous exposure to anaesthetic agents. Premedicated with morphine and scopolamine. At induction, thiopentone, gallamine and suxamethonium were administered intravenously. Severe bronchospasm was noted 3 minutes after the suxamethonium injection; this persisted in spite of hyperventilation with halothane during the course of which the patient developed hypotension. The hypotension resolved when halothane was discontinued, and in an effort to produce further relaxation, a suxamethonium drip was commenced. Isoprenaline introduced via an aerosol spray into the anaesthetic circuit produced a transient improvement, but it was not until the suxamethonium infusion was stopped that improvement occurred. After 15 min of normal ventilation, a challenge dose of suxamethonium produced a recurrence of bronchospasm within 1 min and continued for 12 min before gradual spontaneous resolution. Intradermal skin test performed during the operation using undiluted solution of suxamethonium produced a positive result.

Comment. The result of the intravenous challenge dose provides good evidence that suxamethonium was a causative agent in this reaction. There is insufficient data for further definition of the nature of the reaction.

(e) Bele-Binda and Valeri (1971)

18-year-old female. No history of allergies or asthma. No previous exposure to suxamethonium. Premedicated with atropine and pethidine. Induced with thiopentone and suxamethonium following which, the patient developed severe bronchospasm. This resolved following treatment with aminophylline and dexamethasone. Re-anaesthetised 4 days later. Premedicated with atropine, pethidine and aminophylline suppositories. Induced with Thiamylal and suxamethonium. Bronchospasm again occurred following induction. No tests performed.

Comment. The clinical evidence suggests that suxamethonium was the agent responsible for both reactions. There is insufficient data for differentiation between the different possible mechanisms involved.

Pancuronium

(1) Bronchospasm

(a) Heath (1973)

47-year-old male. History of asthma, but completely free of symptoms and signs at time of operation. Anaesthetised one week previously without exposure to pancuronium. Premedicated with diazepam and atropine. Induced with thiopentone and intubated following suxamethonium. Maintained on halothane-oxygen-nitrous oxide and, on return of muscle tone, pancuronium and pentazocine administered. 2 min following this, developed intense bronchospasm which eventually disappeared following treatment with aminophylline and ephedrine. Further incremental doses of pentazocine produced no further untoward effects. 50 min after the orininal reaction, administration of a small dose of pancuronium resulted in severe bronchospasm within 30 sec. This again resolved on treatment with aminophylline. Several months later, intradermal tests using undiluted solutions of pancuronium and various other agents resulted in wheal and flare reactions which were indistinguishable from each other and from the reactions produced in a "normal" subject.

Comment. The evidence for incrimination of pancuronium rests on the marked reponse to the second dose administered towards the end of the operation. Skin testing was unhelpful, and there is insufficient data for any conclusions to be drawn as to the mechanism underlying the reaction.

(b) Clark (1973)

48-year-old female. Previous uneventful anaesthetic (not exposed to pancuronium). No history of allergies apart from slight swelling of eyelids with certain make-up preparations. Premedicated with papaveratum and haloperidol. Induced with Althesin and pancuronium, and then maintained on nitrous oxide, oxygen and halothane. 2 min after induction, developed bronchospasm. Further dose of Althesin administered and patient intubated. Aminophylline and hydrocortisone given, and bronchospasm gradually resolved over the next 30 min. Pancuronium was administered on 2 further occasions during the same anaesthetic and on both occasions bronchospasm recurred. 3 test doses of Althesin given at the end of the operation failed to elicit a similar reaction. Intradermal testing using diluted solutions of pancuronium and Althesin gave a positive wheal and flare reaction with pancuronium, and only a flare with Althesin.

Comment. The results of intravenous challenge during the operation and the skin tests suggest that pancuronium was the agent responsible. No definite conclusions can be drawn as to the mechanism involved in the reaction.

(2) Bronchospasm and facial flushing

Buckland and Avery (1973)

42-year-old male. History of mild asthma which had developed following the birth of a child 14 years previously. Intermittent therapy with Amesec tablets since then. Uneventful anaesthetic 7 years previously. First anaesthetic – premedicated with atropine. Induced with thiopentone followed by suxamethonium and intubation. Maintained on nitrous oxide-oxygen and phenoperidine uneventfully for 10 min. Pancuronium then administered and intermittent positive pressure ventilation commenced. Mild tachycardia, hypotension and facial flushing were noted, and over the next 10 min, bronchospasm became evident. This responded transiently to aminophylline, but recurred and persisted for 30 min post-operatively before eventually resolving. Skin tests performed intra-operatively with undiluted solutions showed wheal and flare reactions to pancuronium and d-tubocurarine, a milder response to suxamethonium, and negative reactions with saline, pheonperidine, thiopentone and Conray. The patient was re-anaesthetised 2 hours later following premedication with hydrocortisone and promethazine, and a similar anaesthetic sequence was used apart from the substitution of d-tubocurarine for pancuronium. No untoward reactions occurred on this occasion.

Comment. The circumstances of the reaction suggest that pancuronium was the agent responsible, but there is no conclusive evidence to support this. The results of skin testing are not necessarily significant in view of the use of undiluted solutions, and the second anaesthetic was performed under steroid and anti-histamine cover.

(3) Bronchospasm and hypotension

Tweedie and Ordish (1974)

58-year-old male. History of angioneurotic oedema presumed to have resulted from aspirin ingestion. No previous exposure to pancuronium. Premedicated with papaveratum and hyoscine. Induced with Althesin and pancuronium. This was soon followed by bronchospasm, hypotension and tachycardia. The reaction resolved gradually without specific treatment. Skin testing with undiluted solutions gave a minimal response with Althesin and a large wheal and flare reaction to pancuronium.

Comment. Undiluted solutions were used for skin testing the contention that pancuronium was the agent responsible is not necessarily true.

Alcuronium

(1) Circulatory collapse, bronchospasm and cutaneous manifestations

(a) Fisher et al. (1978)

25-year-old male. Allergic to codeine. 5 previous uneventful anaesthetics, alcuronium having been administered on three of these occasions. Anaesthetised with thiopentone and alcuronium; shortly after this, developed bronchospasm, circulatory collapse and widespread erythema. Treated with adrenaline, steroids and fluids with rapid recovery. Intradermal skin testing with dilute solutions revealed a positive wheal and flare reaction with alcuronium, and negative reactions with thiopentone, d-tubocurarine and suxamethonium. Prausnitz-Kustner testing was positive, while passive cutaneous anaphylaxis testing in monkeys was negative at 4 hours and positive at 24 hours for alcuronium.

Comment. Comprehensive testing appears to have been performed and the positive Prausnitz-Kustner reaction is good evidence for an anaphylactic reaction.

(b) Fisher et al. (1978)

38-year-old female. No history of allergies. Three previous uneventful anaesthetics — no exposure to alcuronium during two of these; no details available regarding remaining one. Induction with thiopentone and alcuronium was followed by the development of bronchospasm and severe circulatory collapse requiring external cardiac massage. This was accompanied by the subsequent appearance of a generalised erythematous rash and facial oedema. Treatment with streroids and fluids resulted in partial recovery of the blood pressure, but the circulation only returned to normal after two doses of adrenaline and further fluid infusion. Re-anaesthetised uneventfully two months later using thiopentone and pancuronium. Intradermal skin testing yielded positive reactions with alcuronium and d-tubocurarine, and negative reactions with thiopentone, pancuronium, suxamethonium, gallamine and saline. Prausnitz-Kustner testing was positive, while passive cutaneous anaphylaxis-testing in monkeys yielded a negative result for alcuronium.

Comment. The results of the intradermal tests and the positive Prausnitz-Kustner reaction indicate that this was an anaphylactic reaction to alcuronium.

(2) Circulatory collapse and cutaneous manifestations

(a) Chan and Yeung (1972)

51-year-old female. No previous anaesthetics. No allergies, but two weeks before present episode, had a suspected anaphylactoid reaction to Biligraffin (iodipamide) consisting of cardiovascular collapse and cyanosis. First operation: premedicated with atropine and pethidine. Induction with thiopentone, followed by suxamethonium and intubation. After an uneventful 5 min, given alcuronium. This was followed 4 min later by severe hypotension and the appearance of a generalised erythematous rash. Successful resuscitation with fluids, adrenaline, hydrocortisone and chlorpheniramine. Second operation: re-anaesthetised 4 days later after pethidine and hyoscine premedication. Induced with thiopentone, and then given 2 doses of suxamethonium over a 10-min period with no untoward effect. Alcuronium then injected, and this was followed immediately by a reaction similar to the previous one (hypotension and rash). Treated successfully with fluids, steroids and antihistamines. A further anaphylactoid reaction occurred several hours later following an intravenous dose of ampicillin. Intradermal testing using dilute solutions of thiopentone, suxametonium, alcuronium, and distilled water were all negative 3 weeks after the event.

Comment. There are reasonable grounds for incriminating alcuronium on the basis of the timing of the reactions, but there is no evidence to support the author's conclusion that this was an anaphylactic reaction.

(b) Fisher et al. (1978)

18-year-old female. No history of allergies or asthma. No previous anaesthetics. Induced with thiopentone and alcuronium. Then intubated and maintained on nitrous oxide-oxygen-halothane, during which time moderate hypotension developed and persisted despite withdrawal of halothane. An additional dose of alcuronium was given, and within 2 minutes of this, the patient developed profound circulatory collapse with generalised erythema and angioneurotic oedema. Treated with adrenaline, dexamethasone and fluids with restoration of blood pressure, and gradual resolution of oedema over following 24 hours. An additional feature of this reaction was the development of severe upper abdominal cramp, nausea and vomiting in the first 24 hours post-operatively. Intradermal skin tests were positive for alcuronium and negative for d-tubocurarine and thiopentone. Prausnitz-Kustner testing was positive for Alcuronium, while passive cutaneous anaphylaxis testing in monkeys yielded a negative result.

Comment. There was good evidence to support the conclusion that this was an anaphylactic reaction to alcuronium.

(c) Fisher et al. (1978)

46-year-old male. No previous anaesthetics. No allergies or asthma. Induction with thiopentone and alcuronium was followed immediately by generalised flushing and cardiovascular collapse necessitating external cardiac massage. Treated with fluids, steroids and digoxin, but recovery incomplete until the following day. Skin testing with dilute solutions yielded positieve wheal and flare reactions to alcuronium, and negative reactions to thiopentone, d-tubocurarine and suxamethonium. Prausnitz-Kustner and passive cutaneous anaphylaxis testing were both negative. There were no significant changes in C_3 and C_4 complement fractions.

Comment. The results of the skin tests suggest that alcuronium was the agent responsible, although the aetiological mechanism remains unclear.

(3) Circulatory collapse

Fisher et al. (1978)

68-year-old male. No history of allergies. Induced with thiopentone and alcuronium, following which, the patient developed profound hypotension and a supraventricular tachycardia. Resuscitated with fluids and an infusion of dopamine. The tachycardia was eventually controlled following cardioversion and treatment with lignocaine, digoxin and verapamil. Intradermal skin testing yielded a positive reaction to alcuronium, and negative reactions to thiopentone and d-tubocurarine. Prausnitz-Kustner and passive cutaneous anaphylaxis testing were both negative for alcuronium.

Comment. The intradermal tests suggest that the patient may have reacted to alcuronium, but it should also be borne in mind that the hypotensive episodes could equally have been the result of a primary supraventricular tachycardia precipitated by an unrelated cause.

Fazadinium

Circulatory collapse and cutaneous manifestations

Rowlands and Fidler (1978)

Female patient suffering from scleroderma. Fazadinium administered following induction with Althesin. 5–10 min later developed generalised blotchy redness followed by severe cardiovascular collapse and cyanosis. There was no associated bronchospasm and satisfactory recovery ensued. Intradermal tests with histamine, fazadinium and Althesin performed soon after the event, whilst the patient was still on therapy with chlorpheniramine, were all negative. On repeat testing 10 days later, flare reactions occurred with fazadinium and histamine.

Comment. There is insufficient evidence to form any conclusion about this reaction, but it is possible that fazadinium was the responsible agent.

REFERENCES

Adams, A.K. and Barnett, K.C. (1966): Anaesthesia and intraocular pressure. *Anaesthesia, 21*, 202.
Agoston, S., Vermeer, G.A., Kersten, U.W. and Meijer, D.K.F. (1973): The fate of pancuronium bromide in man. *Acta anaesth. scand., 17*, 267.

Agoston, S., Vermeer, A., Kersten, V.W. and Scaf, A.H.S. (1978): A preliminary investigation of the renal and hepatic excretion of gallamine triethiodide in man. *Brit. J. Anaesth., 50,* 345.

Airaksinen, M.M. and Tammisto, T. (1965): Myoglobinuria after intermittent administration of succinylcholine during halothane anaesthesia. *Clin. Pharmacol Ther., 7,* 583.

Alam, M., Anrep, G.V., Barsoum, G.S., Talaat, M. and Wienginger, E. (1939): Liberation of histamine from the skeletal muscle by curare, *J. Physiol., 95,* 148. .

Ali, H.H., Wilson, R.S., Savarese, J.J. and Kitz, R.J. (1975): The effect of tubocurarine on indirectly elicited train-of-four muscle response and respiratory measurements in humans. *Brit. J. Anaesth., 47,* 570.

Allan, C.M., Cullen, W.G. and Gillies, D.M.M. (1961): Ventricular fibrillation in a burned boy. *Canad. med. Ass. J., 85,* 432.

Alper, M.H., and Flacke, W. (1969): Effects of curare, atropine and halothane on ganglionic transmission in the dog. *Abstracts of Scientific Papers, ASA Annual Meeting*, p 100.

Anand, J.S., Mehta, R.K., Munschi, C.A. and Mulla, D.H. (1972): Reversal of neuromuscular blockade by artificial diuresis: a case report. *Canad. Anaesth. Soc. J., 19,* 651.

Andersen, N. (1962): Changes in intragastric pressure following the administration of suxamethonium: preliminary report. *Brit. J. Anaesth., 34,* 363.

Anderson, E.F. and Rosenthal, M.H. (1975): Pancuronium bromide and tachyarrhythmias. *Crit. Care Med., 3,* 13.

Anderson, I.L. and Jones, E.W. (1976): Porcine malignant hyperthermia. Effect of dantrolene sodium on in-vitro halothane-induced contraction of susceptible muscle. *Anesthesiology, 44,* 57.

Anderson, I.L., Lipicky, R.J. and Jones, E.W. (1978): Dantrolene sodium in porcine malignant hyperthermia: studies on isolated muscle strips. In: *Second International Symposium on Malignant Hyperthermia.* Editor: J.A. Aldrete and B.A. Britt. Grune and Stratton, p. 509.

Arora, M.V., Clarke, R.S.J., Dundee, J.W. and Moore, J. (1973): Initial experience with AH 8165D, a new rapidly acting non-depolarizing muscle relaxant. *Anaesthesia, 28,* 188.

Atkinson, M., Edwards, D.A.W., Honour, A.J. and Rowlands, E.N. (1957): The oesophagogastric sphincter in hiatus hernia. *Lancet, II,* 1138.

Austin, K.L. and Denborough, M.A. (1977): Drug treatment of malignant hyperpyrexia. *Anesth. intens. Care, 5,* 207.

Axelsson, J., Thesleff, S. (1959): A study of supersensitivity in denervated mammalian skeletal muscle. *J. Physiol., 47,* 178.

Baird, W.L.M. and Reid, A.M. (1967): The neuromuscular blocking properties of a new steroid compound, pancuronium bromide. *Brit. J. Anaesth., 39,* 775.

Baldwin, A.C. and Churcher, M.D. (1979): Anaphylactoid response to intravenous tubocurarine. *Anaesthesia, 34,* 339.

Baraka, A. (1964): The influence of carbon dioxide on the neuromuscular blocks caused by tubocurarine chloride in the human subject. *Brit. J. Anaesth., 36,* 272.

Baraka, A. (1967): A comparative study between diallylnortoxiferine and tubocurarine. *Brit. J. Anaesth., 39,* 624.

Baraka, A. (1974): Myasthenic response to muscle relaxants in Von Recklinghausen's disease. *Brit. J. Anaesth., 46,* 701.

Baraka, A. (1977): Self-taming of succinylcholine-induced fasciculations. *Anesthesiology, 46,* 292.

Baraka, A. (1978): Suxamethonium-induced muscle contracture following traumatic denervation in man. *Brit. J. Anaesth., 50,* 195.

Baraka, A., and Gabali, F. (1968): Correlation between tubocurarine requirements and plasma protein pattern. *Brit. J. Anaesth., 40,* 89.

Baraka, A., Haddad, C., Afifi, A. and Baroody, M. (1970): Control of succinylcholine induced myotonia by D-tubocurarine. *Anesthesiology, 33,* 669.

Baraka, A., Haroun, S. and Bassili, M. (1975): Response of the newborn to succinylcholine injection in homozygotic atypical mothers. *Anesthesiology, 43,* 115.

Barrow, M.E.H. and Smethurst, J.R. (1963): Suxamewthonium modified by tetrahydroaminacrine. *Brit. J. Anaesth., 35,* 465.

Basta, J.W., Lichtiger, M. (1977): Comparison of metocurine and pancuronium − myocardial tension-time index during endotracheal intubation. *Anesthesiology, 46,* 366.

Bauld, H.W., Gibson, P.R., Jebson, P.T. and Brown, S.S. (1974): Aetiology of prolonged apnoea after suxamethonium. *Brit. J. Anaesth., 46,* 273.

Becker, L.D. and Miller, R.D. (1976): Clindamycin enhances a non-depolarizing neuromuscular blockade. *Anesthesiology, 45,* 84.

Bele-Binda, N. and Valeri, F. (1971): A case of bronchospasm induced by succinylcholine *Canad. Anaesth. Soc. J., 18,* 116.

Belin, R.P. and Karleen, C.I. (1966): Cardiac arrest in the burned patient following succinyldicholine administration. *Anesthesiology, 27,* 516.

Bennett, A.E. and Cash, P.T. (1943): Myasthenia gravis and curare sensitivity. *Dis. nerv. Syst., 4,* 299.

Bennett, E.J. Ramamurthy, S., Dalal, F.Y. and Salem, M.R. (1975): Pancuronium and the neonate. *Brit. J. Anaesth, 47,* 75.

Bennike, K.A. and Jarnum, S. (1964): Myoglobinuria with acute renal failure, possibly induced by suxamethonium: a case report. *Brit. J. Anaesth, 36,* 730.

Bernhardt, D. and Hoerder, M.H. (1978): Anesthesia induced myoglobinuria without hyperpyrexia − an abortive form of malignant hyperthermia? In: *The Second Intrnational Symposium on Malignant Hyperthermia.* Editor: J.A. Aldrete and B.A. Britt. p. 419.

Birch, A.A. Jr., Mitchell, G.D., Playford, G.A. and Lang, C.A. (1969): Changes in serum potassium response to succinylcholine following trauma. *J. Amer. med. Ass., 210,* 490.

Blitt, C.D., Petty, C.W., Alberternst, E.E. and Wright, B.J. (1977): Correlation of plasma cholinesterase activity and duration of action of succinylcholine during pregnancy. *Anaesth. Analg. Curr. Res., 56,* 78.

Blitt, C.D., Wright, W.A. and Peat, J. (1975): Pancuronium and the patient with myasthenia gravis. *Anesthesiology, 42,* 624.

Blogg, C.E., Savege, T.E., Simpson, J.C., Ross, L.A. and Simpson, B.R. (1973): A new muscle relaxant − AH 8165. *Proc. roy. Soc. Med. 66,* 1023.

Blogg, C.E., Simpson, B.R., Tyers, M.B., Martin, L.E. and Bell, J.A. (1975): Human placental transfer of AH 8165. *Anaesthesia, 30,* 23.

Bodley, P.O., Halwax, K. and Potts, L. (1969): Low serum psudocholinesterase levels complicating treatment with phenelzine. *Brit. med. J., 3,* 510.

Bodman, R.I. (1978): Pancuronium and histamine release. *Canad. Anaesth. Soc. J., 25,* 40.

Bonta, I.L., Goorissen, E.M. and Derkx, F.H. (1968): Pharmacological interaction between pancuronium bromide and anaesthetics. *Europ. J. Pharmacol, 4,* 83.

Booth, P.N., Watson, M.J. and McLeod, K. (1977): Pancuronium and the placental barrier. *Anaesthesia, 32,* 320.

Borden, H., Clarke, M. and Katz, H. (1974): The use of pancuronium bromide in patients receiving lithium carbonate. *Canad. Anaesth. Soc. J., 21,* 79.

Borders, R.W., Stephen, C.R., Nowill, W.K. and Martin, R. (1955): The interrelationship of succinylcholine and the blood cholinesterases during anesthesia. *Anesthesiology, 16,* 401.

Botha, G.S.M., Astley, R. and Carre, I.J. (1957): A combined cineradiographic and manometric study of the gastro-oesophageal junction. *Lancet, I,* 659.

Bourne, J.G., Collier, H.O.J. and Somers, G.F. (1952): Succinylcholine (Succinoylcholine. Muscle relaxant of short duration. *Lancet, I,* 1225.

Bowen, D.J., McGrand, J.C. and Hamilton, A.G. (1978): Intraocular pressures after suxamethonium and endotracheal intubation. The effect of pretreatment with tubocurarine or gallamine. *Anaesthesia, 33,* 518.

Bowen, D.J., McGrand, J.C. and Palmer, R.J. (1976): Intraocular pressures after suxamethonium and endotracheal intubation in patients pretreated with pancuronium. *Brit. J. Anaesth., 48,* 1201.

Brandt, M.R. and Viby-Mogensen, J. (1978): Halothane anaesthesia and suxamethonium III. Atropine thirty seconds before a second dose of suxamethonium during inhalational anaesthesia: effects and side-effects. *Acta anaesth. scand., Suppl. 67,* 76.

Brandus, V., Joffe, S., Benoit, C.V. and Wolff, W.I. (1970): Bronchial spasm during general anaesthesia. *Canad. Anaesth. Soc. J., 17,* 269.

Brandus, V., Joffe, S. and Rubin, J.M. (1973): Histamine-like reaction to tubocurarine. *Brit. J. Anaesth., 45,* 108.

Bridenbaugh, P.O. and Churchill-Davidson, H.C. (1968): Response to tubocurarine chloride and its reversal by neostigmine methylsulfate in man. *J. Amer. med. Ass., 203,* 541.

Bridenbaugh, P.W., Churchill-Davidson, H.C. and Churcher, M.D. (1966): Effects of carbon dioxide on actions of D-tubocurarine and gallamine. *Anesth. Analg. Curr. Res., 45,* 804.

Brim, V.D. (1973): Denervation supersensitivity: the response to depolarizing muscle relaxants. *Brit. J. Anaesth., 45,* 222.

British Medical Journal (1979): Editorial, p. 703.

Britain, R.T. and Tyers, M.B. (1973): The pharmacology of AH 8165: a rapid-acting, short-lasting competitive neuromuscular blocking drug. *Brit. J. Anaesth., 45,* 837.

Britt, B.A. (1972): Recent advances in malignant hyperpyrexia. *Anesth. Analg. Curr. Res., 51,* 841.

Britt, B.A. and Kalow, W. (1970): Malignant hyperthermia: a statistical review. *Canad. Anaesth. Soc. J., 17,* 293.

Britt. B.A., Locher, W.G. and Kalow, W. (1969): Hereditary aspects of malignant hyperthermia. *Canad. Anaesth. Soc. J., 16,* 89.

Britt, B.A., Webb, G.F. and Le Duc, C. (1974): Malignant hyperthermia induced by curare. *Canad. Anaesth. Soc. J., 21,* 371.

Brodsky, J.B. and Brock-Utne, J.G. (1979): Does "self-taming" with succinylcholine prevent post-operative myalgia. *Anesthesiology, 50,* 265.

Brown, B.R., Jr. and Crout, J.R. (1970): The sympathomimetic effect of gallamine on the heart. *J. Pharmacol. exp. Ther., 172,* 266.

Brown, E.M., Smiler, B.G. and Plaza, J.A. (1973): Cardiovascular effects of pancuronium. *Anesthesiology, 38,* 597.

Buckett, W.R., Marjoribanks, C.E.B., Marwick, F.A. and Morton, M.B. (1968): The pharmacology of pancuronium bromide (ORG.NA 97) a new potent steroidal neuromuscular blocking agent. *Brit. J. Pharmacol, 32,* 671.

Buckland, R.W. and Avery, A.F. (1973): Histamine release following pancuronium. *Brit. J. Anaesth., 45,* 518.

Bullough, J. (1959): Intermittent suxamethonium injections. *Brit. med. J., 1,* 786.

Burtles, R. and Tunstall, M.E. (1961): Suxamethonium chloride and muscle pains. *Brit. J. Anaesth., 33,* 24.

Bush, G.H. (1964a): Clinical experiences with diallylnortoxiferine in children. *Brit. J. Anaesth., 36*, 787.

Bush, G.H. (1964b): Use of muscle relaxants in burnt children. *Anaesthesia, 19*, 231.

Bush, G.H. (1965): The clinical comparison between tubocurarine and diallylnortoxiferine in children. *Brit. J. Anaesth., 37*, 540.

Bush, G.H. and Baraka, A (1964): Factors affecting the termination of curarization in the human subject. *Brit. J. Anaesth., 36*, 356.

Bush, G.H. and Roth, F. (1961): Muscle pains after suxamethonium chloride in children. *Brit. J. Anaesth., 33*, 151.

Bush, G.H. and Stead, A.L. (1962): The use of d-tubocurarine in neonatal anaesthesia. *Brit. J. Anaesth., 34*, 721.

Cain, P.A. and Ellis, F.R. (1977): Anaesthesia for patients susceptible to malignant hyperpyrexia. A study of pancuronium and methylprednisolone. *Brit. J. Anaesth., 49*, 941.

Camu, F. and D'Hollander, A. (1978): Neuromuscular blockade of fazadinium bromide (AH 8165) in renal failure patients. *Acta anaesth. scand., 22*, 221.

Carballo, A.S. (1965): Succinylcholine and acetazolamide (diamox) in anaesthesia for ocular surgery. *Canad. Anaesth. Soc. J., 12*, 486.

Carrier, O., Jr. and Murphy, J.C. (1970): the effects of d-tubocurarine and its commercial vehicles on cardiac function. *Anesthesiology, 33*, 627.

Casale, F.F. and Farman, J.V. (1970): Blood loss during hysterectomy associated with the use of tubocurarine or gallamine. *Brit. J. Anaesth., 42*, 65.

Case History, No. 62 (1971): Circulatory collapse following succinylcholine. Report of a patient with diffuse lower motor neuron disease. Anesth. Analg. Curr. Res., 50, 431.

Cavallaro, R.J., Krumperman, L.W. and Kugler, F. (1968): Effect of echothiophate therapy on the metabolism of succinylcholine in man. *Anesth. Analg. Curr. Res., 47*, 570.

Chalstrey, L.J. and Edwards, G.B. (1972): Fatal hyperpyrexia following the use of pancuronium bromide in the pig. *Brit. J. Anaesth., 44*, 91.

Chan, C.S. and Yeung, M.L. (1972): Anaphylactic reaction to alcuronium. *Brit. J. Anaesth., 44*, 103.

Chasapakis, G., Augustaki, O., Kekis, N., Philippou, P., Moraitis, H., Floras, A. and Makkous, A. (1968): The influence of the kallikrein-trypsin inactivator Trasylol on the serum cholineserase. *Brit. J. Anaesth., 40*, 456.

Chatas, G.J., Gottlieb, J.B. and Sweet, R.B. (1963): Cardiovascular effects of d-tubocurarine during Fluothane anaesthesia. *Anesth. Analg. Curr. Res., 42*, 65.

Churchill-Davidson, H.C. (1954): Suxamethonium (Succinylcholine) chloride and muscle pains. *Brit. med. J., I*, 74.

Churchill-Davidson, H.C., Way, W.L. and DeJong, R.H. (1967): The muscle relaxants and renal function. *Anesthesiology, 28*, 540.

Churchill-Davidson, H.C. and Wise, R.P. (1960): Prevention, diagnosis and treatment of prolonged apnoea. *Brit. J. Anaesth., 32*, 384.

Churchill-Davidson, H.C. and Wise, R.P. (1964): The response of the newborn infant to muscle relaxants. *Canad. Anaesth. Soc. J., 11*, 1.

Clarke, I.M.C. and Ellis, F.R. (1975): An evaluation of procaine in the treatment of malignant hyperthermia. *Brit. J. Anaesth., 47*, 17.

Clark, R.M. (1973): Reaction to pancuronium? *Brit. J. Anaesth., 45*, 997.

Cobham, I.G. and Davis, H.S. (1964): Anaesthesia for muscle dystrophy patients. *Anesth. Analg. Curr. Res. 43*, 22.

Cody, J.R. (1968): Muscle rigidity following administration of succinylcholine. *Anesthesiology, 29*, 159.

118

Cohen, E.N., Brewer, H.W. and Smith, D. (1967): The metabolism and elimination of d-tubocurarine H[3]. *Anesthesiology, 28*, 309.

Coleman, A.J., Downing, J.W., Leary, W.P., Moyes, D.G. and Styles, M. (1972): The immediate cardiovascular effects of pancuronium, alcuronium and tubocurarine in man. *Anaesthesia, 27*, 415.

Coleman, A.J., O'Brien, A., Downing, J.W., Jeal, D.E., Moyes, D.G. and Leary, W.P. (1973): AH 8165D: A new non-depolarizing muscle relaxant. *Anaesthesia, 28*, 262.

Coleman, A.J., Walling, P.T., Downing, J.W. and Bees, L.T. (1975): The effect of carbon dioxide on the neuromuscular and haemodynamic effects of AH 8165, a new non-depolarizing muscle relaxant. *Brit. J. Anaesth., 47*, 365.

Collier, C. (1975): Suxamethonium pains and fasciculations. *Proc. roy. Soc. Med., 68*, 105.

Collier, C.B. (1978): Suxamethonium pains and early electrolyte changes. *Anaesthesia, 33*, 454.

Collier, C.B. (1979): Dantrolene and suxamethonium. The effect of preoperative dantrolene on the action of suxamethonium. *Anaesthesia, 34*, 152.

Comroe, J.H. and Dripps, R.D. (1946): the histaminelike action of curare and tubocurarine injected intracutaneously and intra-arterially in man. *Anesthesiology, 7*, 260.

Cook, D.R. and Fischer, C.G. (1975): Neuromuscular blocking effects of succinylcholine in infants and children. *Anesthesiology, 42*, 662.

Cooperman, L.H. (1970): Succinylcholine-induced hyperkalaemia in neuromuscular disease. *J. Amer. med. Ass., 113*, 1867.

Cooperman, L.H., Strobel, G.E., Jr. and Kennel, E.M. (1970): Massive hyperkalaemia after administration of succinylcholine. *Anesthesiology, 32*, 161.

Cowgill, D.B., Mostello, L.A. and Shapiro, H.M. (1974): Encephalitis and a hyperkalaemic response to succinylcholine. *Anesthesiology, 40*, 409.

Crago, R.R., Bryan, A.C., Laws, A.K. and Winestock, A.E. (1972): Respiratory flow resistance after curare and pancuronium measured by forced oscillations. *Canad. Anaesth. Soc. J., 19*, 607.

Craig, H.J.L. (1964): The protective effect of thiopentone against muscular pains and stiffness which follows the use of suxamethonium chloride. *Brit. J. Anaesth., 36*, 612.

Crawford, J.S. (1956): Some aspects of obstetric anaesthesia, Part II: the use of relaxant drugs. *Brit. J. Anaesth., 28*, 154.

Crawford, J.S. (1971): Suxamethonium muscle pains and pregnancy. *Brit. J. Anaesth., 43*, 677.

Craythorne, N.W.B., Rottenstein, H.S. and Dripps, R.D. (1960a): The effect of succinylcholine on intraocular pressure in adults, infants and children during general anaesthesia. *Anesthesiology, 21*, 59.

Craythorne, N.W.B., Turndorf, H. and Dripps, R.D. (1960b): Changes in pulse rate and rhythm associated with the use of succinylcholine in anaesthetized children. *Anesthesiology, 21*, 465.

Crul, J.F. (1970): Studies on new steroid relaxants. In: *Progress in Anaesthesiology. Proceedings of the 4th World Congress in Anaesthesia.* Excerpta Medica, Amsterdam.

Crul-Sluijter, E.J. and Crul, J.F. (1974): Acidosis and neuromuscular blockade. *Acta anaesth. scand., 18*, 224.

Cullen, S.C. (1943): The use of curare for the improvement of abdominal muscle relaxation during inhalational anaesthesia. *Surgery, 14*, 261.

Cullen, D.J. (1971): The effect of pretreatment with non-depolarizing muscle relaxants on the neuromuscular blocking action of succinylcholine. *Anesthesiology, 35*, 572.

Cuthbert, M.F. (1966): The effect of quinidine and procainamide on the neuromuscular blocking action of suxamethonium. *Brit. J. Anaesth., 38*, 775.

Davies, D.D. (1970): Hypertonic syndrome associated with suxamethonium administration. *Brit. J. Anaesth., 42*, 656.

Davies, J.I. (1956): Untoward reactions to succinylcholine. *Canad. Anaesth. Soc. J., 3*, 11.

Day, S. (1976): Plasma potassium changes following suxamethonium and suxemethonium in normal patients and in patients in renal failure. *Brit. J. Anaesth., 48*, 1011.

Del Castillo, J. and Engback, L. (1954): The nature of the neuromuscular block produced by magnesium. *J. Physiol., 124*, 370.

Denborough, M.A. (1977): Malignant hyperpyrexia. *Med. J. Aust. 2*, 757.

Denborough, M.A., Ebeling, P., King, J.O. and Zapf, P. (1970): Myopathy and malignant hyperpyrexia. *Brit. med. J., 1*, 1138.

Denborough, M.A., Forster, J.F.A., Lovell, R.R.H., Maplestone, P.A. and Villiers, J.D. (1962): Anaesthetic deaths in a family. *Brit. J. Anaesth., 34*, 395.

deRoetth, A. Jr., Dettbarn, W.D., Rosenberg, P., Wilensky, J.G. and Wong, A. (1965): Effect of phospholine iodide on the blood cholinesterase levels of normal and glaucoma subjects. *Amer. J. Ophthal., 59*, 586.

De Silva, A.J.C. (1973): Magnesium intoxication: an uncommon cause of prolonged curarization. *Brit. J. Anaesth., 45*, 1228.

DeVasankaraiah, S., Haranath, P.S.R.K. and Krishnamurthy, A. (1973): Passage of intravenously administered tubocurarine into the liquor space in man and dog. *Brit. J. Pharmacol., 47*, 787.

D'Hollander, A.A., Camu, F. and Sanders, M. (1978): Comparative evaluation of neuromuscular blockade after pancuronium administration in patients with and without renal failure. *Acta anaesth. scand., 22*, 21.

Dickmann, P., Goecke, M. and Wiemars, K. (1969): Beeinflussung der intraocularen Drucksteigerung nach succinylcholine durch depolarisationshemmende relaxantien. *Anaesthesist., 18*, 370.

Dillon, J.B., Sabawala, P., Taylor, D.B. and Gunter, R. (1957a): Action of succinylcholine on extraocular muscles and intraocular pressure. *Anesthesiology, 18*, 44.

Dillon, J.B., Sabawala, P., Taylor, D.B. and Gunter, R. (1957b): Depolarizing neuromuscular blocking agents and intraocular pressure in vivo. *Anesthesiology, 18*, 439.

Dobkin, A.B., Arandia, H.Y. and Levy, A.A. (1973): Effect of pancuronium bromide on plasma histamine levels in man. *Anesth. Analg. Curr. Res., 52*, 772.

Dobkin, A.B., Evers, W., Ghanooni, S., Levy, A.A. and Thomas, E.T. (1971): Pancuronium bromide: evaluation of its clinical pharmacology. *Canad. Anaesth. Soc. J., 18*, 512.

Doenicke, A., Gesing, H., Krumey, I. and Schmidinger, S.T. (1970): Influence of aprotinin (Trasylol) on the action of suxamethonium. *Brit. J. Anaesth., 42*, 948.

Doenicke, A., Krunmey, I., Kugler, J. and Klempa, J. (1968): Experimental studies of the break down of epontol: determination of propanidid in human serum. *Brit. J. Anaesth., 40*, 415.

Domench, J.S., Garcia, R.C., Sasiain, J.M.R., Loyola, A.Q. and Oroz, J.S. (1976): Pancuronium bromide: an indirect sympathomimetic agent. *Brit. J. Anaesth., 48*, 1143.

Doughty, A.C. and Wylie, W.D. (1951): An assessment of flaxedil. *Proc. roy. Soc. Med., 44*, 375.

Dowdy, E.G., Dugger, P.N. and Fabian, L.W. (1965): Effect of neuromuscular blocking agents on isolated digitalized mammalian hearts. *Anesth. Analg. Curr. Res., 44*, 608.

Dowdy, E.G. and Fabian, L.W. (1963): Ventricular arrhythmias induced by succinylcholine in digitalized patients. *Anesth. Analg. Curr. Res., 42*, 501.

Dowdy, E.G., Holland, W.C., Yamanaka, I. and Kaya, K. (1971): Cardioactive properties of d-tubocurarine with and without preservatives. *Anesthesiology, 34*, 256.

Dowdy, E.G. and Sullivan, L.J. (1968): Effect of d-tubocurarine on calcium exchange in the myocardium. *Pharmacologist, 10*, 209.

Drabkova, J., Crul, J.F. and van der Kleijn, E. (1973): Placental transfer of ^{14}C-labelled succinylcholine in near-term Macaca Mulatta monkeys. *Brit. J. Anaesth., 45*, 1087.

Duke, P.C., Fung, H. and Gartner, J. (1975): The myocardial effects of pancuronium. *Canad. Anaesth. Soc. J., 22,* 680.

Dundee, J.W. (1951): Gallamine in the diagnosis of myasthenia gravis. *Brit. J. Anaesth., 23,* 39.

Dundee, J.W. and Gray, T.C. (1953): Resistance to d-tubocurarine chloride in the presence of liver damage. *Lancet, II,* 16.

Duvaldestin, P., Agoston, S., Henzel, D., Kersten, U.W. and Desmonts, J.M. (1978): Pancuronium pharmacokinetics in patients with liver cirrhosis. *Brit. J. Anaesth., 50,* 1131.

Edmunds-Seal, J. and Eve, N.H. (1962): Minor sequelae of anaesthesia: A pilot study. *Brit. J. Anaesth., 34,* 44.

Eielsen, O. and Stovner, J. (1978): Dermatomyositis, suxamethonium action and atypical plasmacholine-sterase. *Canad. Anaesth. Soc. J., 25,* 63.

Eisele, J.H., Marta, J.A. and Davis, H.S. (1971): Quantitative aspects of the chronotropic and neuro-muscular effects of gallamine in anaesthetized man. *Anesthesiology, 35,* 630.

Elert, B.T. and Cohen, E.N. (1962): A microspectrophotometric method for the analysis of minute con-centrations of d-tubocurarine chloride in plasma. *Am. J. med. Technol., 28,* 125.

Ellis, F.R., Clarke, I.M.C., Appleyard, T.N. and Dinsdale, R.C.W. (1974): Malignant hyperpyrexia induced by nitrous oxide and treated with dexamethasone. *Brit. med. J., 4,* 270.

Ellis, F.R., Cain, P.A., and Harriman, D.G.F. (1978): Multifactoral inheritance of malignant hyper-thermia susceptibility. In: *The Second International Symposium on Malignant Hyperthermia.* Editors: B.A. Britt and J.A. Aldrete. Grune and Stratton, p. 329.

Enderby, G.E.H. (1959): Muscle relaxation with decamethonium C10. *Anaesthesia, 14,* 138.

Erdos, E.G., Foldes, F.F., Baart, N. and Shanor, S.P. (1956): In vitro effect of chlorpromazine on human cholinesterases. *Fed. Proc., 15,* 420.

Eustace, B.R. (1967): Suxamethonium induced bronchospasms. *Anaesthesia, 22,* 638.

Evans, P.J.D. and McKinnon, I. (1977): An anaphylactoid reaction to gallamine triethiodide. *Anaesth. intens. Care, 5,* 239.

Fahmy, N.R., Gissen, A.J., Savarese, J.J. and Kitz, R.J. (1975): Decamethonium and serum potassium in man. *Anesthesiology, 42,* 692.

Feldman, S.A. (1963): Effect of changes in electrolytes hydration and pH upon the reactions to muscle relaxants. *Brit. J. Anaesth., 35,* 546.

Feldman, S.A., (1973): In: *Muscle Relaxants.* W.B. Saunders.

Feldman, S. (1978a): Neuromuscular Block. In. *A Practice of Anaesthesia* Editors: W.D. Wylie and H.C. Churchill-Davidson. Lloyd-Luke (Medical Books) Ltd., London.

Feldman, S. (1978b): Neuromuscular blocking drugs. In: *A Practice of Anaesthesia,* Edited. W.D. Wylie and H.C. Churchill-Davidson. Lloyd-Luke (Medical Books) Ltd., London.

Fellini, A.A., Bernstein, R.L. and Zauder, H.L. (1963): Bronchospasm due to suxamethonium. Report of a case. *Brit. J. Anaesth., 35,* 657.

Finer, B.L. and Nylen, B.O. (1959): Double cardiac arrest with survival. *Brit. med. J., 1,* 624.

Fisher, M.McD (1975): Severe histamine mediated reactions to intravenous drugs used in anaesthesia. *Anaesth. intens. Care, 3,* 180.

Fisher, M.McD. (1976): Intradermal testing after severe histamine reactions to intravenous drugs used in anaesthesia. *Anaesth. intens. Care, 4,* 97.

Fisher, M.McD. (1978): Anaphylactic reactions to gallamine triethiodide. *Anaesth. intens. Care, 6,* 62.

Fisher, M.McD., Hallowes, R.C. and Wilson, R.M. (1978): Anaphylaxis to Alcuronium. *Anaesth. intens. Care, 6,* 125.

Fleming, W.B., Hueston, J.T., Stubbe, J.L. and Villiers, J.D. (1960): Two episodes of cardiac arrest in one week: full recovery after cardiac massage. *Brit. med. J., 1,* 157.

Foldes, F.F. (1959): Factors which alter the effects of muscle relaxants. *Anesthesiology, 20,* 464.

Foldes, F.F., McNall, P.G., Davis, D.L., Ellis, C.H. and Wnuck, A.L. (1953). Substrate competition between procaine and succinylcholine diiodide for plasma cholinesterase. *Science, 117,* 383.

Foldes, F.F., Rendell-Baker, L. and Birch, J.H. (1956): Causes and prevention of prolonged apnea with succinylcholine. *Anesth. Analg. Curr. Res., 35,* 609.

Foldes, F.F., Brown, I.M., Lunn, J.N., Moore, J. and Duncalf, D. (1963): The neuromuscular effect of diallyl-nortoxiferine in anaesthetized subjects. *Anesth. Analg. Curr. Res., 42,* 177.

Foldes, F.F., Kuze, S. and Erdmann, K.A. (1974): The influence of temperature on the activity of neuromuscular blocking agents. In: *Abstracts of Scientific Papers, Annual meeting of the American Society of Anesthesiologists,* p. 125.

Forrest, T. (1959): A report on two cases of cardiac arrest. *Brit. J. Anaesth., 31,* 277.

Foster, C.A. (1960): Muscle pains that follow administration of suxamethonium. *Brit. med. J., 2,* 24.

Fraley, D.S., Lemoncelli, G.L. and Coleman, A. (1978): Severe hypertension associated with pancuronium bromide. *Anesth. Analg. Curr. Res., 57,* 265.

Fry, E.N.S. (1975): Reduction of post-suxamethonium muscle pains. *Brit. J. Anaesth., 47,* 1342.

Fyke, F.E., Code, C.F. and Schlegel, J.F. (1956): The gastrooesophageal sphincter in healthy human beings. *Gastroenterologia, 86,* 135.

Galindo, A.H. and Davis, T.B. (1962): Succinylcholine and cardiac excitability. *Anesthesiology, 23,* 32.

Gamstorp, I. and Vinnars, E. (1961): Studies in neuromuscular transmission, influence of changes in blood pH and carbon dioxide tension on the effect of tubocurarine and dimethyl tubocurarine. *Acta Physiol. Scand., 53,* 160.

Gerbershagen, H.U. and Bergman, N.A. (1967): The effect of d-tubocurarine on respiratory resistance in anesthetized man. *Anesthesiology, 28,* 981.

Geha, D.G., Blitt, C.D. and Moon, B.J. (1976): Prolonged neuromuscular blockade with pancuronium in the presence of acute renal failure. A case report. *Anesth. Analg. Curr. Res., 55,* 343.

Gertel, M., Fox, G.S., Rabow, F.I. and Graham, D.H. (1972): The cardiovascular effects of pancuronium bromide during halothane anaesthesia. *Canad. Anaesth. Soc. J., 19,* 599.

Gestzes, T. (1966): Prolonged apnoea after suxamethonium injection associated with eye drops containing an anticholinesterase agent. A case report. *Brit. J. Anaesth., 38,* 408.

Ghoniem, M.M. and Long, J.P. (1970): The interaction between magnesium and other neuromuscular blocking agents. *Anesthesiology,32,* 23.

Gibaldi, M., Levy, G. and Hayton, W.L. (1972): Tubocurarine and renal failure. *Brit. J. Anaesth., 44,* 163.

Giesecke, A.H., Morris, R.E., Dalton, M.D. and Stephen, C.R. (1968): Of magnesium, muscle relaxants, toxemic parturients, and cats. *Anesth. Analg. Curr. Res., 47,* 689.

Glauber, D. (1966): The incidence and severity of muscle pains after suxamethonium when preceeded by gallamine. *Brit. J. Anaesth., 38,* 541.

Goat, V.A. (1972): The effect of succinylcholine on the isolated mammalian heart. *Proc. roy. Soc. Med., 65,* 149.

Goat, V.A. and Feldman, S.A. (1972): The effect of non-depolarising muscle relaxants on cholinergic mechanisms in the isolated rabbit heart. *Anaesthesia, 27,* 143.

Goldsmith, E. (1967): An evaluation of succinylcholine and gallamine as muscle relaxants in relation to intraocular tension. *Anesth. Analg. Curr. Res., 46,* 113.

Goodman, L.S. and Gilman, A. (1975): *The Pharmacological Basis of Therapeutics,* 5th edition. Macmillan Publishing Co. Inc., p. 597.

Goonewardene, T.W., Sentheshanmuganathan, S., Kamalanathan, S. and Kanagasunderam, R. (1975): Accidental subarachnoid injection of gallamine. *Brit. J. Anaesth., 47,* 889.

Gordh, T., and Wåhlin, Å. (1961). Potentiation of the neuromuscular effect of succinylcholine by tetrahydro-amino-acridine. *Acta anaesth. scand.*, *5*, 55.

Goudsouzian, N.G. Donlon, J.V. and Savarese, J.J. (1975): Re-evaluation of dosage and duration of action of d-tubocurarine in the pediatric age group. *Anesthesiology, 43*, 416.

Graf, K., Strom, G. and Wahlin, A. (1963): Circulatory effects of succinylcholine in man. *Acta anaesth. scand., 7*, Suppl, XIV.

Greenan, J. (1961): The cardio-oesophageal junction. *Brit. J. Anaesth., 33*, 432.

Griffith, H.R. (1946): Physiological and clinical action of curare. *Anesth. Analg. Curr. Res., 25*, 45.

Grogono, A.W. (1963): Anaesthesia for atrial fibrillation: effect of quinidine on muscular relaxation. *Lancet, 2*, 1039.

Gronert, G.A. and Theye, R.A. (1974): Effect of succinylcholine on skeletal muscle with immobilization atrophy. *Anesthesiology, 40*, 268.

Gronert, G.A. and Theye, R.A. (1975): Pathophysiology of hyperkalaemia induced by succinylcholine. *Anesthesiology, 43*, 89.

Gronert, G.A., Dotin, L.N., Ritchey, C.R. and Mason, A.D. (1969): Succinylcholine-induced hyperkalaemia in burned patients. *Anesth. Analg. Curr. Res., 48*, 958.

Gronert, G.A., Milde, J.H. and Theye, R.A. (1976a) Porcine malignant hyperthermia induced by halothane and succinylcholine: failure of treatment with procaine or procainamide. *Anesthesiology, 44*, 124.

Gronert, G.A., Milde, J.H and Theye, R.A. (1976b): Dantrolene in porcine malignant hyperthermia. *Anesthesiology, 44*, 488.

Gronert, G.A., Milde, J.H. and Theye, R.A. (1977): Role of sympathetic activity in porcine malignant hyperthermia. *Anesthesiology, 47*, 411.

Guernier, S.M. and Mason, J.C. (1952): Undesirable side effects of decamethonium iodide. *Brit. med. J., 1*, 1329.

Gupte, S.R. and Savant, N.S. (1971): Post-suxamethonium pains and vitamin C. *Anaesthesia, 26*, 436.

Gurman, G.M. (1972): Prolonged apnea after succinylcholine in a case treated with cytostatics for cancer. *Anesth. Analg. Curr. Res., 51*, 761.

Guyton, A.C. and Reeder, R.C. (1950): Quantitative studies on the autonomic actions of curare. *J. Pharmacol., 98*, 188.

Hainsworth, A.M. and Bingham, W. (1970): An allergic circulatory collapse following the administration of muscle relaxants. *Anaesthesia, 25*, 105.

Haley, F.C. (1962): Anaesthesia in dystrophia myotonica. *Canad. Anaesth. Soc. J., 9*, 270.

Hall, G.M., Lucke, J.N. and Lister, D. (1975): Treatment of porcine malignant hyperthermia. *Anaesthesia, 30*, 308.

Hall, G.M., Lucke, J.N. and Lister, D. (1977): Treatment of porcine malignant hyperpyrexia. The successful use of dantrolene in the Pietrain pig. *Anaesthesia, 32*, 472.

Haranath, P.S.R.K. (1978): Blood–CSF barrier to d-tubocurarine. *Anesthesiology, 49*, 151.

Haranath, P.S.R.K., Krishnamurthy, A. and Rao, L.N. (1973): Passage of gallamine from blood into liquor space in man and dog. *Brit. J. Pharmacol., 48*, 640.

Harris, H. and Whittaker, M. (1961): Differential inhibition of human serum cholinesterase with fluoride: recognition of two new phenotypes. *Nature, 191*, 496.

Harrison, G. (1966): A case of cardiac arrest associated with bronchospasm and D-tubocurarine. *Aust. N.Z. J. Surg., 36*, 40.

Harrison, G. (1971): Anaesthetic induced malignant hyperpyrexia: a suggested method of treatment. *Brit. med. J., 3*, 454.

Harrison, G. (1972): The cardiovascular effects and some relaxant properties of four relaxants in patients about to undergo cardiac surgery. *Brit. J. Anaesth., 44,* 485.

Harrison, G. (1975): Control of the malignant hyperpyrexia syndrome in MHS swine by Dantrolene sodium. *Brit. J. Anaesth., 47,* 62.

Harrison, G. (1977): The prophylaxis of malignant hyperthermia by oral dantrolene sodium in swine. *Brit. J. Anaesth., 49,* 315.

Hazel, B. and Monier, D. (1971): Human serum cholinesterase: variations during pregnancy and post-partum. *Canad. Anaesth. Soc. J., 18,* 272.

Heath, M.L. (1973): Bronchospasm in an asthmatic patient following pancuronium. *Anaesthesia, 28,* 437.

Hegab, E.S., Schiff, H.I., Smith, D.J. and Tunrdorf, H. (1974): An electron microscopic study of normal and chronically denervated rat skeletal muscle following succinylcholine challenge. *Anesth. Analg. Curr. Res., 53,* 650.

Hegarty, P. (1956): Postoperative muscle pains. *Brit. J. Anaesth., 28,* 209.

Hill, G.E., Wong, K.C. and Hodges, M.R. (1976): Potentiation of succinylcholine neuromuscular blockade by lithium carbonate. *Anesthesiology, 44,* 439.

Hill, G.E., Wong, K.C. and Hodges, M.R. (1977): Lithium carbonate and neuromuscular blocking agents. *Anesthesiology, 46,* 122.

Hodges, R.J.H. (1958): Interaction of suxamethonium and oxytocin. *Brit. med. J., 1,* 1416.

Hodges, R.J.H. and Harkness, J. (1954): Suxamethonium sensitivity in health and disease. A clinical evaluation of pseudocholinesterase levels. *Brit. med. J., 2,* 18.

Hoffmann, H. and Holzer, H. (1953): Die Wirkung von Muskelrelaxantien auf den introkularen Druck. *Klin. Mbl. Angenheilk., 123,* 1.

Hofstee, B.H.J. (1960): Mechanism of action of bivalent metal ions and of phenothiazine derivatives on serum cholinesterase. *J. Pharmacol. exp. Ther., 128,* 299.

Holaday, D.A. (1946): Nitrous oxide-cyclopropane-curare anaesthesia: Review of 200 cases. *Anesthesiology, 7,* 426.

Holmes, R.P., Ross, J.W. and Williams, E.R. (1971): Acute anaphylaxis under anaesthesia. *Anaesthesia, 26,* 363.

Hughes, R. (1970): The influence of changes in acid-base balance on neuromuscular blockade in cats. *Brit. J. Anaesth., 42,* 658.

Hughes, R. and Chapple, D.J. (1976a): Effect of non-depolarizing neuromuscular blocking agents on peripheral autonimic mechanisms in cats. *Brit. J. Anaesth., 48,* 59.

Hughes, R. and Chapple, D.J. (1976b). Cardiovascular and neuromuscular effects of dimethyl tubocurarine in anaesthetized cats and rhesus monkeys. *Brit. J. Anaesth, 48,* 847.

Hughes, R., Ingram, G.S. and Payne, J.P. (1976a): Studies on dimethyltubocurarine in anaesthetized man. *Brit. J. Anaesth., 48,* 969.

Hughes, R., Payne, J.P. and Sugai, N. (1976b): Studies on fazadinium bromide (AH 8165): A new non-depolarizing neuromuscular blocking agent. *Canad. Anaesth. Soc. J., 23,* 36.

Hugin, W. and Kissling, P. (1961): Vorlaufige Mitteilungen uber ein neues kurzwirkenden Relaxans vom depolarisationhindernden Typus, das Ro 4-3816. *Schweiz. med. Wschr., 91,* 455.

Hunter, A.r. (1964): Diallyltoxiferine. *Brit. J. Anaesth., 36,* 466.

Ichiyanagi, K., Ito, Y. and Aoki, E. (1963): Effects of oxytocin on the response to suxamethonium and d-tubocurarine in man. *Brit. J. Anaesth., 35,* 611.

Innes, R.K.R. and Strómme, J.H. (1973): Rise in serum creatine phosphokinase associated with agents used in anaesthesia. *Brit. J. Anaesth., 45,* 185.

Isaacs, H. (1978): Comments on predictive tests for malignant hyperthermia. In: *Second International Symposium on Malignant Hyperthermia.* Editors: J.A. Aldrete and B.A. Britt. Grune and Stratton, p. 351.

Isaacs, H. and Barlow, M.B. (1970a): Malignant hyperpyrexia during anaesthesia: possible association with subclinical myopathy. *Brit. med. J., 1,* 275.

Isaacs, H. and Barlow, M.B. (1970b): The genetic background to malignant hyperpyrexia revealed by serum CPK estimations in asymptomatic relatives. *Brit. J. Anaesth., 42,* 1077.

Ivankovich, A.D., Miletich, D.J. and Albrecht, R.F. (1975): The effect of pancuronium on myocardial contraction and catecholamine metabolism. *J. pharm. Pharmacol, 27,* 837.

Iwatsuki, K. Yusa, T. and Kataoka, Y. (1965): Effects of muscle relaxants on ventricular contractile force in dogs. *Tohuku J. Exp. Med., 86,* 9.

Jacob, J.C. and Varkey, G.P. (1966): Curare sensitivity in ocular myopathy. *Canad. Anaesth. Soc. J., 13,* 449.

Jensen, K., Bennike, K.-Aa, Hanel, H.K. and Olessen, H. (1968): Myoglobinuria following anaesthesia including suxamethonium. *Brit. J, Anaesth., 40,* 329.

Jerums, G., Whittingham, S. and Wilson, P. (1967): Anaphylaxis to suxamethonium: a case report. *Brit. J. Anaesth., 39,* 73.

John, D.A., Tobey, R.E., Homer, L.D. and Rice, C.L. (1976): Onset of succinylcholine induced hyperkalaemia following denervation. *Anesthesiology, 45,* 294.

Johnstone, M. (1955): Relaxant and the human cardiovascular system. *Anaesthesia, 10,* 122.

Johnstone, M. (1956): The human cardiovascular response to Fluothane anaesthesia. *Brit. J. Anaesth. 28,* 392.

Johnstone, M., Hahmoud, A.A. and Mrozinski., R.A. (1978): Cardiovascular effects of tubocurarine in man. *Anaesthesia, 33,* 587.

Kalow, W. (1965): Contribution of hereditary factors to the response to drugs. *Fed. Proc., 24,* 1259.

Kalow, W., Britt, B.A., Terreau, M.E. and Haist, C. (1970): Metabolic error of muscle metabolism after recovery from malignant hyperthermia. *Lancet, II,* 895.

Kalow, W. and Genest, K. (1957): A method for the detection of atypical forms of human serum cholinesterase. Determination of dibucaine numbers. *Canad. J. Biochem, 35,* 339.

Kaniaris, P., Fassoulaki, A., Liarmakopoulou, K. and Dermitzakis, E. (1979): Serum cholinesterase levels in patients with cancer. *Anesth. Analg. Curr. Res., 58,* 82.

Karhunen, U., Heinonen, J. and Tammisto, T. (1972): The effect of tubocurarine and alcuronium on suxamethonium-induced changes in cardiac rate and rhythm. *Acta anaesth. scand., 16,* 3.

Katz, A.M. and Mulligan, P.G. (1972): Bronchospasm induced by suxamethonium. *Brit. J. Anaesth., 44,* 1097.

Katz, B. and Miledi, R. (1965): The effect of calcium on acetylcholine release from motor nerve terminals. *Proc. roy. Soc. B., 161,* 496.

Katz, R.L. and Eakins, K.E. (1969): The action of neuromuscular blocking agents on extraocular muscle and intraocular pressure. *Proc. roy. Soc. Med., 62,* 1217.

Katz, R.L., Eakins, K.E. and Lord, C.D. (1968): The effects of hexafluorenium in preventing the increase in intraocular pressure produced by succinylcholine. *Anesthesiology, 29,* 170.

Katz, R.L., Gissen, A.J. and Karis, J.H. (1965): The effects of hexafluorenium and edrophonium on the neuromuscular blocking actions of succinylcholine, decamethonium, Imbretil and d-tubocurarine. *Anesthesiology, 26,* 154.

Katz, R.L. and Wolf, C.E. (1964): Neuromuscular and electromyographic studies in man: Effects of hyperventilation, carbon dioxide inhalation and d-tubocurarine. *Anaesthesiology, 25,* 781.

Kaufman, L. (1960): Anaesthesia in dystrophia myotonica. Abridged: A review of the hazards of anaesthesia. *Proc. roy. Soc. med.*, *53*, 183.

Keil, A.M. (1962): Effects of oxytocin on the response to suxamethonium in rabbits, sheep and pigs. *Brit. J. Anaesth, 34*, 306.

Kelman, G.R. and Kennedy, B.R. (1971): Cardiovascular effects of pancuronium in man. *Brit. J. Anaesth., 43*, 335.

Kendig, J.J., Bunker, J.P. and Endow, S. (1972): Succinylcholine-induced hyperkalaemia. *Anasthesiology, 36*, 132.

Kennedy, B.R. and Farman, J.V. (1968): Cardiovascular effects of gallamine triethiodide in man. *Brit. J. Anaesth., 40*, 773.

Kennedy, B.R. and Kelman, G.R. (1970): Cardiovascular effects of alcuronium in man. *Brit. J. Anaesth, 42*, 625.

Kepes, E.R. and Haimovici, H. (1959): Allergic reaction to succinylcholine. *J. Amer. med. Ass., 171*, 548.

Kerr, D.D., Wingard, D.W. and Gatz, E.E. (1978): Prevention of porcine malignant hyperthermia by oral dantrolene. In: *Second International Symposium on Malignant Hyperthermia.* Editors: J.A. Aldrete and B.A. Britt. Grune and Stratton, p. 499.

King, H. (1935): Curare alkaloids: I. Tubocurarine. *J. Chem. Soc.*, 1381.

King, J. (1976): Inhibition of cholinesterase by pancuronium. *Brit. J. Anaesth., 48*, 712.

Kivalo, I. and Saarikoski, S. (1976): Placental transfer of ^{14}C-dimethyltubocurarine during Caesarean section. *Brit. J. Anaesth., 48*, 239.

Koide, M. and Waud, B.E. (1972): Serum potassium concentrations after succinylcholine in patients with renal failure. *Anesthesiology, 36*, 142.

Konchigeri, H.N. and Tay, C.H. (1976): Influence of pancuronium on potassium efflux produced by succinylcholine. *Anesth. Analg. Curr. Res., 55*, 474.

La Cour, D. (1969): Rise in intragastric pressure caused by suxamethonium fasciculations. *Acta anaesth. scand., 13*, 255.

Lake, C.L. (1978): Curare sensitivity in steroid-treated myasthenia gravis. A case report. *Anesth. Analg. Curr. Res., 57*, 132.

Lamoureux, L. and Bourgeois-Gavardin, M. (1949): A propos un nouveau curarisant de synthese le Flaxedil 3697 R.P. *Un. méd. Can., 78*, 1164.

Lamoreaux, L.F. and Urbach, K.F. (1960): Incidence and prevention of muscle pain following the administration of succinylcholine. *Anesthesiology, 21*, 394.

Landmesser, C.M., Converse, J.G. and Harmel, M.H. (1952): Quantitative evaluation of the bronchoconstrictor action of curare in the anesthetized patient: A preliminary report. *Anesthesiology, 13*, 275.

Lawson, J.I.M. (1958): Decamethonium iodide. A reappraisal. *Brit. J. Anaesth., 30*, 240.

Lee, C., Chen, D. and Nagel, E.L. (1977a): Neuromuscular block by antibiotics: Polymyxin B. *Anesth. Analg. Curr. Res., 56*, 373.

Lee, C., Yang, E. and Katz, R.L. (1977b): Focal contracture following injections of succinylcholine in patients with peripheral nerve injury. *Canad. Anaesth. Soc. J., 24*, 475.

Lee, D.C. and Johnson, D.L. (1970): Effects of d-tubocurarine and anaesthesia upon cardiac output in histamine depleted dogs. *Fed. Proc., 29*, 2804.

Lee Son, S. and Waud, B.E. (1977): Potencies of neuromuscular blocking agents at the receptors of the atrial pacemaker and the motor endplate of the guinea pig. *Anaesthesiology, 47*, 34.

Lehmann, H. and Liddell, J. (1969): Human cholinesterase (pseudocholinesterase): genetic variants and their recognition. *Brit. J. Anaesth., 41*, 235.

Leigh, M.D., McCoy, D.D., Belton, M.K. and Lewis, G.B. (1957): Bradycardia following intravenous administration of succinylcholine chloride to infants and children. *Anesthesiology, 18*, 698.

Levin, N. and Dillon, J.B. (1971): Cardiovascular effects of pancuronium bromide. *Anesth. Analg. Curr. Res., 50*, 808.

Liddell, J., Lehmann, H. and Silk, E. (1962): A 'silent' pseudocholinesterase gene. *Nature, 193*, 561.

Lincoff, H.A., Ellis, C.H., de Voe, A.G., de Beer, E.J., Impstato, D.J., Berg, S., Orkin, L. and Magda, H. (1955): The effect of succinylcholine on intraocular pressure. *Amer. J. Ophthal., 40*, 501.

List, W.F.M. (1971): Succinylcholine-induced cardiac arrhythmias. *Anesth. Analg. Curr. Res., 50*, 361.

Lister, D., Hall, D.M. and Lucke, J.N. (1975): Malignant hyperthermia. A human and porcine stress syndrome? *Lacet, I*, 519.

Loennecken, S.J., Vanner, G.K., Richard, K.G. and Schmucker, H. (1970): Repeated cardiac arrest following suxamethonium. In: *Progress in Anaesthesiology. Proceedings of the Fourth World Congress of Anaesthesiology.*

Loh, L. (1970): The cardiovascular effects of pancuronium bromide. *Anaesthesia, 25*, 356.

Longnecker, D.E., Stoelting, R.K. and Morrow, A.G. (1970): Cardiac and peripheral vascular effects of d-tubocurarine in man. *Anesth. Curr. Res., 49*, 660.

Longnecker, D.E., Stoelting, R.K. and Morrow, A.G. (1973): Cardiac and peripheral vascular effects of gallamine in man. *Anesth. Analg. Curr. Res.; 52*, 931.

Lopert, H. (1955): Allergic reaction to gallamine triethiodide. *Anaesthesia, 10*, 76.

Lund, I. and Stovner, J. (1962): Experimental and clinical experiences with a new muscle relaxant Ro 4-3816, Diallyl-nor-toxiferine. *Acta anaesth. scand., 6*, 85.

Lupprian, K.G. and Churchill-Davidson, H.C. (1960): Effect of suxamethonium on cardiac rhythm. *Brit. med. J., 2*, 1774.

Lyons, S.M. and Clarke, R.S.J. (1972): A comparison of different drugs for anaesthesia in cardiac surgical patients. *Brit. J. Anaesth., 44*, 575.

Lyons, S.M., Clarke, R.S.J. and Young, H.S.A. (1975): A clinical comparison of AH 8165 and pancuronium as muscle relaxants in patients undergoing cardiac surgery. *Brit. J. Anaesth., 47*, 725.

McArdle, B., (1940): The serum choline esterase in jaundice and diseases of the liver. *Quart. J. Med. 9*, 107.

McCance, R.A., Widdowson, E.M. and Hutchinson, A.O. (1948): Effect of undernutrition and alterations in diet on the choline esterase activity of serum. *Nature, 161*, 56.

McCaughey, T.J. (1962): Hazards of anaesthesia for the burned child. *Canad. Anaesth. Soc. J., 9*, 220.

McComb, R.B., LaMotta, R.V. and Wetstone, H.J. (1964): Studies of cholinesterase activity, VII: kinetic constants of serum cholinesterase in normal populations and those with neoplasms. *J. Lab. Clin. Med., 63*, 827.

McCullough, L.S., Reier, C.E., DeLaunois, A.L., Gardier, R.W. and Hamelberg, W. (1970): The effects of d-tubocurarine on spontaneous postganglionic sympathetic activity and histamine release. *Anesthesiology, 33*, 328.

McCullough, L.S., Stone, W.A. and Delaunois, A.L. (1972): Te effects of dimethyltubocurarine iodide on cardiovascular parameters, postganglionic sympathetic activity and histamine release. *Anesth. Analg. Curr. Res. 51*, 554.

MacDonald, A.G. and Graham, I.H. (1968): Suxamethonium apnoea in a pregnant patient. *Brit. J. Anaesth., 40*, 711.

McDowall, S.A. and Clarke, R.S.J. (1969): A clinical comparison of pancuronium with d-tubocurarine. *Anaesthesia, 24*, 581.

McGavin, D.D.M. (1965): Depressed levels of serum pseudocholinesterase with ecothiophate-iodide eye drops. *Lancet, 2*, 272.

McIntyre, J.W.R. (1962): Succinylcholine-induced bradycardia with reference to methoxyflurane anaesthesia. *Canad. Anaesth. Soc. J., 9*, 408.

McKie, D.D. (1978): Anaphylactic reactions to gallamine. *Anaesth. intens. Care, 6*, 266.

McKlveen, J.F., Sokoll, M.D., Gergis, S.D. and Dretchen, K.L. (1973): Absence of recurarization upon rewarming. *Anesthesiology, 38*, 153.

McLaren, C.A.B. (1968): Myoglobinuria following the use of suxamethonium chloride. *Brit. J. Anaesth., 40*, 901.

McLaughlin, A.P. (1972): Hazards of gallamine in patients with renal failure. *J. Urol., 108*, 515.

McLeod, K., Watson, M.J. and Rawlings, M.D. (1976): Pharmacokinetics of pancuronium in patients with normal and impaired renal function. *Brit. J. Anaesth., 48*, 341.

Macri, F.J. and Grimes, P.A. (1957): The effects of succinylcholine on the extraocular striate muscles and on the intraocular pressure. *Amer. J. Ophthal., 44*, 221.

Magbagbeola, J.A.O. (1970): Abnormal responses to muscle relaxants in a patient with von Recklinghausen's disease (multiple neurofibromatosis). *Brit. J. Anaesth., 42*, 710.

Maier, E.S. and Clark, R.B. (1965): Effect of decamethonium on intraocular pressure in man. *Anesth. Analg. Curr. Res., 44*, 753.

Mandappa, J.M., Chandrasekhara, P.M. and Nelvigi, R.G. (1975): Anaphylaxis to suxamethonium: two case reports. *Brit. J. Anaesth., 47*, 523.

Manser, J. (1970): Abnormal responses in von Recklinghausen's disease. *Brit. J. Anaesth., 42*, 183.

Marbury, B.E., Artusio, J.F. Jr., Wescoe, W.C. and Riker, W.J. Jr., (1951): The effects of a synthetic curare-like compound, the tri-iodo salt of tris (triethylaminoethoxy) 1,2,3 benzene (Flaxedil) on the anaesthetized surgical patient. *J. Pharmacol. exp. Ther., 103*, 280.

Marchand, P. (1955): The gastro-oesophageal 'sphincter' and the mechanism of regurgitation. *Brit. J. Surg., 42*, 504.

Marshall, I.G. (1973): The ganglion blocking and vagolytic action of 3 short-acting neuromuscular blocking drugs in cats. *J. Pharm. Pharmacol., 25*, 530.

Maryellen, E., Balsley, S. and Katz, R.L. (1978): Effecct of diazepam on succinylcholine induced muscle pain, potassium increase and CPK increase. Abstract of Scientific Papers, A.S.A. Annual Meeting, p. 257.

Mathias, J.A. and Evans-Prosser, C.D.G. (1970): An investigation into the site of action of suxamethonium on cardiac rhythm. In: Progress in Anaesthesiology, Proceedings of the Fourth World Congress of Anaesthesiologists, p. 1153.

Mathias, J.A., Evans-Prosser, C.D.G. and Churchill-Davidson, H.C. (1970): The role of the non-depolarizing drugs in the prevention of suxamethonium bradycardia. *Brit. J. Anaesth., 42*, 609.

Matteo, R.S. and Khambatta, H.J. (1978): Blood−CSF barrier to d-tubocurarine. *Anaesthesiology, 49*, 151.

Matteo, R.S., Pua, E.K., Khambatta, H.J. and Spector, S. (1977): Cerebrospinal fluid levels of d-tubocurarine in man. *Anesthesiology, 46*, 396.

Matthews, M.D., Ceglarski, J.Z. and Pabari, M. (1977): Anaphylaxis to suxamethonium − a case report. *Anaesth. Intens. Care, 5*, 235.

Mayrhofer, O. (1959): Die Wirksamkeit von D-Tubocurarin zur Verhutung der Muskelschmerzen nach Succinylcholin. *Anesthesist, 8*, 313.

Mazze, R.I. and Dunbar, R.W. (1968): Intralingual succinylcholine administration in children. An alternative to intravenous and intramuscular routes? *Anesth. Analg. Curr. Res., 47*, 605.

Mazze, R.I., Escue, H.M. and Houston, J.B. (1969): Hyperkalaemia and cardiovascular collapse following administration of succinylcholine to the traumatized patient. *Anesthesiology, 31*, 540.

Mesry, S. and Baradaran, J. (1974). Accidental intrathecal injection of gallamine triethiodide. *Anaesthesia, 29*, 301.

Meyers, E.F., Krupin, T., Johnson, M. and Zink, H. (1978): Failure of non-depolarizing neuromuscular blockers to inhibit succinylcholine-induced increased intraocular pressure: a controlled study. *Anesthesiology, 48*, 149.

Miller, E.D., Jr., Sanders, D.B., Rowlinson, J.C., Berry, F.A., Sussman, M.D. and Epstein, R.M. (1978): Anaesthesia-induced rhabdomyolysis in a patient with Duchenne's muscular dystrophy. *Anesthesiology, 48*, 146.

Miller, R.D. (1975): Factors affecting the action of muscle relaxants. In: *Muscle Relaxants*. Editor: R., Katz, North-Holland Publishing Company, Amsterdam, p. 181.

Miller, R.D. and Cullen, D.J. (1976): Renal failure and post-operative respiratory failure: recurarization? *Brit. J. Anaesth., 48*, 253.

Miller, R.D. and Munger, W.L. (1972) The dependence of d-tubocurarine induced hypotension on the alveolar concentration of halothane and the presence of nitrous oxide. *Abstracts of Scientific Papers, ASA Annual Meeting*, p. 235.

Miller, R.D. and Roderick, L.L. (1978a): Acid-base balance and neostigmine antagonism of pancuronium neuromuscular blockade. *Brit. J. Anaesth., 50*, 317.

Miller, R.D. and Roderick, L.L. (1978b): Diuretic-induced hypokalaemia, pancuronium neuromuscular blockade and its antagonism by neostigmine. *Brit. J. Anaesth., 50*, 541.

Miller, R.D. and Way, W.L. (1971): Inhibition of succinylcholine-induced increased intragastric pressure by non-depolarizing muscle relaxants and lidocaine. *Anesthesiology, 34*, 185.

Miller, R.D., Way, W.L. and Katzung, B.G. (1967): The potentiation of neuromuscular blocking agents by quinidine. *Anesthesiology, 28*, 1036.

Miller, R.D., Way, W.L. and Hickey, R.F. (1968): Inhibition of succinylcholine-induced increased intraocular pressure by non-depolarising muscle relaxants. *Anesthesiology, 29*, 123.

Miller, R.D., Way, W.L., Hamilton, W.K. and Layzer, R.B. (1972): Succinylcholine-induced hyperkalaemia in patients with renal failure? *Anesthesiology, 36*, 138.

Miller, R.D., Stevens, W.C. and Way, W.L. (1973): The effect of renal failure and hyperkalaemia on the duration of pancuronium neuromuscular blockade in man. *Anesth. Analg. Curr. Res., 52*, 661.

Miller, R.D., Eger, E.I., Stevens, W.C. and Gibbons, R. (1975a): Pancuronium-induced tachycardia in relation to alveolar halothane, dose of pancuronium and prior atropine. *Anesthesiology, 42*, 352.

Miller, R.D., Van Nyhuis, L.S., Eger, E.I. and Way, W.L. (1975b): The effect of acid-base balance on neostigmine antagonism of d-tubocurarine-induced neuromuscular blockade. *Anesthesiology, 42*, 377.

Miller, R.D., Van Nyhuis, L.S. and Eger, E.I. (1975c): The effect of temperature on a d-tubocurarine neuromuscular blockade and its antagonism by neostigmine. *J. Pharmacol. exp. Ther., 195*, 237.

Miller, R.D., Sohn, Y.J. and Matteo, R.S. (1976): Enhancement of D-tubocurarfine neuromuscular blockade by diuretics in man. *Anesthesiology, 45*, 442.

Miller, R.D., Agoston, S., Van der Pol, F., Booij, L.H.D.J. and Crul, J.R. (1978): The effect of hypothermia on the pharmacokinetics and pharmacodynamics of pancuronium in the cat. *Abstracts of Scientific Papers, ASA Annual Meeting*, p. 253.

Mitchell, M.M., Ali, H.H. and Savarese, J.J. (1978): Myotonia and neuromuscular blocking agents. *Anesthesiology, 49*, 44.

Mogey, G.A. and Trevan, J.W. (1950): d-tubocurarine salts and derivatives. *Brit. med. J., 2*, 216.

Mone, J.G. and Mathie, W.E. (1967): Quantitative and qualitative defects of pseudocholinesterase activity. *Anaesthesia, 22*, 55.

Moore, W.E., Watson, R. and Summary, J. (1976): Massive myoglobinuria precipitated by halothane and succinylcholine in a member of a family with elevtion of serum creatine phosphokinase. *Anesth. Analg. Curr. Res., 55,* 680.

Morris, D.D.B. and Dunn, C.H. (1957): Suxamethonium chloride administration and post-operative muscle pain. *Brit. med. J., 1,* 383.

Moulds, R.F.W. (1975): Malignant hyperthermia. *Lancet, 1,* 681.

Moulds, R.F.W. and Denborough, M.A. (1974): Biochemical basis of malignant hyperpyrexia. *Brit. med. J., 2,* 241.

Mushin, W.W., Wien, R., Mason, D.F.J. and Langston, G.T. (1949): Curare-like actions of tri(Di-ethylaminoethoxy)-benzene triethyliodide. *Lancet, 1,* 726.

Nana, A., Cardan, E. and Domokos, M. (1973): Blood catecholamine changes after pancuronium *Acta Anaesth. Scand., 17,* 83.

Nana, A., Cardan, E. and Leitersdorfer, T. (1972): Pancuronium bromide – its use in asthmatics and patients with liver disease. *Anaesthesia, 27,* 154.

Nelson, T.E. (1978): Excitation-contraction coupling. A common etiologic pathway for malignant hyperthermia-susceptible muscle. *Second International Symposium on malignant hyperthermia.* Editors: J.A. Aldrete and B.A. Britt. Grune and Stratton, p. 23.

Nelson, T.E. and Flewellen, E.H. (1979): Rationale for dantrolene procainamide for treatment of malignant hyperthermia. *Anesthesiology, 50,* 118.

Newnam, P.T.F. and Loudon, J.M. (1966): Muscle pain following administration of suxamethonium: the aetiological role of muscular fitness. *Brit. J. Anaesth., 38,* 533.

Nightingale, D.A., Glass, A.G. and Bachman, L. (1966): Neuromuscular blockade by succinylcholine in children. *Anesthesiology, 27,* 736.

Norman, J., Katz., R.L. and Seed, R.F. (1970): The neuromuscular blocking action of pancuronium in man during anaesthesia. *Brit. J. Anaesth., 42,* 702.

Okazaki, K., Saito, T., Wakisaka, K., Hirano, T., Kozu, K. and Okazaki, N. (1969): Bronchospasm possibly due to gallamine. A case report. *Tokushima J. exp. Med., 16,* 9.

Older, P.O. and Harris, J.M. (1968): Placental transfer of tubocurarine. *Brit. J. Anaesth., 40,* 459.

Orndahl, G. (1962): Myotonic human musculature: stimulation with depolarising agents. II. A clinico-pharmacological study. *Acta. med. scand., 1721,* 753.

Orndahl, G. and Sternberg, K. (1962): Myotonic human musculature: stimulation with depolarizing agents. *Acta med. scand., 172,* (Suppl. 389), 3.

Oropollo, A.T. (1978): Abnormal pseudocholinesterase levels in a surgical population. *Anesthesiology, 48,* 284.

Pandey, K., Badola, R.P. and Kumar, S. (1972): Time course of intraocular hypertension produced by suxamethonium. *Brit. J. Anaesth., 44,* 191.

Pandit, S.K. Dundee, J.W. and Stevenson, H.M. (1971): A clinical comparison of pancuronium with tubocurarine and alcuronium in major cardiothoracic surgery. *Anesth. Analg. Curr. Res., 50,* 926.

Pandit, S.K., Kothary, S.P. and Cohen, P.J. (1979): Orally administered dantrolene for prophylaxis of malignant hyperthermia. Anesthesiology, 50, 156.

Pantuck, E.J. (1966): Ecothiopate iodide eye drops and prolonged response to suxamethonium. *Brit. J. Anaesth., 38,* 406.

Park, W.Y., Kim, Y.D. and MacNamara, T.E. (1977): Neuromuscular block of gallamine in hypothermia. *Abstracts of Scientific Papers, ASA Annual Meeting, New Orleans,* p. 311.

Park, W.Y. and MacNamara, T.E. (1979): Temperature change and neuromuscular blockade by d-tubocurarine or pancuronium in man. *Anesthesiology, 50,* 161.

Parmentier, P. and Dagnelie P. (1979): Dose-related tachycardia induced by pancuronium during balanced anaesthesia with or without droperidol. *Brit. J. Anaesth. 51,* 157.

Paterson, I.S. (1962): Generalised myotonia following suxamethonium. *Brit. J. Anaesth., 34*, 340.

Paton, W.D.M. (1959): The effects of muscle relaxants other than muscular relaxation. *Anesthesiology, 20*, 453.

Perez, H.R. (1970): Cardiac arrhythmia after succinylcholine. *Anesth. Analg. Curr. Res., 49*, 33.

Porath, A., Acker, M. and Perel, A. (1977): Serum cholinesterase in tetanus. *Anaesthesia, 32*, 1009.

Potts, M.W. and Thornton, J.A. (1961): Abnormal response to suxamethonium in polyarteritis nodosa. *Brit. J. Anaesth., 33*, 405.

Poulton, T.J., James, F.M. and Lockridge, O. (1979): Prolonged apnea following trimetaphan and succinylcholine. *Anesthesiology, 50*, 54.

Powell, D.R. and Miller, R. (1975): The effect of repeated doses of succinylcholine on serum potassium in patients with renal failure. *Anesth. Analg. Curr. Res., 54*, 746.

Powell, J.N. (1970): Suxamethonium-induced hyperkalaemia in a uraemic patient. *Brit. J. Anaesth., 42*, 806.

Raaflaub, J. and Frey, P. (1972): Zur Pharmakokinetik von Diallyl-nor-toxiferin beim Menschen. *Arzneim. Forsch., 22*, 73.

Rack, P.M.H. and Westbury, D.R. (1966): The effect of suxamethonium and acetylcholine on the behaviour of cat muscle spindles during dynamic stretching and during fusimotor stimulation. *J. Physiol. (Lond.), 186*, 698.

Raitt, D.G. and Merrifield, A.J. (1974): Dexamethasone in malignant hyperpyrexia. *Brit. med. J., 4*, 656.

Rathbun, F.J. and Hamilton, J.T. (1970): Effect of gallamine on cholinergic receptors. *Canad. Anaesth. Soc. J., 17*, 574.

Rawlins, M.D. (1978): Drug interactions and anaesthesia. *Brit. J. Anaesth, 50*, 689.

Reitan, J.A., Fraser, A.I. and Eisele, J.H. (1973): Lack of cardiac inotropic effects of gallamine in anaesthetized man. *Anesth. Analg. Curr. Res., 52*, 974.

Relton, J.E.S., Britt, B.A. and Steward, D.J. (1973): Malignant hyperpyrexia. *Brit. J. Anaesth., 45*, 269.

Relton, J.E.S., Creighton, R.E., Conn, A.W. and Nabeta, S. (1967): Generalized muscular hypertonicity associated with general anaesthesia: a suggested anaesthetic management. *Canad. Anaesth. Soc. J., 14*, 22.

Riker, W.F., Jr. and Wescoe, W.C. (1951): The pharmacology of Flaxedil, with observations on certain analogs. *Ann. N.Y. Acad. Sci., 54*, 373.

Riordan, D.D. and Gilbertson, A.A. (1971): Prolonged curarization in a patient with renal failure. *Brit. J. Anaesth., 43*, 506.

Robertson, G.S. (1966): Serum cholinesterase deficiency II: pregnancy. *Brit. J. Anaesth., 38*, 361.

Robertson, G.S. (1967): Serum proteins and cholinesterase changes in association with contraceptive pills. *Lancet, I*, 232.

Robertson, G.S., and Gibson, P.F. (1968): Suxamethonium and intraocular pressure. *Anaesthesia, 23*, 342.

Roizen, M.F. and Feeley, T.,W. (1978): Pancuronium bromide. *Ann. int. Med., 88*, 64.

Ross, R.T. (1963): Ocular myopathy sensitive to curare. *Brain, 86*, 67.

Roth, F. and Wüthrich, H. (1969): The clinical importance of hyperkalaemia following suxamethonium administration. *Brit. J. Anaesth., 41*, 311.

Rouse, J.M., Galley, R.L.A. and Bevan, D.R. (1977): Prolonged curarisation following renal transplantation. A retrospective study. *Anaesthesia, 32*, 247.

Rowlands, D.E. and Fidler, K. (1978): Fazadinium in anaesthesia. *Brit. J. Anaesth, 50*, 289.

Royston, D. and Wilkes, R.G. (1978): True anaphylaxis to suxamethonium chloride. A case report. *Brit. J. Anaesth., 50*, 611.

Ryan, D.W. (1977): Preoperative serum cholinesterase concentration in chronic renal failure. Clinical experience of suxamethonium in 81 patients undergoing renal transplant. *Brit. J. Anaesth, 49*, 945.

Ryan, J.F., Kagen, L.J. and Hyman, A.I. (1971): Myoglobinaemia after a single dose of succinylcholine. *New Engl. J. Med., 285*, 824.

Saint-Maurice, C. Daihl-Dupont, D., Roche, M., Fulin, M. et Viallard, C. (1976): Deux cas de reactions de type anaphylactique en rapport avec l'anesthesie. *Ann. Anesth. franc., 17*, 81.

Salem, M.R., Kim, Y. and El Etr, A.A. (1968): Histamine release following intravenous injection of d-tubocurarine. *Anesthesiology, 29*, 380.

Savarese, J.J. (1975): Histamine, d-Tubocurarine and CSF pressure. *Anesthesiology, 42*, 369.

Savarese, J.J., Hassan, H.A. and Antonio, R.P. (1977): The clinical pharmacology of metocurine: Dimethyl tubocurarine revisited. *Anesthesiology, 47*, 277.

Savarese, J.J. (1979): The autonomic margins of safety of metocurine and d-tubocurarine in the cat. *Anesthesiology, 50*, 40.

Savege, T.M., Blogg, C.E., Ross, L., Lang, M. and Simpson, B.R. (1973): The cardiovascular effects of AH 8165, a new non-depolarising muscle relaxant. *Anaesthesia, 28*, 253.

Saxena, P.R. and Bonta, I.L. (1971): Specific blockade of cardiac muscarinic receptors by pancuronium bromide. *Arch. int. Pharmacodyn. Ther., 189*, 410.

Schaer, H., Steinmann, B., Jerusalem, S. and Maier, C. (1977): Rhabdomyolysis induced by anaesthesia with intra-operative cardiac arrest. *Brit. J. Anaesth., 49*, 495.

Schaner, P.J., Brown, R.L., Kirksey, T.D., Gunther, R.C., Ritchey, C.R. and Gronert, G.A. (1969): Succinylcholine-induced hyperkalaemia in burned patients. *Anesth. Analg. Curr. Res., 48*, 764.

Schoenstadt, D.A. and Whitcher, C.E. (1963): Observations on the mechanism of succinyldicholine-induced cardiac arrhythmias. *Anesthesiology, 24*, 358.

Schuh, F.T. (1975): Influence of ketamine on human plasma cholinesterase. *Brit. J. Anaesth., 47*, 1315.

Schwartz, H. and deRoetth, A. (1958): Effect of succinylcholine on intraocular pressure in human beings. *Anesthesiology, 19*, 112.

Scudamore, H.H., Vorhaus, L.J. and Kark, R.M. (1951): Observations on erythrocyte and plasma cholinesterase activity in dyscrasias of the blood. *Blood, 6*, 1260.

Seed, R.F. and Chamberlain, J.H. (1977): Myocardial stimulation by pancuronium bromide. *Brit. J. Anaesth., 49*, 401.

Shnider, S.M. (1965): Serum cholinesterase activity during pregnancy, labour and the pueperium. *Anesthesiology, 26*, 335.

Simpson, B.R., Savege, T.M., Foley, E.I. Ross, L.A., Strunin, L., Walton, B., Maxwell, M. and Harris, D.M. (1972): An azobis – arylimidaze – pyridinium derivative: a rapidly acting non-depolarizing muscle relaxant. *Lancet, I*, 516.

Singer, M.M. Dutton, R. and Way, W.L. (1971): Prolonged curarization in a patient with renal failure. *Brit. J. Anaesth., 43*, 506.

Sitarz, L. (1974): Anaphylactic shock following injection of suxamethonium. *Anaesth. Resusc. intern. Ther., 2*, 83.

Sklar, G.S. and Lanks, K.W. (1977): Effects of Trimetaphan and sodium nitroprusside on hydrolysis of succinylcholine in vitro. *Anesthesiology, 47*, 31.

Smith, G., Dalling, R. and Williams, T.I.R. (1978): Gastro-oesophageal pressure gradient changes produced by induction of anaesthesia and suxamethonium. *Brit. J. Anaesth., 50*, 1137.

Smith, N.L. (1957): Histamine release by suxamethonium. *Anaesthesia, 12*, 293.

Smith, N.T. and Whitcher, C.E. (1967): Hemodynamic effects of gallamine and tubocurarine administered during halothane anaesthesia. *J. Amer. med. Ass., 199*, 704.

Smith, R.B. and Grenvik, A. (1970): Cardiac arrest following succinylcholine in patients with central nervous system injuries. *Anesthesiology, 33*, 558.

Smith, R.H. and Volpitto, P.P. (1960): Bucking and bronchospasm as problems of anesthesia. *J. Amer. med. Ass., 172*, 1499.

Smith, S.E. (1976): Neuromuscular blocking drugs in man. In: *Handbook of Experimental Pharmacology, New Series.* Editors: G.V.R. Born, O. Eichler, A. Farah, H. Herken and Welch, A.D. Vol. 42, Editors: E. Zaimis. Springer Verlag, 1976.

Sniper, W. (1952): The estimation and comparison of histamine release by muscle relaxants in man. *Brit. J. Anaesth., 24*, 232.

Sniper, W. (1971): Anaphylaxis under anaesthesia. *Anaesthesia, 26*, 527.

Sobel, A.M. (1962): Hexafluorenium, succinylcholine and intraocular tension. *Anesth. Analg. Curr. Res., 41*, 399.

Somogyi, A.A., Shanks, C.A. and Triggs, E.J. (1977): Disposition kinetics of pancuronium bromide in patients with total biliary obstruction. *Brit. J. Anaesth., 49*, 1103.

Stead, A.L. (1955): The response of the newborn infant to muscle relaxants. *Brit. J. Anaesth, 27*, 124.

Stoddart, J.C. (1978): Postoperative respiratory failure: an anaesthetic hazard? *Brit. J. Anaesth., 50*, 695.

Stoelting, R.K. (1972): The hemodynamic effects of pancuronium and d-tubocurarine in anesthetized patients. *Anesthesiology, 36*, 612.

Stoelting, R.K. (1974): Hemodynamic effects of dimethyltubocurarine during nitrous oxide-halothane anesthesia. *Anesth. Analg. Curr. Res., 53*, 513.

Stoelting, R.K. (1977): Comparison of gallamine and atropine as pretreatment before anaesthetic induction and succinylcholine administration. *Anesth. Analg. Curr. Res., 56*, 493.

Stoelting, R.K., Graf, J.P. and Vieira, Z. (1948): Dimethyl ether of d-tubocurarine iodide as an adjunct to anaesthesia. *Proc. Soc. exp. Biol. Med. 69*, 565.

Stoelting, R.K. and Longnecker, D.E. (1972a): Influence of end tidal halothane concentration on d-tubocurarine hypotension. *Anesth. Analg. Curr. Res., 51*, 364.

Stoelting, R.K. and Longnecker, D.E. (1972b): Effect of promethazine on hypotension following d-tubocurarine use in anesthetized patients. *Anesth. Analg. Curr. Res., 51*, 509.

Stone, W.A., Beach, T.P. and Hamelberg, W. (1970a): Succinylcholine – danger in the spinal-cord-injured patient. *Anesthesiology, 32*, 168.

Stone, W.A., Beach, T.P. and Hamelberg, W. (1970b): Succinylcholine-induced hyperkalaemia in dogs with transected nerves or spinal cords. *Anesthesiology, 32*, 515.

Stoner, T.R. and Urbach, K.F. (1968): Cardiac arrhythmias associated with succinylcholine in a patient with phaeochromocytoma. *Anesthesiology, 29*, 1228.

Stovner, J., Theodorsen, L. and Bjelke, E. (1971a): Sensitivity to tubocurarine and alcuronium with special reference to plasma protein pattern. *Brit. J. Anaesth., 43*, 385.

Stovner, J., Theodorsen, L. and Bjelke, E. (1971b): Sensitivity to gallamine and pancuronium with special reference to serum protiens. *Brit. J. Anaesth., 43*, 953.

Stovner, J., Theodorsen, L. and Bjelke, E. (1972): Sensitivity to dimethyltubocurarine and toxiferine with special reference to serum proteins. *Brit. J. Anaesth., 44*, 374.

Stovner, J., Oftedal, N. and Holmboe, J. (1975): The inhibition of cholinesterases by pancuronium. *Brit. J. Anaesth., 47*, 949.

Takki, S. and Tammisto, T. (1973): Effect of pancuronium and tubocurarine on plasma catecholamines. *Ann. Chir. Gynaecol. Fenn., 62*, 260.

Talmadge, E.A. and McKechnie, F.B. (1959): Anaesthetic management of a patient with myotonia dystrophia. *Anesthesiology, 201*, 717.

Tammisto, T. and Airaksinen, M. (1966): Increase of creatin kinase activity in serum as sign of muscular injury caused by intermittently administered suxamethonium during halothane anaesthesia. *Brit. J. Anaesth., 38,* 510.

Tammisto, T. and Welling, I. (1969): The effect of alcuronium and tubocurarine on blood pressure and heart rate: a clinical comparison. *Brit. J. Anaesth., 41,* 317.

Tarkannen, L., Laitinen, L. and Johansson, G. (1974): Effects of d-tubocurarine on intracranial pressure and thalamic electrical impedance. Anesthesiology, 40, 247.

Tashiro, C. and Jordan, W.S. (1976): The effect of diphenhydramine on plasma histamine levels and hemodynamic changes induced by d-tubocurarine. *Jap. J. Anesthesiol., 25,* 768.

Taussig, P.E., Stojak, H.E. and Bennett, N.R. (1979): In vitro interaction of propanidid and suxamethonium with pooled human plasma cholinesterase. *Brit. J. Anaesth., 51,* 181.

Taylor, T.H., Mulcahy, M. and Nightingale, D.A. (1968): Suxamethonium chloride in intraocular surgery. *Brit. J. Anaesth., 40,* 113.

Telford, I. and Keats, A.S. (1957): Succinylcholine in cardiovascular surgery of infants and children. *Anesthesiology, 18,* 841.

Telivuo, L. and Katz, R.L. (1970): The effects of modern intravenous local analgesics on respiration during partial neuromuscular block in man. *Anaesthesia, 25,* 30.

Tewfik, F.I. (1957): Trimetaphan: its effect on the pseudo-cholinesterase level in man. *Anaesthesia, 12,* 326.

Thiel, R.E. (1967): The myotonic response to suxamethonium. *Brit. J. Anaesth., 39,* 815.

Thomas, E.T. (1957): The effect of d-tubocurarine chloride on the blood pressure of anaesthetized patients. *Lancet, 2,* 772.

Thomas, E.T. (1963): The effect of gallamine triethiodide on blood pressure. *Anaesthesia, 18,* 316.

Thomas, E.T. (1969): Circulatory collapse following succinylcholine. Report of a case. *Anesth. Analg. Curr. Res.,* 48, 333.

Thomas, J., Climie, C.R. and Mather, L.E. (1969): The placental transfer of alcuronium. *Brit. J. Anaesth., 41,* 297.

Thomas, J.L. and Holmes, J.H. (1970): Effect of hemodialysis on plasma cholinesterase. *Anesth. Analg. Curr. Res.,* 49, 323.

Thompson, J.C. and Whittaker, M. (1965): Pseudocholinesterase activity in thyroid disease. *J. clin. Path., 18,* 811.

Thompson, J.C. and Whittaker, M. (1966): A study of the pseudocholinesterase in 78 cases of apnoea following suxamethonium. *Acta genet. (Basel), 16,* 209.

Thornton, R.J., Blakeney, C. and Feldman, S. (1976): Presented to the Anaesthetic Research Group, Summary. *Brit. J. Anaesth., 48,* 264.

Tobey, R.E. (1970): Paraplegia, succinylcholine and cardiac arrest. *Anesthesiology, 32,* 359.

Tobey, R.E., Jacobsen, P.M., Kahle, C.T., Clubb, R.J. and Dean M.A. (1972): The serum potassium response to muscle relaxants in neural injury. *Anesthesiology, 37,* 332.

Todrick, A. (1954): The inhibition of cholinesterae by antagonists of acetylcholine and histamine. *Brit. J. Pharmacol., 9,* 76.

Tolmie, J.D., Joyce, T.H. and Mitchell, G.D. (1967): Succinylcholine danger in the burned patient. *Anesthesiology, 28,* 467.

Torda, T.A., Burkhart, J. and Toh, W. (1972): The interaction of propanidid with suxamethonium and decamethonium. *Anaesthesia, 27,* 159.

Tucker, W.K. and Munson, E.S. (1975): Effects of succinylcholine and d-tubocurarine on epinephrine-induced arrhymias during halothane anaesthesia in dogs. *Anesthesiology, 42,* 41.

Tweedie, D.G. and Ordish, P.M. (1974): Reactions to intravenous agents (Althesin and pancuronium) *Brit. J. Anaesth., 46*, 244.

Usubiaga, J.E., Wikinski, J.A. Morales, R.L. and Usubiaga, L.E. (1967a): Interaction of intravenously administered procaine, lidocaine and succinylcholine in anesthetized subjects. *Anesth. Analg. Curr. Res., 46*, 39.

Usubiaga, J.E., Wikinski, J.A., Usubiaga, L.E. and Molina, F. (1967b): Intravenous lidocaine in the prevention of postoperative muscle pain caused by succinylcholine administration. *Anesth. Analg. Curr. Res., 46*, 225.

Verma, R.S., Chatterji, S. and Mathur, Neelu (1978): Diazepam and succinylcholine induced muscle pains. *Anesth. Analg. Curr. Res., 57*, 295.

Verner, J. and Comty, C. (1959): Intermittent suxamethonium injections. *Brit. med. J., 1*, 1239.

Viby-Mogensen, J. and Hanel, H.K. (1978): Prolonged apnoea after suxamethonium. An Analysis of the first 225 cases reported to the Danish Cholinesterase Research Unit. *Acta Anaesth. Scand., 22*, 371.

Viby-Mogensen, J., Hanel, H.K., Hansen, E., Sorensen, B. and Graae, J. (1975a): Serum cholinesterase activity in burned patients. I: Biochemical findings. *Acta anaesth. scand., 19*, 159.

Viby-Mogensen, J., Hanel, H.K., Hansen, E. and Graae, J. (1975b): Serum cholinesterase activity in burned patients. II: Anaesthesia, suxamethonium and hyperkalaemia. *Acta anaesth. scand., 19*, 169.

Viby-Mogensen, J., Wisborg, K., Gabrielsen, J. and Spotoft, H. (1976): Halothane anaesthesia and suxamethonium I: The significance of preoperative atropine administration. A double-blind study. *Acta. anaesth. scand., 20*, 129.

Vitez, T.S. (1978): Potency of metocurine during halothane − nitrous oxide and nitrous oxide-narcotic anaesthesia. *Anesth. Analg. Curr. Res., 57*, 116.

Vorhaus, L.J., Scudamore, H.H. and Kark, R.M. (1950): Mesurement of serum cholinesterase activity in the study of diseases of the liver and biliary system. *Gastroenterology, 15*, 304.

Wåhlin, Å. (1960): Clinical and experimental studies on the effects of succinylcholine. *Acta. anaesth. scand. Suppl. V*, p. 15.

Walmsley, D.A. (1959): Sensitivity reaction to gallamine triethiodide. *Lancet, II*, 237.

Walton, J.D. and Farman, J.V. (1973): Suxamethonium, potassium and renal failure. *Anaesthesia, 28*, 626.

Walts, W.F., Lebowitz, M. and Dillon, J.B. (1967): The effects of ventilation on the action of tubocurarine and gallamine. *Brit. J. Anaesth., 39*, 845.

Walts, L.F. and Prescott, F.S. (1965): The effects of gallamine on cardiac rhythm during general anesthesia. *Anesth. Analg. Curr. Res., 44*, 265.

Wang, R.I.H. and Ross, C.A. (1963): Prolonged apnea following succinylcholine in cancer patients receiving AB-132. *Anesthesiology, 24*, 363.

Ward, M.E., Adu-Gyamfi, Y. and Strunin, L. (1975): Althesin and pancuronium in chronic liver disease, *Brit. J. Anaesth., 47*, 1199.

Waser, P.G. and Harbeck, P. (1962): Pharmakologie und klinische Anwendung des Kurzdauernden Muskelrelaxans Diallyl-nor-toxiferin. *Anesthesist, 11*, 33.

Waterlow, J. (1950): Liver choline-esterase in malnourished infants. Lancet *I*, 908.

Waterman, P.M. and Smith, R.B. (1977): Tobramycin-curare interaction. *Anesth. Analg. Curr. Res., 56*, 587.

Waters, D.J. and Mapleson, W.W. (1971): Suxamethonium pains: hypothesis and observation. *Anaesthesia, 26*, 127.

Watkins, J. (1979): Anaphylactoid reactions to intravenous substances. *Brit. J. Anaesth., 51*, 51.

Watkins, J., and Clarke, R.S.J. (1978): Report of a symposium. Adverse responses to intravenous agents. *Brit. J. Anaesth., 50*, 1159.

Watt, H.K. (1973): Anaphylactic shock from gallamine. *N.Z. Soc. Anaesth. Newsletter, 20*, 21.

Waud, B.E. and Waud, D.R. (1978): Interaction of potassium and calcium with neuromuscular blocking agents. *Abstracts of Scientific Papers, A.S.A. Meeting*, p. 403.

Weintraub, H.B., Heisterkamp, D.V. and Cooperman, L.H. (1969): Changes in plasma potassium concentration after depolarizing blockers in anaesthetized man. *Brit. J. Anaesth., 41*, 1048.

West, R. (1936): Intravenous curarine in the treatment of tetanus. *Lancet, I*, 12.

Westgate, H.D., Gordon, J.R. and Van Bergen, F.H. (1962): Changes in airway resistance following intravenously administered d-tubocurarine. *Anesthesiology, 23*, 65.

Westgate, H.D., Schultz, E.A. and Van Bergen, F. (1961): Urticaria and angioneurotic oedema following d-tubocurarine administration. *Anesthesiology, 22*, 286.

Westgate, H.D. and Van Bergen, F. (1962): Changes in histamine blood levels following d-tubocurarine administration. *Canad. Anaesth. Soc. J., 9*, 497.

White, D.C. (1962): Observations on the prevention of muscle pains after suxamethonium. *Brit. J. Anaesth., 34*, 332.

Whiteacre, R.J. and Fisher, A.J. (1945): Clinical observations of the use of curare in anesthesia. *Anesthesiology, 6*, 124.

Whittaker, M. and Vickers, M.D. (1970): Initial experiences with the cholinesterase research unit. *Brit. J. Anaesth., 42*, 1016.

Wildsmith, J.A.W. (1972): Serum pseudocholinesterase, pregnancy and suxamethonium. *Anaesthesia, 27*, 90.

Williams, C.H. (1976): Some observations on the aetiology of the fulminant hyperthermia-stress syndrome. *Perspect. Biol. Med., 20*, 120.

Williams, C.H., Deutsch, S., Linde, H.W., Bullough, J.W. and Dripps, R.D. (1961): Effects of intravenously administered succinyldicholine on cardiac rate, rhythm and arterial blood pressure in anesthetized man. *Anesthesiology, 22*, 947.

Williams, R.T. and Gain, E.A. (1962): Electrocardiographic changes following repeated injections of decamethonium and subsequent injection of succinylcholine. Canad. *Anaesth. Soc. J., 9*, 263.

Wilson, H.B., Gordon, H.E. and Raffan, A.W. (1950): Dimethyl ether of d-tubocurarine iodide as a curarizing agent in anaesthesia for thoracic surgery. *Brit. med. J., 1*, 1296.

Wilson, S.L., Miller, R.N., Wright, C. and Hasse, D. (1976): Prolonged neuromuscular blockade associated with trimetaphan. A case report. *Anesth. Analg. Curr. Res., 55*, 353.

Wingard, D.W. (1974): Malignant hyperthermia: a human stress syndrome. *Lancet, II*, 1450.

Wisborg, K., Christensen, V. and Viby-Mogensen, J. (1977): Halothane anaesthesia and suxamethonium II. The significance of preoperative gallamine administration. *Acta anaesth. scand., 21*, 266.

Wise, R.P. (1962): A myasthenic syndrome complicating bronchial carcinoma. *Anaesthesia, 17*, 488.

Wislicki, L. and Rosenblum, I. (1967): Effects of propanolol on the duration of action of neuromuscular blocking drugs. *Brit. J. Anaesth., 39*, 939.

Wong, A.L. and Brodsky, J.B. (1978): Asystole in an adult after a single dose of succinylcholine. *Anesth. Analg. Curr. Res, 57*, 135.

Wong, K.C., Wyte, S.R., Martin, W.E. and Crawford, E.W. (1971): Antiarrhythmic effects of skeletal muscle relaxants. *Anesthesiology, 34*, 458.

Wood, G.J. and Hall, G.M. (1978): Plasmapheresis and plasma cholinesterase. *Brit. J. Anaesth., 50*, 945.

Wordsworth, V. (1964): Muscle relaxants. *Lancet, I*, 379.

136

Wretlind, A. and Wåhlin, Å. (1959): The effect of succinylcholine on the orbital musculature of the cat. *Acta anaesth. Scand., 3*, 101.

Wynands, J.E. and Crowell, D.E. (1969): Intraocular tension in association with succinylcholine and endotracheal intubation. A preliminary report. *Canad. Anaesth. Soc. J., 7*, 39.

Yamashita, M. and Matsuki, A. (1975): Muscle relaxant requirements in patients with Von Reckling-haussen's disease. *Brit. J. Anaesth., 47*, 1032.

Zaidan, J., Philbin, D.M., Antonio, R. and Savarese, J. (1977): Hemodynamic effects of metocurine in patients with coronary artery disease receiving propanolol. *Anesth. Analg. Curr. Res., 56*, 255.

Zaimis, E., Cannard, T.H. and Price, H.L. (1958): Effects of lowered muscle temperature upon neuro-muscular blockade in man. *Science, 128*, 34.

Zsigmond, E.K. and Downs, J.R. (1971): Plasma cholinesterase activity in newborns and infants. *Canad. Anaesth. Soc. J., 18*, 278.

Zsigmond, E.K., Matsuki, A., Kothary, S.P. and Kelsch, R.C. (1974): The effect of pancuronium bro-mide on plasma norepinephrine and cortisol concentrations during Thiamylal induction. *Canad. Anaesth. Soc. J., 21*, 147.

Zsigmond, E.K. and Robins, G. (1972): The effect of a series of anticancer drugs on plasma cholinester-ase activity. *Canad. Anaesth. Soc. J., 19*, 75.

5

Mechanisms and factors predisposing towards adverse response to intravenous anaesthetic substances

John Watkins

INTRODUCTION

Despite its undoubted advantages to the clinician, the administration of substances by the intravenous route creates a wide variety of complications. It should be remembered that the so called "hypersensitivity reactions" occupy only a small part in this range of complications. Nevertheless, the majority of untoward reactions, such as microbial contamination of infusion sets, can be avoided and it is the "hypersensitivity type response" which is of increasing importance since at present it cannot be satisfactorily predicted, nor the patient adequately protected.

Incidence, mechanisms and predisposing factors to adverse response are intimately combined. Shakespeare, in the Merchant of Venice, observed "all that glisters is not gold". How true this is for the hypersensitivity-type response, perhaps better described as an anaphylactoid response, since the clinical manifestations alone are not sufficient to define the reaction as immune mediated. The "glister" in all these reactions is provided essentially by histamine release, but quite different mechanisms may be involved in the release of histamine. Fig. 5.1. illustrates three cases which have superficial similarity. Patients (a) and (b) exhibited an anaphylactoid response to gelatin blood plasma substitutes. Both exhibited urticaria and both were hypotensive. Nevertheless, patient (a) showed no *plasma* histamine release whereas significant release was observed with (b). Patient (c) was in fact a fit volunteer in which it was discovered that venepuncture for the withdrawal of blood resulted consistently in marked urticaria. In the latter a small rise of histamine occurred as the urticaria faded, i.e. only as it was released from the skin. Although (c) is not, of course, an "adverse response" one wonders, if she had been receiving

138

an intravenous agent, whether the urticaria might not have been attributed to the injected agent. Clearly (and importantly in cases (a) and (b)) there are different underlying mechanisms for the histamine release in all three cases. Laboratory tests are always necessary to confirm the reaction mechanism whether it be a true Type I immediate hypersensitivity reaction, involving reaginic antibodies or other antibodies, a complement mediated reaction or a reaction caused by the direct release of histamine from mast cells.

FREQUENCY OF ANAPHYLACTOID REACTIONS

The statement of frequency implies that the adverse response can be quantitated in some simple and universally adopted manner. A Symposium held in Sheffield in

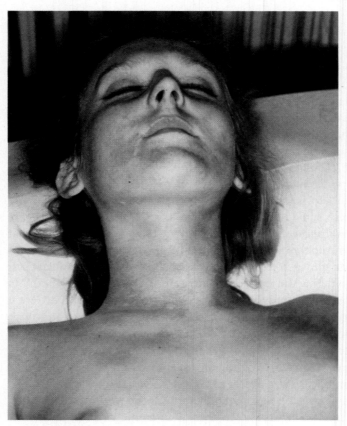

(a) For legend see p. 140

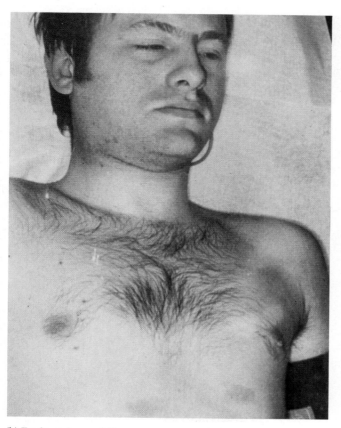

(b) For legend see p. 140

1978 confirmed that this was not the case. While death was an "acceptable" adverse reponse at one extreme of the response spectrum many delegates were accepting minor clinical manifestations, such as "Althesin flush", as normal, despite the fact that the latter might be a harbinger of future problems in a few unlucky individuals (See Watkins and Clarke, 1978). The variability in the literature for anaesthetic drugs, plasma substitutes and radiocontrast media must lie in what the observer regards as a significant response. It seems likely therefore that, like the classical hypersensitivity reactions, Types I–IV, clinically significant anaphylactoid reactions do not represent atypical qualitative effects but only atypical quantitative effects (measured in the overall release of histamine and the organ of its release and effect, i.e. the shock organ). Support for this hypothesis is provided both from the observations of significant, but subclinical, plasma histamine release in patients receiving intravenous hypnotics without obvious untoward effects (Lorenz, 1975),

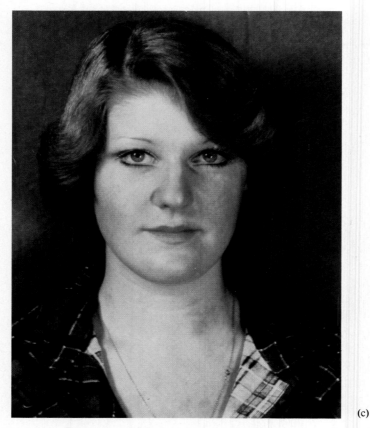

(c)

Fig. 5.1. "Adverse responses" with very different underlying mechanisms in volunteer subjects. Subjects (a) and (b) exhibited serious reactions to gelatin plasma substitutes. Subject (c) exhibits marked urticaria to the simple stimulus of venepuncture alone (see text). Photographs (a) and (b) are reproduced by kind permission of Professors W. Lorenz and A. Doenicke, Universities of Marburg and Munich: photograph (c) reproduced by kind permission of the volunteer.

and also from the marked changes in polymorph concentrations following such administrations (Watkins et al., 1976a, 1977, 1978a).

Measurement of histamine release would be theoretically ideal for defining adverse reactions. Unfortunately, there are two practical disadvantages to this approach (a) the experimental requirements are not really suited to operating theatre conditions, particularly where clinically severe cases are encountered and (b) not all anaphylactoid reactions result in *plasma* histamine release. The latter is particularly true for many of the plasma substitute reactions, where gastric histamine release appears to predominate.

There are several methods for investigating anaphylactoid response (Table 5.1) but only two of these are relevant to the clinical situation; one based on intradermal testing (Fisher, 1976) the other based on the measurement of certain plasma proteins in serial samples of the patient's plasma taken over the 24 hours following reaction (Watkins et al., 1976b). There are advantages and disadvantages to both approaches. Basically, the former approach should lead to identification of the specific agent implicated in a whole battery of drugs given more or less simultaneously, while the latter approach is more likely to elucidate the reaction mechanism rather than its causitive agent. Despite its recent popularity, intradermal testing has two major disadvantages. Firstly, it quite wrongly pre-supposes all reactions are antibody mediated and secondly, several weeks delay are necessary before skin testing can be undertaken following anaphylactoid response, otherwise extremely dangerous challenge reactions may occur in the patient. Although far from perfect the procedure (Watkins et al., 1979a) suggested by this laboratory does not prejudge reaction mechanisms. It merely requires the measurement of the consumption and conversion of complement C3 and C4; C3PA and C1 inhibitor levels, and immunoglobulin IgE involvement in sequential samples of patients

TABLE 5.1.

METHODS FOR INVESTIGATING ANAPHYLACTOID RESPONSE

Technique	Advantages	Disadvantages
Plasma histamine	Direct measure of effector substance	1. Experimental requirements unsuited for clinical response
		2. Not all reactions involve *plasma* histamine
Intradermal testing	1. Simple	1. Must be carried out considerably *after* response
	2. Only *in vivo* test	
	3. Inexpensive	2. Assumes immune medicated response
Cellular tests	High sensitivity	1. Require high technical skill
		2. Assumes immune mediated response
Specific plasma protein Assay	1. Simple	1. Can only identify plasma events
	2. Does *not* assume mechanism of reaction	2. Poor sensitivity for marginal adverse reactions

plasma following reaction (Watkins et al., 1976b). It should remain an essential procedure to be backed up later by intradermal testing only when IgE mediated reactions are indicated.

All laboratory tests must be considered in relation to the clinical features of the case, by themselves, like clinical observations alone, they afford only a limited interpretation of the mechanism. For example, it is necessary to know whether the patient has received the agent before, if so, how frequently. Some indication of his immune status is necessary, for example, if he is recovering from an infection. Based on our own experiences we suggest that four basic mechanisms are involved (Watkins, 1979b) although more than one mechanism may be involved in any given reaction. These reaction mechanisms may be conveniently summarized as follows:

(1) Type I hypersensitivity response. These require previous exposure and involve IgE antibodies. There is direct histamine release from mast cells without the involvement of complement.

(2) Immune reactions. The class of immunoglobulin involved may be in doubt, but histamine release occurs by the classical complement pathway. Immunochemically, serial samples show complement C4 and C3 consumption with varying degrees of C3 conversion, generally less than 30%.

(3) Alternative pathway activation of C3. These involve direct activation of C3 and consequently high levels of C3 conversion may be observed in plasma. Histamine and other vasoactive substances are released from mast cells by the action of the liberated complement fragment, anaphylatoxin, and give rise to the characteristic clinical manifestations of anaphylactoid response. Complement C4 shows no significant consumption or conversion in the reaction. This group appears to contain both individuals apparently sensitized by previous exposure to the substance and first time responders.

(4) Pharmacological or chemical release of histamine. The injected substance causes histamine release directly from the mast cell without antibody or complement involvement. This may reflect drug concentration, speed of injection, the distribution of mast cells in the vascular system, or a combination or these.

At present we can only infer reactions occurring by direct release of histamine by the total lack of involvement of the plasma proteins.

Tale 5.2 shows the analysis of reactions reported to this laboratory between 1974 and 1978. It will be observed that in 1974 and 1975 many samples were received which were totally unsuitable for analysis. More rigorous, but simpler, blood sampling protocols have considerably improved the situation since 1976. A significant feature of Table 5.2 is the increasing frequency of reports implicating thiopentone. This might conceivably represent a genuine increase in such reactions but more probably represents a greater awareness of reactions and reaction

TABLE 5.2

	Cases reported	Mechanism analysis possible	Complement involved		IgE involved	Probably pharmaco-logical
			Classical*	Alternative		
1974						
Althesin	19	5	1	4	2/5	0/5
Thiopentone	1	0	0	0	0	0
Methohexitone	1	1	0	1	1/1	0/1
1975						
Althesin	16	7	3	4	2/7	0/7
Propanidid	1	0	0	0	0	0
Thiopentone	1	1	0	0	0/1	0/1
1976						
Althesin	15	12	4	6	1/10	2/12
Propanidid	2	2	0	2	0/2	0/2
Thiopentone	2	2	1	1	2/2	0/2
1977						
Althesin	12	11	1	5	0/11	5/11
Thiopentone	6	5	3	1	4/5	0/5
Dextran	4	2	0	2	0/2	0/2
1978						
Althesin	20	18	2	14	1/18	3/18
Thiopentone	10	9	1	2	2/9	4/9
Haemaccel	1	1	0	0	0/1	0/1

*Implied immunological memory, often with excessive C3 feedback.

reporting. Reactions were predominantly reported as caused by Althesin and by thiopentone although in several cases co-administered neuromuscular drugs may have influenced the reaction, either directly or synergistically. In this respect Lorenz and Doenicke have reported significant histamine release into the plasma of volunteers following administrations of the intravenous hypnotic etomidate in the presence of suxamethonium (Lorenz and Doenicke, 1978). Etomidate alone did not cause such release (Doenicke et al., 1973).

Supposed reactions to both Althesin and thiopentone involve similar clinical manifestations, amongst which rashes and flushing, hypotension, bronchospasm and oedema are predominant features. However, bronchospasm is apparently more commonly reported in association with thiopentone than with Althesin (Garrett, 1978). Despite the apparent similarity of the clinical reactions there are marked differences in the involvement of the plasma proteins by these two drugs.

COMPLEMENT INVOLVED REACTIONS

Althesin reactions generally involve excessive and direct (alternative pathway) activation of complement C3. In those cases where classical pathway activation was indicated (C4 involvement) the patients had, for the most part, received Althesin uneventfully on a previous occasion. Excessive feedback activation of the C3 pathway was also a feature of the classical response. Approximately 40% of Althesin reactions occur on first exposure (Garrett, 1978). Complement C3 activation following a first exposure to thiopentone has been observed but appears to be a rather unusual mechanism, possibly implicating an underlying immuno-pathology in the patient. However, some degree of classical complement activation does appear to be involved in thiopentone reactions (See Table 5.2). This may reflect antibody involvement other than, or as well as, homocytotropic antibody, possibly the reagin IgG4. Alternatively, this could be a secondary process unrelated to the primary reaction.

Not all reactions involving complement C4 represent classical pathway and implied immunological memory. On two occasions (with Althesin reactions) we are reasonably confident that angioneurotic oedema arose by activation of the second component of complement (C2) via C4C2 complex. The kinin-like peptide released by this mechanism causes vasodilation without the intervention of systemic histamine. The hereditary condition of angioneurotic oedema involves a defect in the esterase inhibitor (C1 inhibitor), often manifest by low levels of this protein. Both our reactants had low C1 inhibitor levels and both exhibited C4 involvement in the *absence* of C3 consumption or conversion. The clinical symptoms appeared to be confined to facial oedema and there was no previous record of anaesthesia with this drug.

Complement and coagulation

Disseminated intravascular coagulation may be triggered by several mechanisms including hypoxia, trauma and infection (See Preston, 1979).

Stress and or shock are undoubtedly associated with both anaesthetic and surgical trauma and it would be surprising if the extreme case of anaphylactoid shock did not result in some degree of intravascular coagulation. The association between complement and coagulation systems in man is at present ill defined. There is evidence that the "analogue" of complement C3 in the coagulation pathway, Factor XII, can activate C1 either directly or through the intermediary action of plasmin (Donaldson, 1967; Ratnoff, 1967). It has been shown that coagulation abnormalities occur in rabbits congenitally deficient in C6 (Zimmerman et al., 1971) and that complement activation by inulin causes marked enhancement of the coagulation activity of rabbit platelets. Experiments in man have been less convincing but a similar enhanced coagulation activity may also be induced by complement proteins in human platelets.

Our own studies have repeatedly shown dramatic and rapid falls in platelet counts in some subjects receiving intravenous anaesthetic substances, frequently in the absence of clinical manifestations (Fig. 5.2). These falls were reversed within 20 min of onset and appear to occur in patients who have received the anaesthetic drug on at least one previous occasion. In some minor cases clinical manifestations also occurred and the fall in platelet count was accompanied by measureable C3 conversion, margination, followed by accumulation, of polymorphonuclear leucocytes (Watkins et al., 1978a), and increased vascular permeability. These are all features of anaphylatoxin release. Additionally, the reactions possess attributes of antigenic memory and we have previously speculated upon their possible relevance to thrombotic episodes observed in patients receiving surgery under general anaesthesia. It is possible that at least a proportion of the haematological problems associated with anaesthesia and surgery have an immunological basis.

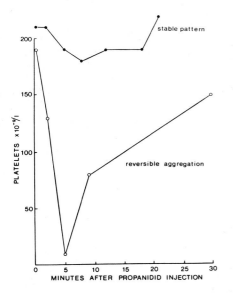

Fig. 5.2. Platelet movements in patients exhibiting no obvious untoward clinical manifestations to intravenous anaesthetic drugs. One patient exhibits a very marked primary (reversible) platelet aggregation phenomenon.

REAGIN INVOLVED REACTIONS

Definite IgE involvement is an uncommon feature of Althesin reactions although some type of short term immunological memory, perhaps cellular, does appear to be associated with this drug. This contrasts sharply with thiopentone reactions where IgE involvement following uneventful previous exposures to the drug (potential sensitization) is quite frequent.

Although IgE is the major reaginic antibody, other antibodies such as IgG subclass 4 (IgG 4) may also possess reaginic characteristics (Berrens et al., 1977). Additionally, these antibodies may also activate complement. In this situation the patient may well have normal IgE levels, the only indication of antibody involvement being the consumption of complement C4.

TABLE 5.3.

INTER-RELATIONSHIP OF IgD AND IgE LEVELS IN FAMILIES OF PATIENTS EXHIBITING HYPERSENSITIVITY RESPONSES

	IgD (I.U./ml)	IgE (I.U./ml)
Family "T"		
Patient (Age, 5, F)	60*	15
Mother	70*	8
Father	42	>1000*
Sister (Age, 9)	90*	49
Family "W"		
Patient (Age, 12, F)	206*	220*
Mother	1	5
Father	13	400*
Sister (Age, 15)	1	110
Sister (Age, 17)	1	450*
Atopy (Asthma) Family "H"		
Patient (Age, 7, M)	942*	650*
Father	94*	150
Mother	132*	13
Sister	16	—
Brother	174*	25

Patients in families T and W exhibited adverse response to Althesin. The family (H) of the child with extrinsic asthma (established hypersensitivity) makes an obvious comparison "control"! Allen and Watkins unpublished observations.

*Values exceeding 95th centile.

Althesin behaves anomalously in that reactions are often observed when a second exposure to the drug occurs 1 –4 weeks after the administration. Preliminary studies (Watkins et al., 1978b) suggest that either the patients themselves or their families may have increased IgD concentration, with one or more of the family displaying concentrations of IgE consistent with hypersensitivity (Table 5.3). IgD is a lymphocyte receptor and may have memory characteristics for short term response. An analagous situation in the miniature pig model has been reported in detail by Glen et al. (1978, 1979). A second exposure to Althesin less than three weeks after the first, produces marked anaphylactoid distress in more than half of the pigs tested. This response decreases rapidly or is lost completely if either the "challenge" dose or a third dose is injected more than three weeks after the first. Other similarities with the human response include marked polymorph margination, indicative of complement activation, although the latter is unproven. Although one is tempted to regard this as a "model" for Althesin response, the very high frequency of response is, of course, atypical of adverse response manifestations in man and suggests caution in extrapolating the findings. This is borne out by the observation of these workers that the same sequence and frequency of events could be observed in the miniature pig using the detergent Cremophor EL and the active constituent of the formulation, alphaxalone, separately. Although Cremophor EL releases histamine directly and fatally, in dogs (Lorenz et al., 1976) such release in man is always subclinical.

SPEED OF RESPONSE

While the majority of anaphylactoid reactions are "immediate" resembling classical Type I hypersensitivity responses, there are numerous cases of delayed response occurring one to two hours after exposure to the agent. Such reactions are in all probability non-specific and represent physicochemical changes induced into harmless circulating immune complexes, converting them into complement activating entities. In a recent case (see p. 160) a patient was found to react similarly with methohexitone and Althesin, administered on separate occasions, three months apart. On both occasions the patient developed urticaria, hypotension, tachycardia and mild bronchospasm, one and half hours after induction. This was clearly not a specific drug effect. A death has been reported to Althesin following such delay (Vanezis, 1979). Type II and Type III hypersensitivity reactions may also be somewhat delayed but the evidence for these is somewhat conjectual. Immediate reactions to human serum albumin, used as a plasma substitute, usually correlate with old or badly stored material in which critically sized aggregates or polymers of albumin have been produced (Ring, 1976; Richter et al., 1978). A similar situation was recently observed with intravenous inulin used in a medical trial (unpublished observations). Delayed reactions to albumin (two to three days after administration) are effectively transfusion reactions caused by antibody formation against "foreign" albumin allotypes in the administered preparation (Weitkamp et al., 1973).

Delayed (Type IV) hypersensitivity reactions to anaesthetic drugs are again largely a matter of conjecture. Even the "short lived" intravenous anaesthetic drugs or their metabolites can be shown to persist in the body for quite long periods (>24 hours, Watkins et al., 1976a), leading to potential immunisation either against these or against the carrier, whether it be cell or protein. Such antibody production may, or may not, be destructive to the host, indeed in many classical auto-immune diseases there is little to substantiate the role of the autoantibody in the direct pathogenesis of the disease. Nevertheless, this is a possibility and certain organs, particularly the liver, may well suffer auto-immune attack. This is a very tempting mechanism to explain the so-called halothane hepatitis but the reader should proceed with caution since the contribution of surgical trauma and genetic features of the host, e.g. α_1-antitrypsin deficiency, cannot be overlooked.

THE DURATION OF ANAPHYLACTOID RESPONSE

There is a marked difference in the duration of anaphylactoid response between antibody mediated barbiturate reactions and complement mediated, or pharmacological reactions. Clinical manifestations of the former may persist for one or more days while the latter disappear rapidly in a few hours, probably irrespective of therapy.

The rapid clearance of complement mediated reactions should not be taken to indicate that such mechanisms are relatively harmless but only that they are likely to be harmless if the precipitating factor (i.e. the drug or other agent) is rapidly removed by biological degredation, or even by dilution. Agents like Althesin and propanidid are rapidly deactivated pharmacologically and if the patient survives the initial impact, then all appears to be well. In contrast, the rare complement C3 mediated reactions to dextrans and other plasma substitutes, and more frequent C3 mediated reactions to radio-contrast media (Witten, 1975), have a high mortality, probably related to the persistance of these substances in the vascular system.

Reagin mediated reactions to the barbiturates are likely to be particularly dangerous since the characteristics of these drugs leads to prolonged retention in the body and hence continued challenge. Although the short-lived hypnotic and neuromuscular drugs may elicit true immediate hypersensitivity reactions of great severity, the reaction is not ongoing.

SIGNIFICANCE OF REACTION MECHANISM

Reactions effectively fall into two groups, complement mediated and immune mediated responses with a considerable degree of overlap between the groups. Although we have considered the reactions as "mediated" by these mechanisms it must be stated that our acceptance that they are involved directly in the tissue damaging, life threatening, anaphylactoid response is based almost entirely on the analogy with immunopathological reactions associated with established disease conditions. For complement involved reactions the analogy is with generalised immediate hypersensitivity or allergic airways disease, to established allergens. In certain reactions even plasma histamine release may represent a very subsidiary function and other "chemical" effectors of immune response, such as anaphylatoxins, kinins, prostaglandins, slow reacting substance anaphylaxis (SRA-A), and serotin may have far greater significance to the anaphylactoid response than we appreciate at the present time.

Although our measurements of plasma protein involvement may not always reveal the true underlying reaction mechanism, the differentiation into complement and immune mediated reactions must conclusively establish two quite different, fundamental, reaction mechanisms and as such they acquire practical significance. Any reaction involving immunological memory will, of necessity, be exacerbated if the causative agent, or a related cross reacting antigen/hapten, is presented to the patient at some future time. In contrast, complement involved reactions, particularly to short acting anaesthetic drugs, are most unlikely to be exacerbated by further exposure of the patient who later will probably show little specificity for the supposed causative agent. He may, in fact, either react in a similar fashion to a different type of drug at a later date or even not react at all to the original drug, if a temporary causitive factor, e.g. underlying infection, has disappeared.

The degree of plasma complement C3 activation does appear to correlate quite well with the clinical severity of the anaphylactoid response, see Fig. 5.3. In general, reactions involving less than 10% C3 conversion, produce subclinical manifestations, particularly leucocyte taxis and primary aggregation of platelets: those producing 30% C3 conversion show minor clinical manifestations such as urticaria or flushing while reactions producing more than 70% C3 conversion are generally associated with life threatening siuations. We have stressed that the pharmaco-kinetic behaviour of the drug or other substance then influences the outcome of the reaction but nevertheless anomalies do abound. The author is aware of cases of extreme C3 conversion to Althesin on first exposure which resulted in only minor clinical manifestations, while the same level of conversion ($\geq 70\%$) was observed in a rare death following Althesin (Vanezis, 1979). In the former cases it

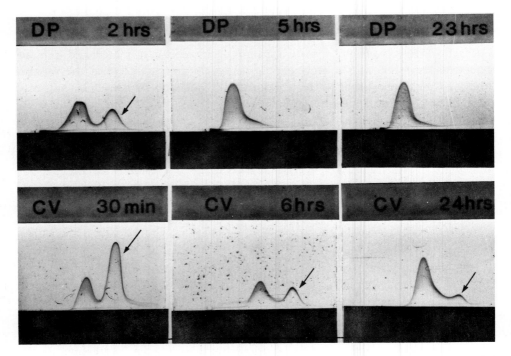

Fig. 5.3. Laurell immunoelectrophoresis patterns of C3 components in plasma taken from patients DP and CV showing anaphylactoid response after induction with Althesin for identical minor surgical procedures. Sample times after injection are indicated. Note the initial high degree of conversion (twin peaks): the C3c inactive products are indicated by the arrows. The surgical procedure had to be abandoned in the case of patient CV in whom significant conversion persisted for 24 hours. Patient DP exhibited a lower degreef of conversion and it was possible to continue surgery. Photograph reproduced by the author, with permission from: Adverse Response to Intravenous Drugs (1978). Academic Press, London, New York. p. 75.

seemed possible that despite complement activation the histamine release (but not complement activation) might have been modulated by premedication e.g. by diazepam, or by disodium cromoglycate, while in the latter both the reaction sequence and the laboratory data indicated an underlying immunopathology as the prime cause of the response (Watkins et al., 1978c).

SUBCLINICAL MANIFESTATIONS

Although the clinically severe anaphylactoid reactions which may hazard the patient's life are happily few, reactions of lesser severity (e.g. skin flushing and urticaria) are more frequently found and there may be other, subclinical, reactions

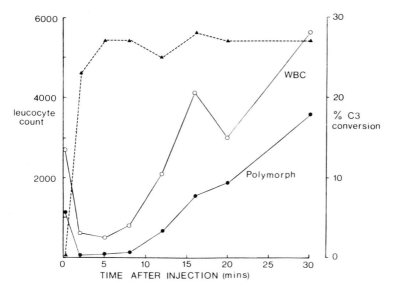

Fig. 5.4. Rapid changes in white blood cell numbers and complement conversion in a patient showing a minor, but clinically significant, adverse response following a second exposure to Althesin. This is a memory response. Photograph reproduced by the author, with permission from Adverse Response to Intravenous Drugs (1978). Academic Press, London, New York. p. 74.

without significant clinical manifestations.

Our experience of clinically significant response to intravenous local anaesthetic drugs and plasma substitutes has indicated the widespread involvement of complement in these reactions. An important feature of complement C3 activation is the chemotactic effect upon white cells, predominantly on polymorphs and other phagocytic cells, and changes in white cell numbers and types may be used as a very sensitive indicator of such action. Complement mediated reactions attract white cells into the circulation, probably initially from the margination pool. Nevertheless, two white cell patterns are observed, a slight but continuing rise in number over some 20 min or so, or a dramatic fall and recovery over the same period (Watkins et al., 1976a). Reactions of the latter type (Fig. 5.4) are invariably associated with previous exposure of the patient to the specific agent (i.e. immunological memory) and probably involve C3 activation (Watkins et al., 1976a). The fall, which is due to margination of the polymorphs, reverses rapidly and cells flood into the vascular system over the next 12 hours or so, giving overall rises in polymorphs 200% to 300% above "basal levels" of the patient (Watkins et al., 1977). The fall in white cells is often paralleled by a similar fall in platelets (primary aggregation). Similar polymorph effects have been observed in the mini pig model (Glen et al., 1978, 1979). In man such changes can sometimes be measured for several years after previous exposure to the agent but possibly less than 1 in 10 patients with such drug history exhibits this pattern.

Table 5.4

SIGNIFICANCE OF THE CHANGES IN PERIPHERAL BLOOD LEUCOCYTES FOLLOWING ANAESTHESIA AND SEDATION

Treatment	No. of Patients	Signification of change at various times (min) after cannulation* (P from T-test)			
		10	13	16	28
Etomidate + N_2O/O_2/Halothane	30	*<0.05*	*<0.05*	*<0.01*	*<0.001*
N_2O/O_2/Halothane	11	*<0.05*	*<0.05*	*<0.05*	>0.05
Diazepam	16	>0.05	*<0.05*	*<0.01*	*<0.001*
Cannulation alone	10	*<0.01*	*<0.01*	*<0.05*	ND

*Cannulation for blood sampling preceeded drug administration by 8 min.

Statistically significant values appear in italics: the data should be viewed in conjunction with Fig. 5.5.

Rising white cell patterns on first or subsequent exposure are more common. It is essential to isolate these reactions from the initial *chemical* response (Modgil et al., 1977) to the injection of the drug which reflects the direct chemotactic effect of the agent itself. The former reactions involve the activation of natural mediators, e.g. complement, kinins, prostaglandins, and reach a maximum some 5–10 min after drug injection (Watkins et al., 1976a). As such they have marked analogy with the subclinical histamine release studies of Lorenz and Doenicke (1978). Rising white cell patterns were frequently observed with the intravenous hypnotics, Althesin, Epontol, methohexitone, thiopentone, etomidate and also inhalational anaesthesia (nitrous oxide/oxygen/halothane). Changes in white cell numbers in the last two groups were shown to have high statistical significance in comparison with the initial pretreatment sample (Fig. 5.5; Table 5.4). However, white cell changes following either vein cannulation alone or the administration of intravenous diazepam were in the opposite direction to those observed with the anaesthetic drugs, suggesting a different mechanism (Fig. 5.5 and Table 5.4). This could be due to prostaglandin release since both procedures are associated with a degree of pain and stress. Changes in the individual lymphocyte and polymorph counts respectively parallel those in the total white cell counts (Watkins, Thornton, Padfield and Bennett, unpublished observations).

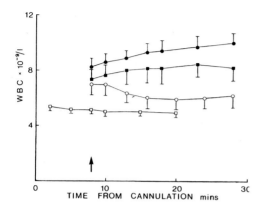

Fig. 5.5. Changes (Means ± SEM) in total white blood cell numbers following first exposure of groups of patients and volunteers to various procedures. See also Table 5.4. Treatments, •——•, etomidate induction, maintenance with $N_2O/O_2/Halothane$; ■——■, $N_2O/O_2/Halothane$ anaesthesia alone; ∘——∘, intravenous diazepam; □——□, cannulation alone (control group). Times are measured from time of insertion of the blood sampling cannula in the antecubital vein. Drugs administered, where applicable, 8 min later (arrowed).

TABLE 5.5

	Number of surgical patients	Patients reacting (Clarke et al., (1975)
Number questioned	5,500	86
Eczema, hay fever or asthma	9	14
Drug or food allergies	14	19
Previous anaesthesia	66	61
Same anaesthetic previously	0	47

Reproduced with permission from Clarke, Fee and Dundee (1978) In: Adverse Response to Inravenous Drugs. Academic Press, London, New York.

The changes observed in our investigations provide strong evidence for some form of subclinical response in the *majority* of subjects undergoing anaesthetic procedures. However, individual response varies widely, indicating that the subclinical response, like the clinical response, has a similar degree of patient variability. At the present moment we are unable to say whether or not subclinical manifestations of this type are harbingers of future clinically severe reactions.

FACTORS PREDISPOSING TO ADVERSE RESPONSE

Several major factors predisposing to anaphylactoid response have emerged from our investigations into reaction mechanisms. These may be summarized:

(a) Genetic features of the patient such as allergy, atopy or hypersensitivity and inherited complement system anomalies.

(b) Frequency of exposure to the agents, with anomalous behaviour to Althesin.

(c) Underlying immune processes leading to complement C3 instability and possible activation of other secondary immune effectors, such as prostaglandins.

(d) Pharmacological effects.

A fifth factor, stress, should also be added to these. This we have not considered previously but there is no doubt that anaesthetic and surgical trauma indirectly combine to produce marked alterations in cell metabolism and in both the cellular and the humoral "limbs" of specific immune response.

We shall examine some of these factors in greater detail.

Allergy, atopy and hypersensitivity

The correlation between immunological hypersensitivity and incidence of anaphylactoid response is complex. The fact that many subjects respond on first exposure to some substance, effectively precludes reagin mediated response. Champions of anaphylactic response as a fundamental mechanism of all these reactions suggest the presence of cross-reacting antibodies. While this is undoubtedly a possibility in classical immunology involving full "antigens" this seems most unlikely with the small haptenic molecules which comprise the drugs used in anaesthetic practice. Even in the dextran reactions, where cross-reacting antibodies (presumably raised against infective microorganisms) can be shown to be present in the patient's blood (Hedin et al., 1976) their significance to anaphylactoid response remain obscure. Quite certainly titres of such antibodies fall in subjects reactive to dextrans: however, they also fall in subjects who exhibit no clincial manifestations to adverse response (Richter et al., 1977). The so-called antibodies to gelatin substitutes are now thought to be euglobulins or possibly non-classical rheumatoid factor immunoglobulins which combine with the gelatin substitutes in a non-specific manner. The reaction may thus reflect immune complex activation of complement in the manner we have previously suggested for certain anaesthetic drugs.

The work of Clarke, Dundee and their colleagues (1975, 1978) suggests that atopy is a predisposing factor to anphylactoid response and more particularly, previous exposure (Fee et al., 1978) to the same (precipitating) agent (Table 5.5). This is now widely accepted despite the fact that the majority of reactions do not possess immunological memory characteristics. Equally, the classification of hypersensitivity in their patients is based essentially on answers to a questionaire, without recourse to a laboratory parameter, such as IgE level. Drs. Clarke, Fee, Dundee and myself decided to carry out a small trial in which we measured the plasma IgE levels (Pharmacia, PRIST technique) of two groups of 50 patients, one group attributed with hypersensitivity characteristics as a result of the standard questionaire, the other "normal". Significance of IgE level was based on values above the 95th centile of the normal population (>200 I.U./ml) Although the normal, control, group produced one patient above this level (this is approximately correct for the incidence of "atopy" within the population as a whole), the hypersensitive ascribed group produced only 25/50 patients with such levels. This was a much lower proportion than we expected and even more perplexing, several of the socalled hypersensitivity patients had extremely *low* levels of IgE, below 5 I.U./ml. There would thus appear to be two populations within the ascribed hypersensitive population of Clarke et al., one with classically raised IgE levels, the other with low or normal levels. We must now ask which of these two subgroups, or whether both, are represented in the *clinical* responders to intravenous agents.

Extrapolating our own studies makes it seem unlikely that both are represented equally since the bulk of the responses to hypnotic drugs investigated are to Althesin, which are predominantly complement mediated. It would thus appear that the two sides of Table 5.5 are not necessarily related either to each other or to the classical definition of atopy. Although irritating to the immunologist on theoretical grounds, we appear to have here a most useful practical test. The patient who *says* he is sensitive to any substance, however, apparently trivial e.g. zinc oxide plaster, and has received anaesthetic drug(s) on at least one previous occasion, must be considered "at risk". Perhaps we shall discover the significance of this strange phenotyping later.

Type I hypersensitivity reactions. There appears to be little doubt that the barbiturate hypnotics do preferentially activate classical Type I hypersensitivity reactions. Direct C3 activation is uncommon. Relatively few Althesin reactions involve the classical response mechanism while the muscle relaxants for the most part would also appear to involve either C3 activation or direct histamine release from mast cells, e.g. d-tubocurarine. The plasma substitutes (Johnson and Laurell, 1974) and radio-contrast media (Lang et al., 1976), similarly appear to involve the complement pathway at some point or other.

Reactions to barbiturate drugs are hence likely to be enhanced if the patient receives the drug again: "amplification" is a characteristic of immune mediated

156

reactions, but not of complement mediated reactions. The difference in basic mechanism is the most likely explanation to the observation (Clarke et al., 1975) that although Althesin reactions are reported in the literature more frequently than those to thiopentone only one death was reported in 90 cases of Althesin reaction: there were six deaths reported in 45 reactions following thiopentone. The data can be interpreted to indicate that, although the patient is more likely to have a reaction to Althesin than to thiopentone, *under theatre conditions* any reaction to the former is unlikely to be fatal.

Complement system anomalies

These can be divided into primary and secondary anomalies. Primary anomalies

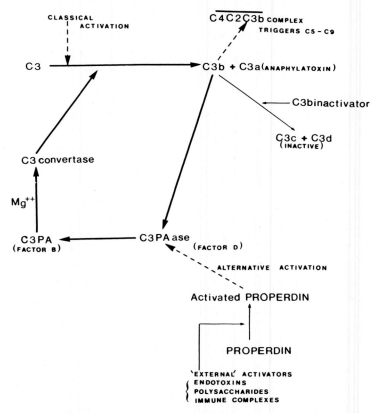

Fig. 5.6. Diagramatic representation of alternative pathway mechanism showing the various enzymes involved, their activators and their inhibitors.

comprise inherited anomalies of concentration or of function, or of both, within this system of enzymes, while secondary anomalies may arise as a result of ongoing immune or auto-immune processes disturbing the normal equilibrium of the complement system. Either situation may lead to complications with administered intravenous substances.

Primary anomalies

Complement C3 acts as a central factor for both the classical and the alternative pathways of activation and it is with this protein and its associated activator and inactivator enzymes that most of the problems appear to arise. Examination of the schematic alternative pathway mechanism (Fig. 5.6) reveals several factors which can either trigger or enhance the contribution of this cycle. The rate controlling step is the concentration of the active species C3b. Below a certain level this may take part either in the classical sequence or be harmlessly absorbed by the vascular tissues. The safety threshold is again likely to be genetic and may vary between individuals.

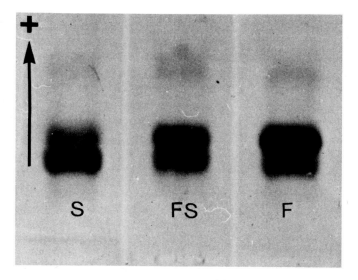

Fig. 5.7. Extended electrophoresis on agarose gels of the third component of human complement (C3). Plasma samples from patients exhibiting the three common C3 types. Patterns fixed specifically with anti C3 antiserum (immunofixation) after electrophoresis, the gel washed free from non-fixed plasma proteins and then stained with conventional protein stain. The common heterozygous phenotype FS appears as two distinct, equal intensity staining, bands.

Four factors which may increase the concentration beyond the safety threshold are (a) a genetic instability of complement C3, reflecting allotypic differences (b) an increased and abnormal rate of C3 conversion particularly following stimulation, again possibly genetic, but also due to activating species e.g. immune complex, (c) blocking of the inactivating protease for C3b (d) increased C3 convertase activity.

(a) Allotypic varieties of C3. Three electrophoretic distinct varieties of C3 have been established using prolonged agarose electrophoresis techniques (Fig. 5.7). These are usually considered to represent two homozygous allotypes S (slow) and F (fast) respectively and one heterozygous situation, FS. More than 20 rarer, apparently genetically controlled electrophoretic variants of C3 have been described (Rittner and Rittner, 1974) but whether or not all of these are true antigenically distinct allotypes or whether they represent precursors or conformational modifications of a few native C3 species is open to speculation. Nevertheless, there is some reason to believe that these electrophoretic patterns may tie up with C3 stability (see Table 5.6). Investigation has until now been hampered by the relatively small number of clinical cases usually available for analysis but it should now be possible to find a definite answer.

TABLE 5.6

GENETIC POLYMORPHISM IN HUMAN C3:
CORRELATION WITH ANAPHYLACTOID RESPONSE

Phenotype	Reported frequency (Switzerland)		Measured frequency			
			Controls		Anaphylactoid	Response
	n	%	n	%	n	%
F	129	4.4%	8	35%	9	82%
S	1865	63.0%	12	52%	1	9%
FS	939	32.0%	3	13%	1	9%

(b) rate of C3 conversion. It should be remembered that all the plasma proteins are in *dynamic* equilibrium and are not *static* entities. Amongst other factors they reflect the equilibrium between synthesis and catabolism and the distribution between vascular and extravascular pools. Low complement C3 and C4 levels, those which are within normal population range and non-pathological, may reflect an inherent tendency to breakdown as much as the inability of the individual to

synthesise higher levels. Many of the patients exhibiting complement mediated anaphylactoid reactions to Althesin have complement anomalies of this type, although the picture is often complicated by secondary utilization of the complement proteins in underlying immunopathological conditions (e.g. infection, immune complex disease). It is also obvious from Fig. 5.6 that these immunopathological features may stimulate C3 conversion by activating plasma properdin, thus amplifying both the classical and alternative pathways for the activation of C3–C9.

Other enzymes such as plasmin, trypsin and lysomal cathepsins may cleave C3 directly without the intervention of immune processes. Activation of these enzymes in inflammatory conditions may generate appreciable quantities of the anaphylatoxin, (C3a), and C3b. In vitro plasmin conversion is, of course, a problem in the analysis of patient plasma samples, often taken of necessity under less than ideal conditions.

(c) C3b inactivator activity. Unlike the other important protease inactivator of the complement system, C1 esterase inhibitor, *inherited* defects of the C3b inactivator are rare in man (Alper et al., 1972). In the absence of direct confirmation this is the most likely rate controlling step for the alternative pathway.

It is interesting to note that the two hypnotic drugs Althesin and Epontol, although very dissimilar chemically, have a similar predisposition to cause complement activation. The answer may lie, as many people suspect, in the detergent, Cremphor EL, used in both formulations.

(d) C3 convertase activity. This will, of course directly influence the rate of C3 conversion as in (b). The only established "activator" of this enzyme is a component of cobra venom, (CVF), which combines with the inactive enzyme precursor to form a convertase for C3 and the alternative pathway. The convertase formed by CVF action differs structurally from "native" convertase and may modify anaphylatoxin release. This should be remembered when examining animal models of anaphylactoid response and using cobra venom factor to activate C3. Conversion, measured experimentally in terms of the terminal product of C3b, C3c, gives no direct measure of anaphylatoxin (C3a) release activity.

Other involved complement components

Activation of the C2 kinin-like peptide, giving rise to vasodilation and oedema in the absence of histamine release appears relatively uncommon with the intravenous anaesthetic drugs. In the *inherited defect* (hereditary angioneurotic oedema, HANE) which is surprisingly widespread, the fault lies in either too low, or functionally inactive, C1 esterase inhibitor. It would seem a wise precaution, however, not to use drugs known to activate any part of the complement system, on patients with a history, or family history, of this condition. Low plasma levels of C1 inhibitor in otherwise healthy individuals have been reported to predispose to reactions with intravenous contrast media (Lasser, personal communication).

Secondary anomalies

Major disturbances of the complement system may arise as a result of chronic infection or of immune complex disease. The latter may exhibit appreciable degree of complement C3 conversion ($\leq 30\%$) in vivo. Synthetic immune complexes, e.g. albumin–antialbumin or heat aggregated IgG, will readily activate fresh serum samples in vitro and those reactions are frequently enhanced in the presence of "anaesthetic drugs". In vivo, reactions against the gelatin plasma expanders (e.g. Haemaccel) supposedly against antigelatin antibodies, may actually involve non-classical rheumatoid factors and euglobulins in the collagenosis patient (Richter et al., 1977). Many of the reactions to anaesthetic drugs examined in this laboratory involve patients whose immunoglobulin, complement and other plasma protein levels provide clear evidence of ongoing immune processes. These situations may will lead to increased properdin activity and the reactions in such patients are unlikely to be drug specific but more "patient specific". This is well illustrated by two recent case histories.

Case 1. The patient, a 21-year-old male student, had suffered from chronic otitis media since infance. This had necessitated a number of surgical procedures involving general anaesthesia over a period of 12 years. An initial exposure to Althesin was uneventful but his second exposure caused angio-oedema, peripheral vaseodilation and sweating. Following appropriate treatment, recovery progressed smoothly. Two further procedures over the next 4 years were carried out uneventfully with methohexitone. However, a further procedure (at age 21) involving thiopentone again produced angio-oedema. Neither reaction showed evidence of immunological hypersensitivity, only direct complement C3 conversion was involved, i.e. these were not drug specific hypersensitivity reactions.

Case 2. The patient, a 33-year-old male, was suffering from recurrent axillary abcesses, required incision drainage under general anaesthesia. A previous exposure to anaesthetic (methohexitone) had been uneventful but a second produced a delayed reaction, involving body rash, hypotension and some bronchospasm, one and a half hours after administration. Unfortunately, this reaction was not monitored by laboratory tests. Four months after this event, Althesin was used for induction and again a *delayed* anaphylactoid reaction occurred, apparently paralleling the methohexitone reaction. This reaction was shown to be C3 mediated.

The laboratory features of these two cases are summarised in the Table 5.7. The cases have overall similarity. Both patients possess chronic infection or secretion states which would be expected to make them more susceptible to complement C3 activation, particularly with potential "complement activating" drugs like Althesin. In either of these two subjects the absence of laboratory tests might have led the anaesthetist to believe that the patient was allergic to the first administered drug and excluded this on subsequent occasions. Later there would have been surprise and dismay when the patient again reacted adversely but to a totally unrelated drug.

Adverse pharmacological effects

An understanding of mechanisms of adverse response to intravenous agents is incomplete without an appreciation of pharmacological factors influencing drug

TABLE 5.7

PLASMA CHEMISTRY AT TIME OF ADVERSE RESPONSE

Incident	Anaesthetic	IgG (g/l)	IgA (g/l)	IgM (g/l)	IgE (I.U./ml)	C3 (g/l)	C4 (g/l)	C3 conversion (%)
Patient 1 (M; Age at first reaction, 18)								
Anaphylactoid response Oct. 1974	Althesin N$_2$O/O$_2$/ Halothane	10.1	2.6	0.6	260	0.42	0.12	>50
Lip swelling Jan., 1978	Thiopentone Sux. N$_2$O/O$_2$/Halothane	10.6	2.6	0.2	18	1.10	0.35	≤30
Patient 2 (M; Age, 33)								
Delayed anaphylactoid Dec., 1978	Methohexitone N$_2$O/O$_2$/Halothane				Reaction not monitored			
Delayed anaphylactoid April, 1979	Althesin N$_2$O/O$_2$/Halothane	8.3	1.6	0.4	98	0.85	0.32	≤50

Note:

Patient 1, first reaction, shows clear laboratory evidence of immunoglobulin and complement involvement in an underlying immune reaction; complement conversion arising from the intravenous agent is very obvious.

Patient 2, shows some evidence of underlying complement utilization in an immune process but again marked C3 conversion from the intravenous drug.

activity. A detailed study of these factors is beyond the scope of this chapter (see Tucker, 1978), but we can consider briefly the impact of immediate and of delayed pharmacological effects.

Immediate effects. These may be divided into local and systemic manifestations. The most important manifestations of the former are (a) thrombosis (b) extravasation necrosis and (c) sepsis. The systemic manifestations may involve speed of drug administration (whether bolus or continuous perfusion), operator error and interactions of solutions of inappropriate acidity or ionic strength. Some of these may in turn cause histamine release, prostaglandin release, and indeed, activation of several other *secondary* effectors of the inflammatory response at both local and systemic level. Many drugs release histamine directly from histamine containing cells without intermediary action. This may reflect both patient "sensitivity", in terms of the numbers of available histamine containing cells, specific chemical effects and either drug concentration or rate of drug administration.

Distribution of the injected substance to various body tissues is in proportion to their share of the cardiac output and in this respect the lung has a unique position since it receives all of this output initially and can then modify output. It is conceivable that the buffering effect of the lung can be severely modified by the appreciable (0.25–0.5 ml) test doses of drugs often given by the anaesthetist. This might well modify the pharmacokinetics sufficiently to predispose towards *pharmacological* response rather than exclude the far less likely anaphylactoid response.

Immediate vasodilation and hypotension is not uncommon following rapid injection of many substances, including narcotics, barbiturates and even radiocontrast media. This may well represent direct action on vascular smooth muscle and nerve endings (Blair, 1975). Reactivity may be exacerbated by underlying renal and liver disease, particularly with thiopentone (Ghoneim and Kortilla, 1977). This may in part reflect altered plasma protein binding in these pathological conditions. While albumin remains the major plasma binding protein for many drugs used in anaesthetic practice, lipoproteins and α_1 acid glyoprotein are also involved (Piafsky and Borga, 1977). The latter is particularly influenced by underlying inflammatory conditions, pregnancy and the use of oral contraceptives (Piafsky and Borga, 1977).

Delayed effects. Delayed effects may be considered as those occurring a day or more after administration of a drug or of some procedure. Although many drugs used by the anaesthetist are inactivated in the plasma, these metabolites may require further metabolism to polar products in the liver before they can be excreted through the kidneys. Clearance by the liver will obviously be impaired in liver disease. Metabolites may, in any case, be toxic to some degree in the liver and produce post-operative complications. Halothane hepatitis is frequently considered a manifestation of such catabolism although the combined effects of surgical, anaesthetic and other trauma must not be excluded. Even more delayed effects refer to ill-defined changes in the immune status of the patient measured perhaps in an increased predisposition to infection and perhaps to metastatic spread of tumour in the cancer patient. Many factors control such changes, none more so than the stress response linked to both surgical and anaesthetic trauma.

The stress response

This may be considered to be the sum of the bodies response to noxious stimuli and includes the contribution of surgical and anaesthetic trauma and the patient's psychological and physiological status. The stress response is expressed directly by changes in the hormone balance mediated through the central, hypothalmic and pituitary axis of the brain (Oyama, 1973; Van Brunt and Ganong, 1963). In turn, the hormone inbalance influences many other parameters including blood sugar (Clarke, 1970), cell metabolism and immune responsiveness. (Bruce and Wingard, 1971; Moudgil and Wade 1976).

Anaesthetic drugs and surgical trauma stimulate adrenocorticotrophine, cortisol, catecholamine and growth hormone (George et al., 1974): the influence of surgical trauma is probably greater than the drug effect. Catecholamine levels affect white cell levels and distributions and many anaesthetic gases used for prolonged periods may severely interrupt white cell maturation and function (Doenicke and Kropp, 1976); Moudgil and and Wade, 1976). Influences on the immune system are generally considered to be mediated by alteration of cell metabolism. However, there is little doubt that this can be brought about directly both by inhalational agents and by intravenous induction drugs in vitro. There seems to be some evidence that premedication with diazepines may selectively suppress T-lymphocytes populations (Allen and Watkins, unpublished work), further modifying the immune responsiveness of the host. The effects of anaesthetic agents directly, and stress overtly, on the immune responsiveness of the host are intricately interwoven. The presence of these drugs in patients makes conventional assessment of immune responsiveness in terms of PHA lymphocyte responsiveness (Bruce, 1975) almost valueless. However, it is difficult to believe that the changes which do occur will effectively reduce immune responsiveness of the host in the absence of grossly pathological conditions. The situation may well be different in patients maintained immobilized for long periods in intensive care under perfused anaesthetic drugs. Interference with immune responsiveness may well be a serious adverse response in such situations, directly attributable to the anaesthetic agent.

Psychological factors are even more difficult to define although they undoubtedly play a role in adverse reactions. The lady in Fig. 5.1c is clearly exhibiting some type of emotional response and it seems likely that some reported cases of similar minor clinical manifestations following anaesthetic induction involve these apparently harmless mechanisms. Nevertheless, many anaesthetists think that unpremedicated patients, particularly those in distressed emotional states, are most likely subjects for adverse response than premedicated patients. This may well be so, but it should be remembered that premedication may also pharmacologically protect against, or minimise, histamine release actions by the drugs used in anaesthetic practice. For example, the diazepines may encourage systemic prostaglandin release, acting directly on mast cell metabolism to prevent degranulation, while the use of disodium cromoglycate (Intal) in the ashmatic patient may also protect in an analagous manner. This would appear to be a fertile area for original investigation.

CONCLUSIONS

Immunological hypersensitivity, by definition, implies memory (antibody) mediated events which may be either immediate (Type I) or delayed (Type IV). The Type II and III hypersensitivity reactions may occupy intermediate positions in response timing: the life threatening situation with Type I reactions is brought about by gross release of systemic histamine and it is this (and related substances) which causes the clinical manifestation of the anaphylactoid (histaminoid) response. Such histamine, or other mediator, release can also be brought about by reactions in which antibodies are not involved at all and the clinical manifestations are quite indistinguishable from the true antibody mediated reactions.

The majority of the immediate anaphylactoid reactions to the drugs used in anaesthesia do not involve antibodies or other immunological memory mediated mechanisms, but are brought about by direct activation of secondary mediators, particularly complement, which release histamine or kinins with vasodilatory activity. Unlike true antibody mediated reactions the clinical situation in such responding patients is unlikely to be exacerbated if the drug(s) is used again by chance on some later occasion. Antibody mediated reactions will be exacerbated and may lead to death, irrespective of any resuscitative procedure used by the anaesthetist. It is important, therefore, to establish the mechanism for anaphylactoid response in a particular patient.

Non-immune mediated reactions to anaesthetic drugs may also be life theatening, the extent of reaction reflecting the pharmacokinetics of the drug (or drug interactions) and physiological and psychological features of the patient.

We cannot, as yet, satisfactorily predict definite reactivity but we can define patients at greater risk to anaesthetic drugs than the population as a whole. Genetic features of the immunoglobulin and complement systems are obvious high risk factors but the role of "atopy" is probably exaggerated. Nevertheless, repeated exposures to the same drug or drugs should be avoided if at all possible. Relatively temporary features such as infection and stress should also be considered when selecting anaesthetic drugs. They may contra-indicate certain drugs e.g. Althesin and suggest the inclusion of others, e.g. the use of Fentanyl in "stress".

Finally, the problem of anaphylactoid response should be put into perspective for the anaesthetist. Radiological control media has probably the highest potential risk with a mortality rate of 1 in 40,000 patients, about 15 patients in the United Kindom per year. Anaphylactoid response resulting in death from anaesthetic drugs and plasma substitutes is far less frequent.

REFERENCES

Alper, C.A., Rosen, F.S. and Lachman, P.J. (1972): Inactivator of the third component of complement as an inhibitor in the properdin pathway. *Proc. nat. Acad. Sci. (Wash.), 69*, 2910-2913.

Berrens, L., Koers W.J. and Bruynzeel, P.L.B. (1977): IgE and IgG$_4$ antibodies in specific allergies. *Lancet, 2*, 92.

Blair, M.R. (1975): Cardiovascular pharmacology of local anaesthetics. *Brit. J. Anaesth., 47*, 247-252.

Bruce, D.L. (1975): Halothane inhibition of RNA and protein synthesis of PHA-treated human lymphocytes. *Anaesthesiology, 42*, 11-14.

Bruce, D.L. and Wingard, D.W. (1971): Anaesthesia and the immune response. *Anaesthesiology, 34*, 271-277.

Van Brunt, E.E. and Ganong, W.F. (1963): The effects of preanaesthetic medication, anaesthesia and hypothermia on the endocrine response to injury. *Anaesthesiology, 24*, 500-513.

Clarke, R.S.J. (1970): The hyperglycaemic response to different types of surgery and anaesthesia. *Brit. J. Anaesth., 42*, 45-53.

Clarke, R.S.J., Dundee, J.W., Garrett, R.T., McArdle, G.K. and Sutton, J.A. (1975): Adverse reactions to intravenous anaesthetics: a survey of 100 reports. *Brit. J. Anaesth. 47*, 575-585.

Doenicke, A. and Kropp, W. (1976): Anaesthesia and the reticuloendothelial system: Comparison of halothane-nitrous oxide and neuroleptanalgesia. *Brit. J. Anaesth., 48*, 1191-1195.

Doenicke, A., Lorenz, W., Beigl, R., Bezecny, H., Uhlig, G., Kalmar, L., Praetorius, B. and Mann, G. (1973): Histamine release after intravenous application of short acting hypnotics. A comparison of etomidate, Althesin CT 1341 and propanidid. *Brit. J. Anaesth., 45*, 1097-1104.

Donaldson, V.H. (1967): Mechanisms of activation of C1 esterase in hereditary angioneurotic edema plasma in vitro. The role of Hageman factor, a clot promoting agent. *J. exp. Med., 127*, 411-429.

Dundee, J.W., Fee, J.P.H., McDonald, J.R. and Clarke, R.S.J. (1978): Frequency of atopy and allergy in an anaesthetic patient population. *Brit. J. Anaesth., 50*, 793-798.

Fee, J.P.H., McDonald, J.R., Dundee, J.W. and Clarke, R.S.J. (1978): Frequency of previous anaesthesia in an anaesthetic patient population. *Brit. J. Anaesth., 50*, 917-920.

Fisher, M. McD. (1976): Intradermal testing after severe histamine reactions to intravenous drugs used in anaesthesia. *Anaesth. Intens. Care, 4*, 97-104.

Garrett, R.T. (1978): The clinical manifestations of adverse reactions following Althesin and thiopentone. In: *Adverse Response to Intravenous Drugs*. Editors: J. Watkins and A.M. Ward. Academic Press, London, New York. pp. 37-40.

George, J.M., Reier, G.E., Lanese, R.R. and Rower, J.H. (1974): Morphine anaesthesia blocks cortisol and growth hormone response to surgical stress in humans. *J. clin. Endocr. Metab., 38*, 736-741.

Ghoneim, M.M. and Kortilla, K. (1977): Pharmacokinetics of intravenous anaesthetics: Implications for clinical use. *Clin. Pharmacokin., 2*, 344-372.

Glen, J.B., Davies, G.E., Thomson, D.S., Scarth, S.C. and Thompson, A.V. (1978): Adverse reactions to intravenous anaesthetics in animals. In: *Adverse Response to Intravenous Drugs*. Editors: J. Watkins and A.M. Ward. Academic Press, London, New York, pp. 129-135.

Glen, J.B., Davies, G.E., Thomson, D.S., Scarth, S.C. and Thompson, A.V. (1979): The response of the mini-pig to repeated injections of Cremophor-containing and non-Cremophor containing intravenous anaesthetics. *Brit. J. Anaesth., 51*, 819-827.

Hedin, H., Richter, W. and Ring, J. (1976): Dextran induced anaphylactoid reactions in man. Role of dextran reactive antibodies. *Int. Arch. Allerg. appl. Immunol., 52*, 145-159.

Johnson, U. and Laurell, A.B. (1974): Activation of complement in anaphylactoid reactions in connection with infusion of dextran. *Scand. J. Immunol., 3*, 673-676.

Lang, J.H., Lasser, E.C. and Kolb, W.P. (1976): Activation of serum complement by contrast media. *Invest. Radiol., 2*, 303-308.

Lorenz, W. (1975): Histamine release in man. *Agents Actions, 5*, 402-416.

Lorenz, W. and Doenicke, A. (1978): Anaphylactoid reactions and histamine release by intravenous drugs used in surgery and anaesthesia. In: *Adverse Response to Intravenous Drugs*. Editors: J. Watkins and A.M. Ward. Academic Press, London, New York. pp. 83-112.

Lorenz, W., Reimann, H.J., Schmal, A., Dorman, P., Schwarz, B., Neugebauer, E. and Doenicke, A. (1977): Histamine release in dogs by Cremophor EL and its derivatives: oxethylated oleic acid is the most effective constituent. *Agents Actions, 7*, 63-67.

Moudgil, G.C., Allan, R.B., Russell, R.J. and Wilkinson, P.C. (1977): Inhibition by anaesthetic agents of human leucocytes locomotion towards chemical attractants. *Brit. J. Anaesth., 49*, 97-105.

Moudgil, C.C. and Wade, A.G. (1976): Anaesthesia and immunocompetence. *Brit. J. Anaesth., 48*, 31-39.

Oyama, T., (1973): Endocrine responses to anaesthetic agents. *Brit. J. Anaesth., 45*, 276-281.

Preston, F.E. (1979): Haematological problems associated with shock. *Brit. J. Hosp. Med., 21*, 232-245.

Piafsky, K.M. and Borga, O. (1977): Plasma protein binding of basic drugs. II. Importance of α_1 acid glycoprotein for interindividual variation. *Clin. Pharmacol. Ther., 22*, 545-549.

Ratnoff, O.D. and Naff, G.B. (1967): The conversion of C1s to C1 esterase by plasmin and trypsin. *J. exp. Med., 125*, 337-358.

Richter, W., Hedin, H. and Ring, J. (1977): Immunological findings in infusions of colloid solutions. *Med. Welt, 28*, 1717-1719.

Richter, W., Messmer, K., Hedin, H. and Ring, J. (1978): Adverse reactions to plasma substitutes: incidence and pathomechanisms. In: *Adverse Response to Intravenous Drugs*. Editors: J. Watkins and A.M. Ward. Academic Press, London, New York. pp. 49-70.

Ring, J. (1976): *Habitationsschrift*, Universität München.

Rittner, C. and Rittner, B. (1974): Report 1973-1974 of the reference laboratory for the polymorphism of the third component (C3) of the human complement system. *Vox. Sang., 27*, 464-472.

Tucker, G.T. (19787: Pharmacokinetic aspects of the intravenous bolus. In: *Adverse Response to Intravenous Drugs*. Editors: J. Watkins and A.M. Ward. Academic Press, London, New York. pp. 1-15.

Vanezis, P. (1979): Death after Althesin. *The Practitioner, 222*, 259-251.

Watkins, J. (1979b): Anaphylactoid reactions to i.v. substances. *Brit. J. Anaesth., 51*, 51-60.

Watkins, J., Allen, R. and Ward, A.M. (1978b): Adverse response to alphadolone/alphaxalone: possible role of IgD. *Lancet, 2*, 736.

Watkins, J. and Clarke, R.S.J. (1978): Report of a symposium. Adverse responses to intravenous agents. *Brit. J. Anaesth., 50*, 1159-1164.

Watkins, J., Clark, A., Appleyard, T.N. and Padfield, A. (1976): Immune mediated reactions to Althesin (alphaxalone). *Brit. J. Anaesth., 48*, 881-886.

Watkins, J., Padfield, A. and Alderson, J.D. (1978c): Underlying immunopathology as a cause of adverse responses to two intravenous agents. *Brit. Med. J., 1*, 1180-1181.

Watkins, J., Thornton, J.A. and Clarke, R.S.J. (1979a): Adverse reactions to i.v. agents. *Brit. J. Anaesth., 51*, 469.

Watkins, J., Udnoon, S., Appleyard, T.N. and Thornton, J.A., (1976b): Identification and quantitation of hypersensitivity reactions to intravenous anaesthetic agents. *Brit. J. Anaesth., 48*, 457-461.

Watkins, J., Udnoon, S. and Taussig, P.E. (1978a): Mechanisms of adverse response to intravenous agewnts in man. In: *Adverse Response to Intravenous Drugs*. Editors: Academic Press, London. New York. pp. 71-82.

Watkins, J., Ward, A.M., and Appleyard, T.N. (1977): Changes in peripheral blood leucocytes following i.v. anaesthesia and surgery. *Brit. J. Anaesth., 49*, 953.

Weitkamp, L.R., Salzano, F.M., Neel, J., Porta, F., Geerdinf, R.A. and Tanoky, A.L. (1973): Human serum albumin: twenty-three genetic variants and their population distribution. *Ann. hum. Genet., 36*, 381-392.

Witten, D.M. (1975): Reactions to urographic contrast media. *J.A.M.A., 231*, 974-977.

Zimmerman, T.S., Arroyave, C.M. and Müller-Eberhard, H.J. (1971): A blood coagulation abnormality in rabbits deficient in the sixth component of complement (C6) and its correction by purified C6. *J. Exp. Med., 134*, 1591-1600.

6

The role of histamine in adverse reactions to intravenous agents *

W. Lorenz, A. Doenicke, B. Schöning and E. Neugebauer

1. INTRODUCTION

Since Alam et al. (1939) first directed histamine release by curare several thousand studies have been devoted to the questions of whether or not histamine plays any significant role in adverse reactions to intravenous agents, and whether this role can be distinctly defined – qualitatively and quantitatively. Excluding the numerous reviews and books on type I, antigen-antibody anaphylaxis (Gell and Coombs, 1975) and without any real attempt to be complete we have found about 40 surveys on this subject, some of these merely collect data more or less comprehensively (first group), some of them stress special hypotheses or points of view from a large spectrum of opinions (second group).

Examples of the first group of surveys were produced by Rocha e Silva (1955), Wolstenholme and O'Connor (1956) as the editors of the famous Ciba Foundation symposium, Paton (1957, 1958, 1959), Rothschild (1966), Giertz and Hahn (1966), Mota (1966), Goth (1972), Maslinski (1975) and Beaven (1978). The majority of their data referred to animal and in-vitro experiments, and since all these authors were educated as basic research scientists the readers will find little emphasis on the clinical relevance and on urgent therapeutic consequences of the findings reported in these surveys.

On the other hand reviews have been published in recent years which were compiled by clinicians who were concerned about anaphylactoid events in their daily work. These surveys dealt mainly with the clinical incidence, diagnosis and therapy

*Supported by grant of Deutsche Forschungsgemeinschaf (Lo 199/10).

of adverse reactions to intravenous agents in which histamine was assumed to be involved. Examples of such reviews still belonging in the first group of surveys are those produced by Murphy (1962), Dundee and Wyant (1974), Clarke et al. (1975), Fisher (1975), Doenicke (1977), Langrehr et al. (1977), Walton (1978) and Ahnefeld et al. (1979).

Examples of the second group of surveys (reviews on smaller facets of the rather complicated problems) were also published by numerous investigators. Studies on isolated mast cells were comprehensively described by Kazimierczak and Diamant (1978) and Fantozzi et al. (1978), those on the cardiovascular system by Levi et al. (1977), Altura and Halevy (1978a, b), Reinhardt (1979) and Pavek and Wegmann (1980), those on plasma histamine assays by Lorenz and Doenicke (1973), Lorenz (1975), Beaven (1976), Lorenz and Doenicke (1978a,b) and those on the mechanisms of active substance release in adverse reactions to intravenous agents by Ring and Messmer (1977b), Ring (1978), Watkins and Ward (1978) as the editors of the first Sheffield meeting on adverse reactions to drugs, by Richter et al. (1978), Watkins and Clarke (1978) and by Watkins (1979).

This impressive number of papers, however, does *not* produce a convincing answer to the question of whether the role of histamine can be distinctly defined in adverse reactions to intravenous agents in *clinical states* — except in the case of the anaesthetic drug propanidid (Epontol[R]) (Lorentz et al., 1972a; Lorenz, 1975) and the plasma substitute Haemaccel (Messmer et al., 1970; Lorenz et al., 1974a,b,c; Lorenz et al., 1976, 1977a, 1980; Lorenz and Doenicke, 1978a). The numerous reasons for this disappointing finding will be analysed in the following sections.

2. DEFINITION OF THE TYPE OF ADVERSE REACTIONS TO DRUGS AS "ANAPHYLACTOID" AND "ALLERGOID"

Instead of "adverse reaction" the terms "anaphylactoid reaction" and "allergoid reaction" are used to describe more precisely which type of adverse reactions to drugs is considered to be associated with free, biologically active histamine. In the past the definition of such reactions has been a matter of vehement discussion, but an agreement was obtained by most of the research workers in the field (Lorenz et al., 1977a, 1978b; Watkins and Clarke, 1978; Kazimierczak and Diamant, 1978; Lorenz et al., 1980):

(a) According to the participants of the second Sheffield meeting on adverse reactions to drugs (Watkins and Clarke, 1978) the term "anaphylactoid" merely defines clinical manifestations (cutaneous, pulmonary and cardiovascular) which resemble those of immediate, immune-mediated hypersensitivity reactions. The term "allergoid" to describe clinical manifestations restricted to the skin was also acceptable to the participants.

(b) According to Kazimierczak and Diamant (1978) mast cells and basophils can be triggered to release histamine and other mediators by various non-reagin-mediated stimuli. The clinical signs and symptoms elicited in this way are the effects of the same mediators and thus cannot be distinguished from those of the immediate allergic (anaphylactic) reaction. In contrast to the IgE-specific anaphylactic state these non-reaginic reactions are denoted as "anaphylactoid".

(c) According to Lorenz et al. (1978b) reactions to drugs or surgical treatment which cause various combinations of clinical symptoms (Table 6.1) mimicing anaphylaxis or allergy were defined as "anaphylactoid" or "allergoid", if they could not unequivocably be *demonstrated* to be caused by defined immunological processes involving reaginic antibodies (e.g. IgE or IgG4).

The functional or operational aspect which is emphasized by the last definition enforced Lorenz et al. (1977a, 1978a, 1980) to particularly differentiate between "anaphylactoid" and "allergoid" reactions since elevated plasma histamine levels

TABLE 6.1

CLINICAL SYMPTOMS AND BIOLOGICAL REACTIONS OBSERVED IN ANAPHYLACTOID AND ALLERGOID REACTIONS IN MAN

Items obtained from case reports in the literature (cf. Lorenz et al., 1972a, 1976; Fisher, 1975) and from a controlled trial in 40 volunteers receiving i.v. histamine and Haemaccel (Lorenz et al., 1978a, and data later on in this communication).

(1) Skin	*(2) Gastrointestinal tract*	*(3) Respiratory tract*
– Sensation of heat	– Metallic taste	– Sneezing
– Red ears	– Salivation	– Snuffling
– Erythema	– Heartburn	– Stuffed-up nose
– Flush	– Epigastric fullness	– Nasal catarrh
– Hives (wheals)	– Nausea	– Narrowness in the throat
– Pruritus	– Vomiting	– Narrowness in the chest
– Conjunctivitis	– Gastrointestinal pain	– Coughing
– Blepharoedema	(cramps, colics)	– Respiratory distress
– Swollen ears	– Straining	– Bronchospasm
– Quincke's oedema	– Defecation	

(4) Head and nervous system	*(5) Heart and circulation*
– Tinnitus	– Tachycardia (rare: bradycardia)
– Congestion in the head	– Arrhythmia
– Pulsation in the temporal region	– Disturbed atrioventricular conduction
– Headache	– Hypotension (rare: Hypertension)
– Drowsiness	– Circulatory and cardiac insufficiency
– Dizziness	and arrest
– Sensation of hang-over	

could be predicted with a high efficiency only in the case of the former (Lorenz et al., 1978a, 1980). For this reason "anaphylactoid" reactions were classified by the criteria of generalized urticaria (more than 5 wheals in different regions of the body), discomfort (nasal catarrh, narrowness of the throat, blepharoedema, nausea or vomiting, diarrhoea), bronchospasm, tachycardia, hypotension, cardiac arrest. At least generalized urticaria *plus* discomfort (except dermal pruritus) were necessary for classifying an adverse reaction to drugs or operations (Lorenz et al., 1973a; Meyer-Burgdorff et al., 1973; Thermann et al., 1977) as "anaphylactoid". Generalized urticaria plus tachycardia, but also bronchospasm, cardiac arrhythmia, hypotension or cardiac arrest with or without urticaria were other combinations of clinical findings being classified as "anaphylactoid". "Allergoid" reactions were classified by erythema, urticaria and dermal pruritus *only* (Lorenz et al., 1977a, 1980).

(d) According to Dúkor et al. (1980) unexpected adverse responses to drugs, the signs and symptoms of which mimic those of an allergic section of any type (type I–IV according Gell and Coombs, 1975) were denoted as *pseudo-allergic*, anaphylactoid and allergoid (= antineurons anaphylactoid) reactions are in agreement with that definition if they are considered as pseudo-allergic reactions of type I.

Only the clinician in his day-to-day practice in anaesthesia, surgery, or intensive care knows how difficult it is to detect and record all these symptoms or combinations of symptoms in clinical states leading to the diagnosis of an "anaphylactoid" or "allergoid" reaction. Moreover in addition, special precautions have to be taken to acchieve high specificity in medical decision making (Lusted, 1968). The numerous errors in recording "bronchospasm" were listed comprehensively by Fisher (1975). Short or long lasting tachycardia occurs for many reasons such as the primary disease state, surgical or psychological trauma, or by drug effects. Atropine or muscle relaxants may induce tachycardia by mechanisms other than release of histamine (Rothschild, 1966; Lorenz et al., 1974d, 1978b). In addition we have recently learnt to improve the sensitivity of our clinical decision making: Life-threatening cardiac arrhythmias, tachycardia and/or hypotension may be recorded without significant skin manifestations and may not be accepted as anaphylactoid reactions despite the fact that mediator release could be demonstrated (Cohen et al., 1979; Lorenz et al., 1980). The same is true of gastrointestinal manifestations of adverse reactions to dextran (Lorenz et al., 1976) or headache and the metallic taste in the case of Haemaccel (Lorenz et al., 1977a, 1978a).

Misleading definitions of "anaphylactoid" and "allergoid reactions" (mainly by highly sophisticated basic research scientists) have caused considerable confusion and − to the grave disadvantage of patients! − have excluded clinical syndromes in day-to-day practice which clearly should be diagnosed and treated as anaphylactoid reactions, for instance heart and gastrointestinal manifestations. The misleading definitions have masked the true incidence of anaphylactoid reactions to intravenous agents (for a discussion of this problem see Schöning and Koch, 1975; Ring and Messmer, 1977a; Lorenz et al., 1980). Finally this is one of the major reasons why the role of histamine could not be clearly elucidated in the causation of clinically significant adverse reactions to intravenous agents.

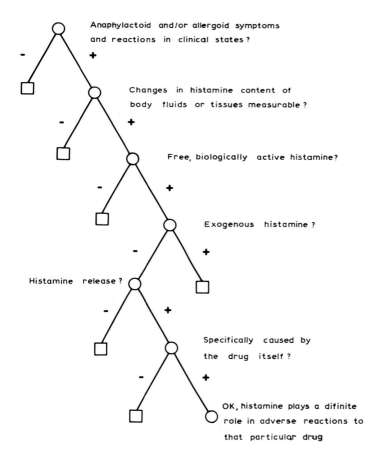

Fig. 6.1. Decision tree defining an intravenous agent as a chemical histamine liberator in clinical states. The structure includes 7 test nodes and 6 binary branches of which 5 were positive. According to Lusted, 1968.

3. DECISION TREE FOR DEFINING AN INTRAVENOUS AGENT AS HISTAMINE LIBERATOR IN CLINICAL STATES

Incorrect logistics is one of the main obstacles against the assessment of a definite role for histamine and other candidates for active substances (mediators) in adverse reactions to drugs (Fig. 6.1).

3.1. Anaphylactoid and/or allergoid symtoms and reactions in clinical states?

Following administration of a particular drug the clinical symptoms and biological reactions usually observed in anaphylactoid and allergoid reactions in man (Table 6.1) must be detected and recorded in agreement with their definitions. For many subjective and practical reasons it is not always easy to recognize the real incidence. The observer variation is very high.

As an example, the anaesthetic drug propanidid was reported to be free of allergic side-effects in 35 000 or 40 000 applications (Harrfeldt, 1970; Rasche and Harrfeldt, 1973) whereas in other studies (Dannemann and Lübke, 1970; Kay, 1972; Doenicke, 1974) the incidence of anaphylactoid reactions was 1 in 750, 1 in 1700 and 1 in 540 (for a survey see Clarke et al., 1978).

Similarly, the plasma substitutes based on chemically modified gelatin were originally described as free from anaphylactoid incidents (Lundsgaard-Hansen, 1969) whereas in a controlled clinical trial the incidence of those reactions was more than 1 per cent (Schöning and Koch, 1975). Until now only the plasma substitute Haemaccel has been subjected *repeatedly* to strict and meticulous randomized trials in patients and human volunteers (Table 6.2). The comparison of the incidence of adverse reactions to this drug in controlled trials with that in an occasional survey (Ring and Messmer, 1977a) showed an incredible 200–300 times difference. However, the same extraordinary discrepancy occurred in the case of "modified fluid gelatin" (incidence 0.07% (Ring and Messmer, 1977a) versus 15 and 31% (Schöning and Koch, 1975 and 1980)) and in the case of oxypolygelatin (0.25% (Ring and Messmer, 1977a) versus 19 and 8(3–18)% (Schöning and Koch, 1975)). It is impossible to define the role of histamine in adverse responses to drugs administered in clinical states if they are not recognized at all, or only so extremely rare and with such an observer variation as shown in Table 6.2.

In addition, it must be demonstrated in clinical states that the drug *itself* is responsible for an adverse reaction, and not the exposure to a solvent or the insertion of a needle. For this reason the drug again has to be tested in a comparative clinical trial against its solvent mixture in exactly the same composition as used for drug delivery. Examples of clinical symptoms of adverse reactions to sodium muriate and concomitant histamine release were published by Lorenz and

TABLE 6.2

INCIDENCE OF ANAPHYLACTOID AND ALLERGOID REACTIONS TO HAEMACCEL
COMPARISON OF FIVE PROSPECTIVE TRIALS

The studies of Schöning and Koch (1975) and Lorenz et al. (1980) were executed in patients and were prolective, cohort, randomized controlled trials. The trials of Lorenz et al. (1977a) and Lorenz et al. (1978a) were performed in human volunteers using the high infusion speed of 500 ml in 3 min (pressure infusion). Ring and Messmer's (1977a) report was an occasional survey.

Number of infusions (n_1)	Number of infusions complicated by reactions (n_2)	Incidence (n_2/n_1) (%)	Trial
150	45	30	Schöning and Koch (1975)
6151	9	0.15	Ring and Messmer (1977a)
25	9	36	Lorenz et al. (1977a, 1980)
40	21	53	Lorenz and Doenicke (1978a)
600	187	31	Lorenz et al. (1980)

Doenicke (1978b) and Lorenz et al. (1980). J. Watkins (personal communication) observed the full clinical picture of an adverse reaction in a young lady just after inserting a needle and Schöning counted five vagal syncopes and one bronchospastic reaction in the 600 patients of our trial (Lorenz et al., 1980) in the time between inserting the braunula and starting the infusion of Haemaccel. It is quite easy to imagine that in a clinical situation other than a meticulously performed controlled trial these 6 clinical incidents would have been classified as "anaphylactoid reactions" to the drug given a few seconds later, blood taken for histamine assay, *no* histamine release detected and a new hypothesis on the pathomechanism of the adverse response to that particular drug published a few months later.

The importance of anaphylactoid and allergoid reactions to an intravenous agent in clinical conditions can be illustrated by the case of atropine. As an intravenous premedication in anaesthesia this drug caused histamine release in human subjects with the same incidence and similar severity as sodium chloride (Lorenz et al., 1974d; Lorenz and Doenicke, 1978b). However, injected into the human skin or applied to cats and dogs in doses upto 15 mg/kg it was clearly demonstrated to be a histamine liberator (Rothschild, 1966). It would be incorrect logistics if in the event of an adverse reaction to atropine premedication one would assume that this was caused by its effect as a *chemical* histamine releaser. The last step cannot be done before the first.

3.2. **Are changes in histamine content of body fluids or tissues measurable?**

The second step in the decision tree (Fig. 6.1) considers the question of whether, in patients or test persons, any changes in mediator concentrations in body fluids or tissues (such as the skin) can be measured in association with the observed adverse reaction. Some important characteristics of a mediator are given in Table 6.3. There are numerous candidates for mediators (active substances) (Table 6.4). In this article and especially in this section on logistics we restrict ourselves to the role of histamine and ask whether changes in the histamine content of body fluids or tissues are measurable.

The answer to this question depends mainly on four conditions: (1) reliable assay of histamine (2) in samples of the relevant organ system or tissue (3) at the right time (4) under correct in-vivo (clinical) conditions.

TABLE 6.3

SOME CHARACTERISTICS OF A MEDIATOR (ACTIVE SUBSTANCE)

- its effects are either observable in categories or measurable continuously in a biological system
- it is an endogenous, chemically defined compound, not a phenomenon
- it acts at a receptor which characterizes the type of its effects (dose-response relation, mass-action law)
- it releases, forms or influences the metabolism of a substance acting at a receptor
- it stimulates or modulates a second messenger system

TABLE 6.4

GROUPS OF CANDIDATES FOR ACTIVE SUBSTANCES (AS) IN CLINICAL CONDITIONS
5-HT serotonin, SRS-A slow-reacting substance of anaphylaxis, ECF-A eosinophil chemotactic factor of anaphylaxis, NCF-A neutrophil chemotactic factor of anaphylaxis, PAF platelet-activating factor. For a survey see also Kazimierczak and Diamant (1978).

AS acting at receptors	Histamine, catecholamines, 5-HT, kinins, anaphylatoxins SRS-A, ECF-A, NCF-A, PAF, prostaglandins, thromboxanes
Releaser or former of AS	Anaphylatoxins (C3a and C5a) arginine esterase, C1-esterase
Stimulator or modulator of second-messenger systems	Acetylcholine, ATP, cyclic nucleotides, Ca^{2+}

3.2.1. *The reliable assay of histamine*

To show changes in histamine content samples of plasma, whole blood, urine, gastric juice, saliva, blister fluid or biopsies of skin, gastrointestinal and respiratory tract can be taken from human subjects under in-vivo conditions. The histamine assay can be performed by three methods, the bio-assay, the fluorometric assay and the radioenzymatic assay (Table 6.5). It can, however, not be predicted whether one of these assays will be reliable for measuring histamine in a particular body fluid or tissue under correct in-vivo conditions, for example after injection of intravenous agents, during operation or in a state of disease.

TABLE 6.5

METHODS USED TODAY FOR DETERMINING HISTAMINE IN TISSUES AND BODY FLUIDS
The fluorometric assay of Lorenz et al. (1970, 1972b) is denoted in the text as fluorometric-fluoroenzymatic since the identification of the substance measured in the assay among other procedures is carried out with purified histamine methyltransferase (Lorenz et al., 1972b; Barth et al., 1973, 1980). The distinction between fluorometric and fluoroenzymatic has become necessary because of the repeatedly proposed argument of a low sensitivity and specificity against the fluorometric assay (Beaven et al., 1972; Beaven, 1976; Domschke et al., 1977; Taylor et al., 1980) which is true for the Shore procedure, but definitely *not* for the assay of Lorenz et al. (1970, 1972b).

Principle	First publication	Optimum development till today regarding reliability*
Bio-assay on the terminal isolated guinea-pig ileum	Guggenheim and Löffler, 1916	Adam et al., 1957
Fluorometric assay following condensation with o-phthaldialdehyde	Shore et al., 1959	Lorenz et al., 1970, 1972b, Lorenz and Doenicke, 1978b
Enzymatic double isotope dilution assay using histamine methyltransferase	Snyder et al., 1966	Beaven et al., 1972; Taylor and Snyder, 1972; Beaven and Horáková, 1978

* Reliability: Sensitivity, specificity, precision and accuracy.

This controversial subject has been treated comprehensively in several reviews and original articles (Lorenz et al., 1974a; Lorenz, 1975; Beaven, 1976; Horáková et al., 1977; Beaven and Horáková, 1978; Lorenz and Doenicke, 1978a; Lorenz et al., 1978a; Rohde et al., 1980) and can be summarized at present: The original fluorometric assay of Shore et al. (1959) has the most limitations, the bio-assay the

178

second-most. The fluorometric-fluoroenzymatic assay (Lorenz et al., 1970, 1972b) and the enzymatic double-isotope dilution assay (Beaven et al., 1972) are *equally* suitable for measuring histamine in many conditions. For human plasma histamine determination at present the modified fluorometric-fluoroenzymatic assay (Lorenz and Doenicke, 1978b, Lorenz et al., 1978b) is the most sensitive test available. Using this method the normal plasma histamine concentration was found to be only 245 pg/ml on the average (Fig. 6.2).

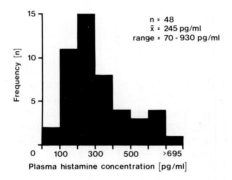

Fig. 6.2. Histogram of normal plasma histamine concentrations in human subjects. Plasma histamine levels determined by the modified fluorometric assay of Lorenz et al. (1978b); Lorenz and Doenicke, 1978b. Single values obtained from plasma samples of 50 orthopedic patients (Lorenz et al., 1980). 2 samples were lost during the extraction step. Calculation of the median and range.

In certain circumstances, however, both the fluorometric-fluoroenzymatic assay and the radioenzymatic assay give unreliable results (Lorenz et al., 1974a,b; Lorenz and Doenicke, 1978a; Beaven and Horáková, 1978; Subramanian et al., 1978). Tests after administration of intravenous agents are an example, especially the plasma substitues (Figs. 6.3 and 6.4; Table 6.6 and 6.7). For this reason it is mandatory to test the reliability of any histamine assay whenever a new drug, operation, disease etc. is investigated. It is irrational to develop theories about any pathomechanism of histamine release (such as following injection of contrast media!) before this possible error has been carefully excluded.

3.2.2. *Sample-taking from the relevant organ system or tissue*

From the theory that histamine elicits anaphylactoid and allergoid reactions mainly by binding to and acting at receptors (at present H_1- and H_2-receptors (Black

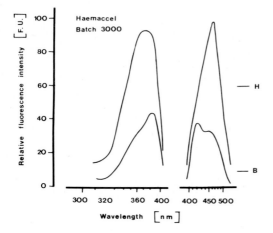

Fig. 6.3. Fluorescence excitation and emission spectra of the O-phthaldialdehyde-reactive substances demonstrated in Haemaccel. H = Haemaccel; B = reagent blank. For further conditions see Lorenz et al. (1974b).

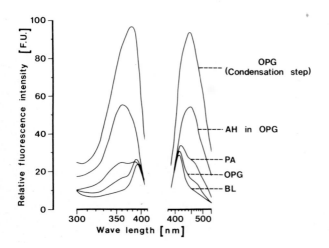

Fig. 6.4. Fluorescence excitation and emission spectra of the O-phthaldialdehyde-reactive substances demonstrated in oxypolygelatin (Gelifundol(R)). OPG (condensation step) = oxypolygelatin, diluted 1:2000 with 0.1 M HCl, used as native plasma substitute for the condensation step. OPG = extract of 6 ml OPG following the combined method (negligible fluorescence, but only for the batches used in Table 6.6!). AH in OPG = authentic histamine (30 ng) added to 6 ml OPG, thereafter combined method. Bl = reagent blank. PA = plasma from a patient suffering from an anaphylactoid reaction to OPG. Note the histamine which can be clearly demonstrated in the plasma (about 2 ng/ml plasma).

TABLE 6.6

SUBSTANCES IN PLASMA SUBSTITUTES WHICH INTERFERE WITH THE FLUOROMETRIC
PLASMA HISTAMINE ASSAY

All values are arithmetic means obtained from a pair of estimations on two different days. For
measurement the native plasma substitute was diluted with 0.1 M HCl (initially 0.1 ml plus 1.9 ml hydro-
chloric acid) and then underwent the usual condensation step at 21° C (Lorenz et al., 1972b). The extract
after the combined method (Dowex 50 + butanol extraction) was obtained from 6 ml plasma substitute
treated by 2 ml 2 M HClO$_4$ in the same way as human plasma (Lorenz et al., 1972b). Haemaccel
(polyurea gelatin) batch 1 = Op 3000, batch 2 = Op 3812. Gelifundol[(R)]S (oxypolygelatin) batch 1 = 29056,
batch 2 = 41056. Neoplasmagel[(R)] (gelatin cross-linked by succinic acid anhydride) batch 1 = 614 361,
batch 2 = 615 462. Macrodex[(R)] (dextran-60) batch 1 = G 320 C 6, batch 2 = G 321 C 6. Plasmasteril[(R)]
(Hydroxyethyl starch, 400/0.7) batch 1 = AE 146/K5, batch 2 = AE 147/K7. Following the combined
method interfering substances are reasonably separated from histamine in all cases except Haemaccel.

Drug	Batch	Fluorescence intensity in ng histamine equivalent 5ml solution	
		Native plasma substitute	Extract after combined method
Haemaccel[(R)]	(1)	3072	30.8
	(2)	3648	45.2
Gelifundol[(R)]	(1)	16320	1.4
	(2)	17280	2.0
Neoplasmagel[(R)]	(1)	422	0.6
	(2)	394	0
Macrodex[(R)]	(1)	0.3	0.7
	(2)	0.3	0.4
Plasmasteril[(R)]	(1)	12	0.6
	(2)	10	0

et al., 1972)) the conclusion can be drawn that changes in histamine content are
expected to occur in organ systems or tissues where the clinical symptoms and/or
biological reactions are observed. Examples confirming this hypothesis in human
subjects are measurements of histamine in blister fluid of the skin during uticaria
(Kaplan et al., 1978) or in gastric juice during stimulation of acid secretion by
exogenous histamine (Adam et al., 1954). Anaphylactoid symptoms and reactions
can also indirectly be mediated by histamine, such as by central effects on the blood
pressure, via biophysical effects on the circulatory system (splanchnic pooling) or
by releasing other mediators such as catecholamines from the adrenal medulla
which in turn may effect the heart rate and contribute to tachycardia. Those indirect
effects of histamine may not be associated with changes of histamine concentrations

TABLE 6.7

COMPARISON OF PHYSICAL AND CHEMICAL PROPERTIES OF THE CONDENSATION PRODUCT BETWEEN O-PHTHALDIALDEHYDE AND PLASMA HISTAMINE AND OF LUMINESCENT COMPOUNDS IN PLASMA SUBSTITUTES

Mean values from 5 determinations. All wave-lengths correspond to those at maximum fluorescence intensities. From Macrodex (Knoll, Ludwigshafen) no spectra were obtained (see Table 6.6). Gelifundol (Biotest, Frankfurt) showed two maximum excitation wave lengths − 360 nm following the combined method, 380 nm with the native plasma substitute. 0 = no increase in luminescence compared to the reagent blank, + increase in luminescence. Note that Haemaccel (Behringwerke, Marburg) can be distinguished from histamine by its luminescence in the reversed blank and by the persistence of the luminescence following heating. This is important for the histamine identification following Haemaccel infusion. For Neoplasmagel (Braun, Melsungen) and Plasmasteril (Fresenius, Bad Homburg) note the wave-lengths different from plasma histamine. For further conditions see Table 6.6.

Luminescent compounds	Physical and chemical properties			
	Excitation wave-length (nm)	Emission wave-length (nm)	Luminescence in the reversed blank	Demonstrable after 2h heating
Plasma histamine	360	450	0	0
Haemaccel[R]	370	460	+	+
Gelifundol[R]	360/380	450	0	0
Neoplasmagel[R]	375	440		0
Macrodex[R]	−	−	0	0
Plasmasteril[R]	355	475	0	0

in reacting organs or tissues, but evidence for such processes until now has been obtained predominantly from animal experiments.

However, it is mainly the pharmacokinetics of histamine in the human organism which allows the determination of the most important alterations of the histamine content in the course of anaphylactoid reactions (Lorenz et al., 1972a,c; Lorenz, 1975; Lorenz and Doenicke, 1978a). The intravenous injection of a small dose of histamine (600 ng/kg) which elicited most of the clinical symptoms and biological responses of an anaphylactoid and allergoid reaction (except the wheals which need an intradermal injection (Lorenz and Doenicke, 1978a, b; Table 6.8)) led to an measurable increase in peripheral venous plasma histamine levels of the arm opposite to that where the injection was done in all human subjects tested even after elapse of one or more circulation times (Fig. 6.5). *Thus by the highly sensitive assay of histamine in human plasma the technical and physiological possibility exists of measuring alterations of the peripheral venous plasma histamine levels even after*

TABLE 6.8

INCIDENCE OF CHANGES IN PERIPHERAL VENOUS PLASMA HISTAMINE LEVELS, CHANGES IN PULSE RATE AND BLOOD PRESSURE AND SEVERAL CLINICAL SYMPTOMS OF AN ANAPHYLACTOID REACTION AFTER I.V. INJECTION OF HISTAMINE IN HUMAN VOLUNTEERS

Injection of histamine as an intravenous bolus (600 ng/kg) into the left cubital vein. Blood samples were taken from the right cubital vein via a braunula. Pulse rate, blood pressure and plasma histamine were measured according to Lorenz et al., 1972a, the clinical symptoms according to Lorenz et al., 1977a (see also Table 6.1). For further conditions see Fig. 6.5.

Parameters or symptoms		Incidence
Increase in plasma histamine	(>0.4 ng/ml)	39/39
Increase in pulse rate	(>5 beats/min)	30/40
Changes in blood pressure	(>5 mm Hg)	0/40
Flush		36/40
Metallic taste		32/40
Headache		21/40

release of only very tiny amounts of histamine from any organ or tissue of the body into the systemic circulation.

Against this statement several objections may be raised which mainly deal with findings and hypotheses obtained and developed in the relatively long history of histamine:

(a) Order of magnitude for histamine doses, plasma histamine levels and clinical reactions. It is difficult to believe that such a small intravenous dose of histamine (600 ng/kg) can produce measurable increases in peripheral venous plasma histamine levels in man and concomitantly such well-known symptoms and responses of anaphylactoid and allergoid reactions as shown in Fig. 6.5 and Table 6.8. Studies were performed 30–40 years ago (Rose, 1940; Rose and Browne, 1938; Rose et al., 1950) in which even doses of histamine in the milligram range were unable to induce a reasonable increase in the blood histamine levels in animals and in man.

However, both the *sensitivity* and *specificity* of the histamine assay has been drastically improved and because the techniques of sample-taking proved critical in earlier studies (Adam et al., 1957; Lindell and Westling, 1966) they have been meticulously studied (Lorenz et al., 1972b; Lorenz, 1975) to achieve a highly reliable plasma histamine determination.

The finding that small increases in plasma histamine levels are associated with

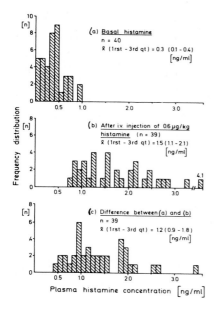

Fig. 6.5. Peripheral venous plasma histamine concentrations in human volunteers before and after injection of exogenous histamine. Basal histamine levels as means from two determinations, those after histamine injection as single values (maximum increase, sample taken always 1 min after injection). 40 test persons (32 males, 8 females, age 21-37). 1 plasma was lost during preparation. Histamine was injected as a bolus into the arm opposite to that where the blood samples were taken for plasma histamine assay. From Lorenz and Doenicke, 1978a.

symptoms and biological responses similar to anaphylaxis and allergy is highly important. It is crucial for the acceptance of a role of histamine in adverse responses to intravenous agents since, following administration of these drugs, increases in plasma histamine levels and clinical reactions were observed which resemble those of injected and infused histamine in small doses (Lorenz et al., 1972a,b; Lorenz and Doenicke, 1978a). For this reason we have also performed studies with a 10-times higher histamine dose, but for ethical reasons only in dogs. Even the comparatively small dose of 6 μg histamine/kg in these animals which are similar to human subjects in their plasma histamine levels (Fig. 6.6a) and their sensitivity to histamine in the cardio-vascular system (Thermann et al., 1977) elicited increases in plasma histamine levels and circulatory disturbances very similar (Fig. 6.6b) to those observed in *severe* adverse reactions in man in clinical conditions (Lorenz et al., 1972a, 1976) (See also Tabel 6.14, Fig. 6.14). Further studies on the relationship

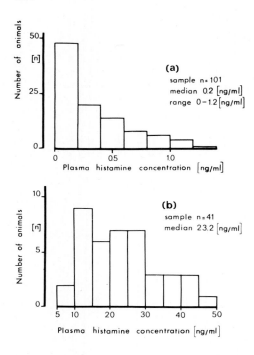

Fig. 6.6. Histograms of canine plasma histamine concentrations under "basal" conditions and following administration of exogenous histamine. (a) Basal plasma histamine values. Blood was taken from the V. cava inferior 30 min after having inserted the polyethylene catheter. (b) Plasma histamine values following i.v. injection of 6 μg/kg histamine into the V. cava inferior. The catheter was carefully washed after the injection of the bolus. 30 sec later blood was taken via the same catheter to measure the plasma histamine values reported in the figure. The mean fall in systolic arterial blood pressure measured at the time of highest plasma histamine levels (30 sec after injection) was 68 ± 9 mm Hg ($\bar{x} \pm$ S.D.). For further conditions see Lorenz et al. 1974a, c.

between plasma histamine levels and circulatory symptoms and reactions in dogs were published by Lorenz et al., 1973b and Thermann et al., 1977a. From these findings it can easily be seen that histamine doses, elevation of plasma histamine levels and the severity of clinical reactions to histamine and to various drugs causing adverse responses are not any longer in themselves contradictory.

(b) Blood and plasma histamine levels. It is difficult to believe that whole blood histamine levels in man and animals show such marked alterations in hypersensitivity reactions, when changes in plasma histamine levels are so small (for a review see Lindell and Westling, 1966; Altura and Halevy, 1978b).

However, there are several possible explanations of these apparent contradictions. Many of the histamine determinations in whole blood are unreliable, especially those in the whole blood of dogs which are used for many studies on adverse responses to intravenous agents (cremophor El, tween, PVP, Haemaccel, dextran etc.). Our values which have been vigorously tested for specificity (Lorenz et al., 1974c; Lorenz and Doenicke, 1978a) are lower by 1 or 2 orders of magnitude (Fig. 6.7) than those of the other workers in this field (see Table 6.9 and values collected by Altura and Halevy, 1978b) including those of authors using the radio-enzymatic assay (Shaff and Beaven, 1979). Moreover changes in whole blood histamine levels reflect also alterations in the content of basophilic granulocytes as well as histamine release from these cells (decrease in whole blood histamine content) or histamine uptake into erythrocytes (Lindell and Viske, 1961) and elevation of histamine concentrations in plasma (increase in whole blood histamine content). Examples of such alterations in white blood cell counts were given by Lindell and Westling (1966) in various disease states by Doenicke et al. (1973) and Watkins et al. (1976) following injection of althesin and by Lorenz et al. (1972a,c, 1976) following administration of propanidid, thiopentone and Haemaccel. Finally, considerable alterations of histamine concentrations in whole blood following

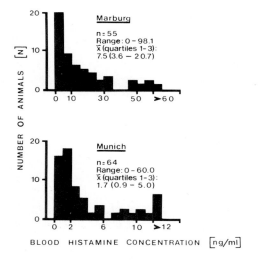

Fig. 6.7. Histograms of histamine content in canine whole blood obtained from animals in two different communities. Single values obtained from each of the dogs. Histamine as free base, combined method according to Lorenz et al. (1972b). Identification of histamine in each of the samples by fluorescence spectra before and after heating, in the pool of blood samples from all the animals by various tests including thin-layer chromatography, histamine methyltransferase and diamine oxidase incubations and determination of PA$_2$-values on the isolated guinea-pig ileum (Lorenz and Doenicke, 1978a).

TABLE 6.9

HISTAMINE CONTENT IN CANINE WHOLE BLOOD MEASURED BY VARIOUS AUTHORS
OVER A PERIOD OF MORE THAN 30 YEARS

Values as mean values, ranges or medians (interquartile range) calculated as far as possible from the
original literature. Histamine as free base.

Histamine content [ng/ml]	References
280-410	Kadykov and Federowa, 1956
110 (50-180)	Zeppa et al., 1961
140-190	Hahn and Wellmann, 1952
40-90	Emmelin et al., 1941
40-75	Barsoum and Gaddum, 1935
50 (30-80)	Anrep et al., 1939
50	Shore et al., 1959
40	Halpern et al., 1956
30	Code and Mitchell, 1957
25-35	Minard, 1941
25-33	Anrep and Barsoum, 1935
19-37	Magazinović et al., 1966
23 (20-40)	Behrmann et al., 1945
0-100	Hinshaw et al., 1961
16 (0-40)	Code, 1939
14	Thompson and Walton, 1963
0-20	Tinel et al., 1938
9	Mundy et al., 1967
0-18	Code and Jensen, 1941
0-16	Code, 1937

application of several intravenous agents were caused by a considerable enhanced
histamine uptake (and therefore inactivation) by the cellular histamine stores in the
blood (Tauber et al., 1975).

(c) Extraction of histamine from plasma in various capillary beds. It is difficult to
believe that significant amounts of histamine released from single organs or tissues
can be measured in plasma of the systemic circulation since histamine is removed
quickly from blood during its transit through various capillary beds.

Arterio-venous differences of histamine contents in human whole blood and
plasma have been demonstrated in various organs by reliable isotopic and non-
isotopic methods (Table 6.10), but systematically the question could again only be
investigated in dogs for ethical and technical reasons (Table 6.11; Fig. 6.8). With
four catheters placed in four circulatory regions it could be shown that basal plasma

TABLE 6.10

STUDIES ON ARTERIO-VENOUS DIFFERENCES OF HISTAMINE LEVELS IN WHOLE BLOOD
AND PLASMA OF HUMAN SUBJECTS

0 = no change; — = decrease of histamine values in the venous blood compared to those of the
corresponding arteries.

Organ, body fluid		Qualitative changes of histamine levels	References
Lung,	blood	0	Rose et al., 1950
Liver,	blood	—	Arnoldsson et al., 1962
	blood	—	Helander et al., 1965
	plasma	—	Stopik et al., 1974, 1977, 1978
	plasma	—	Beger et al., 1975
Kidney,	blood	—	Arnoldsson et al., 1962
	blood	—	Helander et al., 1965
Uterus,	blood	—	Lindberg, 1963
Placenta,	blood	—	Marcou et al., 1938
	blood	—	Wicksell, 1949
	blood	—	Bjurö et al., 1961

histamine levels were similar though slightly higher values could be detected in the
portal vein (Table 6.11). However, following intracaval injection of 6 µg/kg
histamine (Fig. 6.8) the highest plasma histamine levels were measured in the aorta,
lower in the v. cava inferior and the portal vein and the lowest in the hepatic veins.
Apparently the periphery of the body and kidneys, the gastrointestinal tract and the
liver were capable of eliminating some histamine from the circulation as it was also
shown in man (Table 6.10). Our findings in dogs and those of Beger et al. (1975) in
man, however, to do not support the opinion that even relatively small increases of
plasma histamine in one circulatory region could not be detected by measuring
venous plasma histamine in the systemic circulation. The contrary is true. Therefore
we conclude *histamine release into the venous outflow of any organ is always likely
to be detected by a histamine assay of cubital venous blood.* For quantitative
considerations, however, the particular organ and the circulatory regions in which
the histamine release occurs have to be taken into account.

*(d) Differences between intravenous application of exogenous histamine and release
of endogenous histamine by histamine releasers.* It may be possible that injection of
exogenous histamine into the circulation can be detected easily by a plasma
histamine assay. But histamine release occurs in the connective tissue and therefore,
perhaps, endogenous histamine liberated into the interstitial space may be detected

TABLE 6.11

PLASMA HISTAMINE CONCENTRATIONS IN 4 CIRCULATORY REGIONS OF DOGS UNDER "BASAL" CONDITIONS

Blood was collected from the blood vessels 30 min after completing the operation described in Methods. In the Wilcoxon test only the differences between III/IV were statistically significant ($p < 0.05$). For further conditions see Lorenz et al., 1974c.

Animal No.	Plasma histamine concentration (ng/ml)			
Abdominal aorta (I)	V. cava inferior (II)	Portal vein (III)	Hepatic vein (IV)	
1	1.4	1.2	1.3	1.2
2	0.4	0.4	0.4	0.3
3	0.4	0	0.4	0.3
			0.4	
4	0.3	0.4		0.2
5	0.3	0.3	0.3	0.2
6	0.3	0.3	0.2	0.2
7	0.3	0.8	0	0
8	0.3	0.2	0	0.3
9	0.1	0.2	0.6	0.3
10	0.1	0.1	0	0
11	0.1	0.4	0.6	0.4
12	0.1	0	0.3	0.2
13	0	0	0.6	0.4
Median (lower−upper quartiles)	0.3 (0.1-0.4)	0.3 (0-0.4)	0.4 (0.2-0.6)	0.3 (0.2-0.4)

with less reliability, and in particular with much less sensitivity, than exogenous histamine.

Two examples of adverse responses to intravenous agents, however, show in experiments in dogs and in clinical incidents that if anaphylactoid reactions occur increases in plasma histamine levels can be measured (Lorenz and Doenicke, 1978a; Lorenz et al., 1980).

The first example deals with the plasma substitute *Haemaccel*. In dogs histamine contents were determined in various tissues before and after infusion of this drug (Table 6.12). By this well-accepted technique (Rothschild, 1966) it could be demonstrated that Haemaccel released histamine mainly in the skin, the skeletal muscle and the liver whereas the intestine took up large amounts of the released

TABLE 6.12

HISTAMINE CONTENT OF VARIOUS TISSUES OF DOGS BEFORE AND AFTER ADMINIS-
TRATION OF HAEMACCEL

Mean values ± S.D. since tissue histamine contents in human subjects and dogs are usually normally distributed. Histamine as dihydrochloride. The data were obtained from the same 10 dogs whose changes in whole blood histamine content were shown in Fig. 6.10. Thus these data are and should be to some extent complementary to the others. The tissues were taken 20 min after maximum decrease in arterial blood pressure. Statistical evaluation was performed by the t-test for paired data. NS = not significant ($\alpha = 0.05$). For further conditions see Lorenz et al. (1974c).

| Tissue | Histamine content in μg/g fresh weight | | Changes | Significance |
	before infusion	after infusion	($\pm$ %)	
Reacting animals (n = 6)				
Skin, neck	36.2 ± 18.0	27.6 ± 14.5	− 24	$p < 0.05$
abdomen	30.5 ± 15.2	15.6 ± 12.4	− 49	$p < 0.05$
Muscle, diaphragm	18.1 ± 13.8	12.2 ± 10.6	− 33	$p < 0.05$
Stomach, fundus	90.5 ± 38.2	91.2 ± 40.7	0	NS
corpus	66.0 ± 27.1	62.9 ± 21.8	− 5	NS
antrum	45.7 ± 15.9	41.3 ± 11.7	− 10	NS
Ileum	45.8 ± 8.5	65.7 ± 18.0	+ 43	$p < 0.05$
Liver	66.6 ± 24.7	36.2 ± 17.0	− 46	$p < 0.05$
Lung	45.6 ± 21.4	47.8 ± 25.1	+ 5	NS
Non-reacting animals (n = 4)				
Skin, neck	37.1 ± 12.7	36.1 ± 10.5	0	
abdomen	15.4 ± 9.8	17.6 ± 10.1	+ 14	
Muscle, diaphragm	12.8 ± 3.6	12.3 ± 3.7	0	NS
Stomach, fundus	107 ± 23.5	108 ± 46	0	in all
corpus	103 ± 32	97 ± 31	− 6	cases
antrum	55.2 ± 9.6	53.5 ± 10.3	0	
Ileum	49.0 ± 13.8	48.1 ± 5.3	0	
Liver	51.0 ± 9.8	56.0 ± 10.6	+ 10	
Lung	52.9 ± 13.5	61.9 ± 16.9	+ 17	

amine. These findings could clearly be confirmed by plasma histamine assays both in the canine plasma (Fig. 6.9) and whole blood (Fig. 6.10). In animals which did not show any clinical symptoms or blood pressure responses and any changes of histamine contents in tissues also no increase in plasma histamine concentration could be detected in the *corresponding* or any of the other circulatory regions tested. In contrast to human subjects the histamine assay in whole blood of dogs is a sensitive test for histamine release since about 20–30 times less histamine is stored in the whole blood of this species than in that of man.

Of course, in man histamine contents in various tissues could not be determined

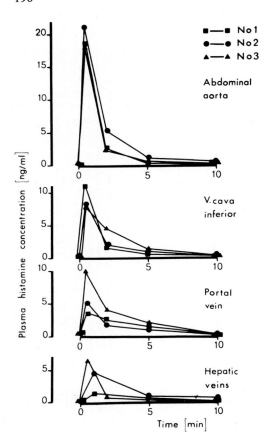

Fig. 6.8. Plasma histamine concentrations in 4 circulatory regions of dogs following intravenous injection of exogenous histamine. Single values from 3 dogs with the exception of the histamine concentration at 0 min (immediately before the injection of 6 μg/kg histamine (base)) which was determined in 2 samples. ■—■, dog No. 1; ●—●, dog No. 2; ▲—▲, dog No. 3. For further conditions see Lorenz et al., 1974c.

before and during adverse responses to Haemaccel to show the sensitivity and reliability of the plasma histamine assay in states of histamine release by this drug. All clinicians, however, and hopefully also the pharmacologists will accept that the plasma histamine assay is sufficiently sensitive to demonstrate histamine release by

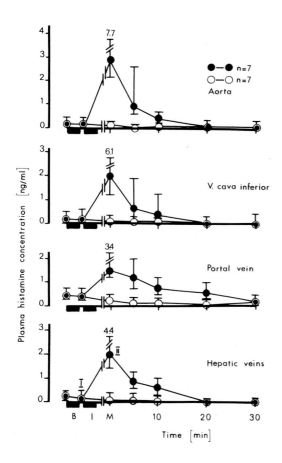

Fig. 6.9. Plasma histamine concentrations in four circulatory regions of dogs before and after adminis-tration of Haemaccel[(R)]. Medians and interquartile ranges obtained from 7 animals showing an adverse reaction to Haemaccel, batch 3123 (hypotension, hyperventilation, erythema of the skin etc.) ($\bullet$—$\bullet$) and from those showing no such reaction ($\circ$—$\circ$) to the same batch in a continuous series of experi-ments (n of the sample = 14, reactions happened by chance, incidence = 50%). B = bleeding; I = infusion; M = maximum hypotension. Significance in the Wilcoxon test: reacting animals $PI/II < 0.01$ in all circulatory regions, non-reacting animals PI/II not significant. For further conditions see Lorenz et al. (1974c).

Haemaccel in man if even the mildest type of anaphylactoid reaction as defined in section 2, can be predicted by the plasma histamine assay in the peripheral venous blood. Several clinical trials have been performed both in human volunteers (Lorenz

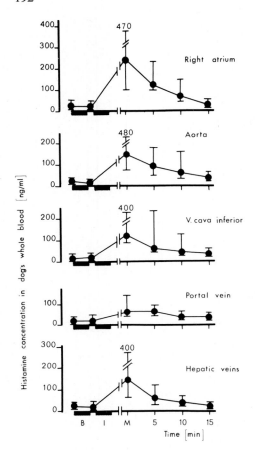

Fig. 6.10. Whole-blood histamine concentrations in five circulatory regions of dogs before and after administration of Haemaccel[(R)]. Medians and interquartile ranges obtained from 6 animals showing an adverse reaction to Haemaccel, batch 2559 (n of the sample = 10, incidence 60%). For further conditions see Fig. 6.9. The medians of blood histamine concentrations in the non-reacting 4 animals were the same before and at any time after the Haemaccel[(R)] infusion. Significance in the Wilcoxon test: $PI/M < 0.05$ in all circulatory regions. Histamine usually in this communication and also in this figure is given as free histamine base, but in few cases due to the reproduction of figures or tables from previous articles in histamine dihydrochloride. The mass ratio between the dihydrochloride and the free base is 10:6. M = time of maximum hypotension from Lorenz et al. (1974c).

et al., 1978c; Lorenz and Doenicke, 1978a,b) and in patients (Lorenz et al., 1980; Schöning and Lorenz, 1980) to answer this question. Sophisticated methods in clinical decision making (Lusted, 1968; Galen and Gambino, 1975) were applied

(Table 6.13) as well as simple descriptions of individual cases were performed in whom adverse reactions to Haemaccel occurred and concomitantly plasma histamine assays were performed (Table 6.14; Fig. 6.11). All these studies showed

TABLE 6.13

EFFICIENCY OF THE PLASMA HISTAMINE ASSAY FOR PREDICTING ANAPHYLACTOID REACTIONS FOLLOWING HAEMACCEL INFUSION

PV positive: 100 (%); PV negative: 97.5 (%); incidence: 16.2 (%); efficiency: 97.8 (%). According to Lorenz et al. (1980).

	Plasma histamine		Totals
	>1 ng/ml	<1 ng/ml	
Anaphylactoid reaction	26	4	30
No anaphylactoid reaction	0	155	155
Totals	26	159	185

TABLE 6.14

PLASMA HISTAMINE LEVELS, CLINICAL SYMPTOMS AND BIOLOGICAL RESPONSES IN 5 PATIENTS WITH ANAPHYLACTOID REACTIONS TO HAEMACCEL[R]

For details of the clinical trial see Lorenz et al. (1980). Blood was taken at maximum development of the reaction (plateau of the pulse rate). All patients were males.

No.	Patient age (years)	Clinical symptoms and biological reactions	Plasma histamine level after infusion (ng/ml)
1	43	Erythema in the upper half of the body, coughing, urticaria, oedema in the face, tachycardia (68→105 beats/min 5 min after the infusion) hypotension at the same time (115/70→ <40 mm Hg)	14.0
2	30	Erythema in the face and neck, abdominal pain, tachycardia (64→79 beats/min 5 min after the infusion).	6.8
3	38	Erythema and urticaria in the face, chest and femur. Tachycardia slight (only 72→80 beats/min).	4.6
4	36	Erythema in the upper half of the body, oedema in the face, coughing, tachycardia (65→86 beats/min).	3.1
5	31	Erythema in the face, Urticaria on both groins and back. Coughing, tachycardia slight (only 78→85 beats/min).	2.1

194

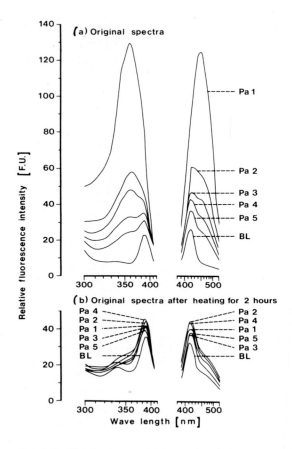

Fig. 6.11. Fluorescence excitation and emission spectra of the isolated substances from plasma of 5 patients with anaphylactoid reactions to the infusion of Haemaccel[(R)]. Original registration. (a) Patients 1-5 in Table 6.14. Bl = blank. (b) Heating test for 2 hours. The histamine-induced fluorescence was no longer detectable. Therefore the substances measured in plasma were identified by these criteria as hista-mine. Even the slightest reaction occuring in patient 5 was measurable by the plasma histamine assay in the peripheral venous blood. Time of blood collection at the maximum development of the anaphylactoid reaction.

convincingly that in human subjects the plasma histamine assay in the peripheral venous blood is so sensitive and so reliable that in anaphylactoid reactions to Haemaccel of all degrees of severity an increase of the plasma histamine content was demonstrated.

The second example – even more interesting – deals with the solubilizer *cremophor El.* In various concentrations and in different compositions because of its complex composition (Fig. 6.12) this mixture is used for solubilizing propanidid (Epontol[R]), althesin (alphaxalone[R]), diazepam (Valium[R]) (mainly in England and in the Scandinavian countries), flunitrazepam (Rohypnol[R]) and lorme-thazepam, various vitamin preparations for i.v. application etc. It causes anaphylactoid reactions and histamine release in dogs and cats (Lorenz et al., 1971a, 1973b, 1977b) and in pigs which have previously exposed (Glen et al,., 1978, 1979).

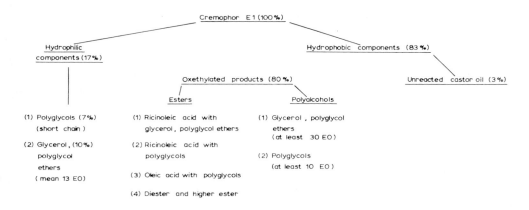

Fig. 6.12. Chemical composition of the detergent cremophor El. According to Lorenz et al. (1977b).

Again we have determined the histamine content in various tissues of the *dog* before and after injection of this drug (Table 6.15). The spectrum of organs, however, in which changes of the histamine contents were observed, was different from that with Haemaccel: The gastrointestinal tract was severely affected whereas the lungs and liver and the diaphragm did not show any significant alterations of their histamine content. However, the skin reacted to the drug as it did to Haemaccel by a considerable decrease of the histamine concentration. As far the clinical signs in the animals are concerned, the picture of the anaphylactoid reaction to cremophor El showed a remarkable difference from the adverse response to Haemaccel: The animals regularly suffered from immediate *diarrhoea*. This reaction correlated well with the altered histamine content of the gut.

As in the case of Haemaccel, these finding could be confirmed by measuring histamine in the plasma of the v. cava inferior and in the whole blood of four circulatory regions (Fig. 6.13). In contrast to Haemaccel where the portal histamine levels were low, but those in the hepatic veins were high supporting the findings in

TABLE 6.15

HISTAMINE CONTENT OF VARIOUS TISSUES OF DOGS WITH AND WITHOUT TREATMENT
WITH CREMOPHOR El

Mean values ± S.D. (for a comment see Table 6.11). Histamine as dihydrochloride. 6 pairs of dogs were used as pairs of the same litter. The sequence of applications (A = saline, B = 0.4 ml/kg cremophor El in the same composition as in Fig. 6.13) was performed at random using random digits. The animals were chosen for the experiment before the random number was obtained from a notice in an envelope. Data were analysed by the student t-test. For further conditions see Lorenz et al. (1973b).

Tissue	Histamine content in $\mu g/g$ ($\bar{x} \pm$ S.D.)		Change $\pm$ (%)	Significance
	Untreated	Treated		
(a) Gastrointestinal				
Submandibular gland	31.9 ± 9.8	23.2 ± 5.3	− 27	$p < 0.1$
Parotid gland	7.4 ± 1.7	5.8 ± 1.5	− 22	$p < 0.1$
Gastric mucosa				
Fundus	101 ± 15	81 ± 22	− 20	$p < 0.1$
Corpus	117 ± 37	102 ± 24	− 13	−
Antrum	69 ± 25	44 ± 18	− 36	$p < 0.1$
Gastric musculature				
Fundus	40.8 ± 12.6	40.1 ± 9.5	−	−
Corpus	39.0 ± 12.7	36.0 ± 12.7	− 8	−
Antrum	28.4 ± 5.5	13.0 ± 7.1	− 54	$p < 0.005$
Jejunum	145 ± 26	38 ± 21	− 39	$p < 0.005$
Ileum	84 ± 17	57 ± 19	− 32	$p < 0.05$
Colon	77 ± 19	49 ± 18	− 37	$p < 0.05$
Pancreas	11.4 ± 3.6	2.8 ± 2.1	− 75	$p < 0.001$
(b) Others				
Lung	63.8 ± 25.4	64.7 ± 17.8	−	−
Liver, capsule	45.1 ± 17.2	41.4 ± 19.2	− 10	−
parenchyma	41.0 ± 15.3	45.4 ± 16.7	+ 10	−
Spleen	20.9 ± 10.5	31.6 ± 16.9	+ 50	$p < 0.3$
Diaphragm	12.1 ± 4.7	11.3 ± 4.3	− 7	−
M.quadriceps	5.4 ± 2.2	3.7 ± 0.9	− 32	$p < 0.1$
Abdominal skin	18.5 ± 7.0	3.2 ± 0.3	− 83	$p < 0.001$

the tissues in the case of cremophor E1 the portal histamine content was even higher than that in the aorta whereas in the hepatic veins the lowest histamine contents of all circulatory regions were measured − again in agreement with the findings in the tissues.

In *man* anaphylactoid reactions to cremophor E1 *alone* have not yet been

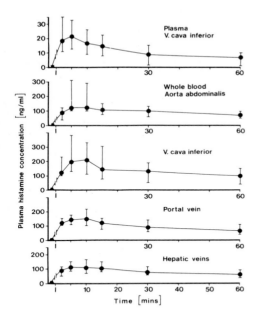

Fig. 6.13. Plasma and whole-blood histamine concentrations in four circulatory regions of dogs before and after i.v. injection of cremophor El. Medians and interquartile ranges obtained from 8 dogs showing an adverse reaction to cremophor El including diarrhoea, skin erythema and hypotension. The medians of plasma and blood histamine concentrations in 4 non-reacting animals were the same before and at any time after cremophor El injection. Dose of cremophor El (Micellophor): 0.4 ml/kg in exactly the same dilution and composition of the mixture as used for propanidid injection (Doenicke et al., 1973). Significance in the Wilcoxon-test: BI versus 1 min after Ip < 0.01 in all circulatory regions. Histamine as free base.

observed (Lorenz et al., 1972a,c,; Doenicke et al., 1973), but only to cremophor El in combination with drugs such as propanidid, althesin, diazepam (see section 3,1; Clarke et al., 1975; Padfield and Watkins, 1977). It is very interesting to note that anaphylactoid responses to diazepam were not published as long as the drug was dissolved in a mixture with propylene glycol (Benke et al., 1979) whereas following marketing of ampoules with valium[R]) dissolved in cremophor El several of such reports *immediately* could appear (Milner, 1977; Blatchley, 1977; Falk, 1977; Padfield and Watkins, 1977). Plasma histamine assays in the periopheral venous blood for predicting anaphylactoid reactions to cremophor in combination with a drug have never been studied so systematically in so many patients as in the case of Haemaccel. But again individual cases have been described where an adverse reaction

198

to propanidid (Epontol[R]) occurred and concomitantly plasma histamine assays could be performed (Fig. 6.14). Once again the plasma histamine assay in the peripheral venous blood was so sensitive and so reliable that in anaphylactoid reactions to propanidid of all degrees of severity (one case was a so-called "border-line" case) (Lorenz et al., 1972a; Doenicke and Lorenz, 1973, 1976) an increase of the plasma histamine content was measured.

In the case of *althesin* we know only about a slight adverse reaction where plasma histamine levels were simultaneously determined (Doenicke et al., 1973). Again

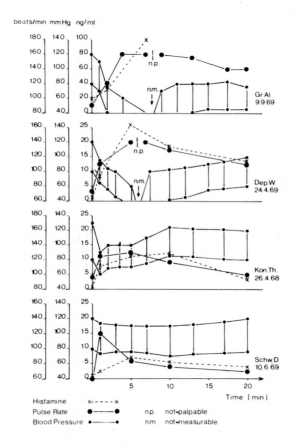

Fig. 6.14. Correlation between plasma histamine concentration, pulse rate and blood pressure in four cases of anaphylactoid reactions to propanidid (Epontol[R]). Note that the "borderline" case No. 4 reacts only by a prolonged tachycardia and by an erythema of the face and neck (See Lorenz et al., 1972a). The first case, however, had a cardiac arrest, but could be successfully reanimated. For further conditions see Lorenz et al. (1972a).

elevated plasma histamine concentrations were found in this case. The same agreement between occurrence of symptoms and changes in plasma histamine levels was obtained in two test subjects who received flunitrazepam (Rohypnol[R]) and developed slight adverse reactions. In both cases elevated plasma histamine levels were undoubtedly shown (Lorenz et al., 1978b).

3.2.3. Sample-taking at the right time

To assess the role of histamine in adverse reactions to intravenous agents it is extremely important to choose the right time for taking blood for the plasma histamine assay. Exogenous histamine is eliminated very rapidly (Fig. 6.15) the half-life being about 2 min in man which is very similar to that in dogs (Lorenz et al., 1974a,c). The pharmacokinetics resemble those of first-order kinetics corresponding

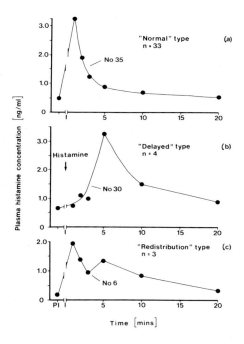

Fig. 6.15. Histamine elimination curves following i.v. injection of exogenous histamine (600 ng/kg). Single values obtained from human volunteers in the trial on comparison of the effects of exogenous histamine and endogenous histamine released by Haemaccel[R] in the same subject (Table 6.8, Fig. 6.5). In a sample of 40 volunteers three types of elimination curves could be differentiated. Their number (n) is registered in the figure. For further details see also Lorenz and Doenicke (1978a).

200

to a one-compartment model for elimination, but in dogs it could be demonstrated that elimination and catabolism are both involved in the clearance of histamine from plasma (Lorenz et al., 1973b, 1974c). In addition to the "normal" type of disappearance of histamine from plasma (Fig. 6.15a) which was observed in about 80 per cent of the cases, a few test persons showed a "delayed" type (Fig. 6.15b) or a "redistribution" type (Fig. 6.15c) of curve. The most likely interpretation for

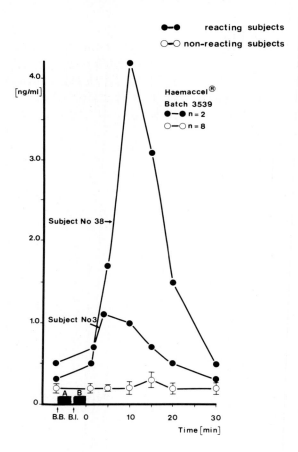

Fig. 6.16. Increase in plasma histamine levels in volunteers following rapid infusion of Haemaccel[(R)]. Single histamine values are shown for the "responders", but x̄ ± S.E.M. for the "non-responders". The trial comprised 40 male subjects. The sequential trial numbers of the reacting individuals are given in the figure. Plasma histamine level in ng/ml. B.B. = before blood donation (A) (500 ml); B.I. = before infusion of the plasma substitute (B) (500 ml). For further conditions see Lorenz et al. (1978c) and Lorenz and Doenicke (1978b).

these apparent elimination curves is difficulty with histamine bolus injection, but their occurrence is interesting from a clinical point of view. Difficulties with drug application including varying speeds of injection or infusion may cause adverse responses to the particular substance and may led to an onset and duration of clinical symptoms as well as to atypical histamine elimination curves which may easily cause a misinterpretation concerning the mediator involved in the particular adverse reaction. For illustration individual cases with adverse responses to plasma substitutes and anaesthetic drugs will be shown.

Following *Haemaccel*[(R)] infusion the maximum plasma histamine level usually is reached 5 (1–10) min (median (range)) after the end of infusion (Fig. 6.16). A mere 30 min later, no increased plasma histamine concentration was demonstrable. This finding is crucial for all kinds of sample-taking following clinically suspected adverse reactions. By the time a suitable syringe for plasma preparation is available

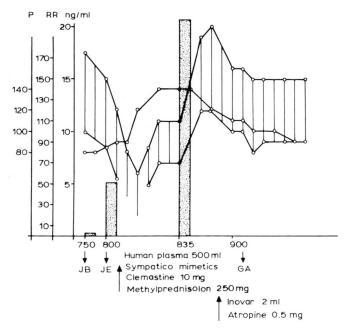

Fig. 6.17. Record of a severe anaphylactoid reaction to Haemaccel[(R)] in an orthopedic patient. Random number No. 26451 in the controlled clinical trial No. 1 published by Lorenz et al. (1980). P = pulse rate (O—O), RR = systolic and diastolic arterial blood pressure (□□□), ng/ml = plasma histamine concentration (■). IB = start of infusion, IE = end of infusion, GA = general anaesthesia. Both anaesthesia and operation run without any clinical complication. For further conditions see Lorenz et al. (1980). Note the long time interval between start of infusion and the highest plasma histamine level measured!

to the clinician (Lorenz et al., 1972b; Lorenz and Doenicke, 1978b) all the released histamine may already have been eliminated from plasma. However, there are individual patients in whom extremely high plasma histamine levels can also be measured 45 min after starting the Haemaccel infusion (Fig. 6.17) indicating some variability in the time-curve of histamine invasion into the plasma and its subsequent elimination. A useful marker for the best time to take blood plasma histamine assay is the severity of the symptoms which should reach a plateau or should just start to diminish (see tachycardia in Fig. 6.17). However, if only a small histamine release occurs without the eruption of clinical symptoms it may be difficult to detect the optimum time for blood-sampling. In one series of experiments we were unable to show any histamine release by the plasma substitute hydroxyethyl starch (Lorenz et al., 1975). However, in a second series of infusions we detected two cases of elevated plasma histamine levels which occurred quite a long time after the end of infusion (Fig. 6.18).

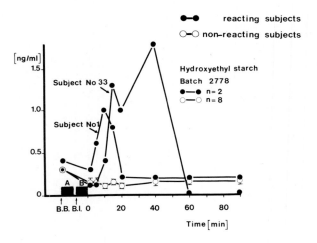

Fig. 6.18. Increase in plasma histamine levels in volunteers following rapid infusion of hydroxyethyl starch. Single histamine values are shown for the "responders", but $\bar{x}\pm$S.E.M. for the "non-responders". For further conditions see Fig. 6.16.

It is interesting to note that as in dogs where the elevated plasma and blood histamine levels persisted for a relatively long time following injection of cremophor E1 (Fig. 6.13) in man increased plasma histamine concentrations could also be measured for a relatively long time following injection of anaesthetic drugs dissolved in cremophor El (Fig. 6.19 and 6.20).

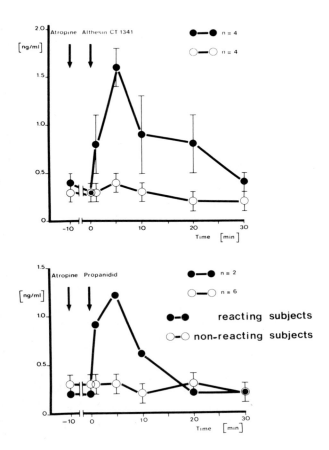

Fig. 6.19. Elevated plasma histamine levels in human volunteers following i.v. administration of althesin CT 1341 and propanidid (Epontol[(R)]). x̄ ± S.E.M. Data obtained from a published study (Doenicke et al., 1973; Lorenz et al., 1974d; Lorenz and Doenicke, 1978b).

3.2.4 *Histamine determination under correct in-vivo (clinical) conditions*

It has been suggested that in many pathological processes evoked by drugs or cellular systems the release of active substances, such as histamine, plays a key role

204

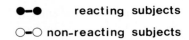

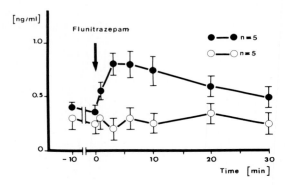

Fig. 6.20. Elevated plasma histamine levels in human volunteers following i.v. administration of flunitrazepam (Rohypnol(R)). x̄±S.E.M. Data according to Lorenz and Doenicke, 1978b; Doenicke and Lorenz, 1978.

— but is it significant in clinical conditions? The reasons for the discrepancy between experimental and clinical findings concerning histamine release are listed in Table 6.16. In this review and especially in this section which is concerned with logical sequences (logistics) the first statement in Table 6.16 will be explained in more detail (Table 6.17).

(a) If anaphylactoid reactions to drugs dissolved in *cremophor El* were observed in patients receiving these drugs, conclusions were drawn by analogy with findings obtained with detergents in several animal species such as tween in dogs (Giertz

TABLE 6.16

REASONS FOR THE DISCREPANCY BETWEEN EXPERIMENTAL AND CLINICAL FINDINGS CONCERNING ACTIVE SUBSTANCE RELEASE

- Experiments are designed for extreme conditions
- Principles of controlled clinical trials are neglected in planning animal and human studies
- Methods for measuring active substances in clinical situations are unreliable
- Correlations regarding extent and time-course of incidents and release cannot be shown convincingly. Predictive values are not calculated (causality?)
- Adverse reactions to a given drug are caused by more than *one* mechanism

TABLE 6.17

EXAMPLES FOR THE FIRST STATEMENT IN TABLE 6.16: EXPERIMENTS ARE DESIGNED
FOR EXTREME (NON-CLINICAL) CONDITIONS

- Species selected regarding incidents (dogs for solvents and proteins, rats for dextran)
- Species selected regarding sensitivity to active substances (rats for serotonin and kinins, guinea-pigs for histamine)
- Species strains selected for non-reactivity (rat strains for dextran)
- Doses and pharmacokinetics selected for maximum incidence and severity
- Incubation medium selected for optimum release of active substances

and Hahn, 1966) and octylamine in guinea-pigs (Rothschild, 1966). Histamine release by these drugs due to a cytotoxic action on mast cells is considered to be the mechanism of action, but apparently this is not true in man in doses used for solubilizing the particular lipophilic drugs (Lorenz et al., 1972a,c; Doenicke et al., 1973). Histamine release in pigs following a second exposure to cremophor E1 seems to be a more suitable model for the reactions to drugs recorded in man (Glen et al., 1978, 1979), but it is far from clear whether the involvement of complement is the only or even the predominant mechanism of action in patients after medical treatment.

In dogs protein hydrolysates *("peptone")* were for a long time the classical histamine liberators in many studies (for a survey see Rocha e Silva, 1955). It was assumed that Haemaccel[R] could probably act in dogs and in patients in the same way, but the infusion of gelatin hydrolysate did not cause a significant histamine release whereas the cross-linking process with hexamethylene – diisocyanate developed the full activity of this fluid as histamine releaser (Lorenz et al. (unpublished results)).

In rats *dextran* was shown to be a classical histamine releaser in numerous experimental studies (Hahn and Wellmann, 1952; Halpern, 1956; Giertz and Hahn, 1966) and in combination with phosphatidylserine also in isolated rat peritoneal mast cells (Goth, 1972). In man, however, it always appeared only a weak histamine releaser in test persons (Fig. 6.21). There was no correlation between the appearance and severity of clinical symptoms and the increase in plasma histamine levels (Table 6.18). In life-threatening conditions (Fig. 6.22) or even in a case of death (Table 6.19) *no* histamine release at all could be measured. Since in the previous section 3.2.2 it was extensively explained how easily changes in plasma histamine concentration can be detected in a *systemic* reaction to drugs it seems almost unthinkable and impossible that histamine

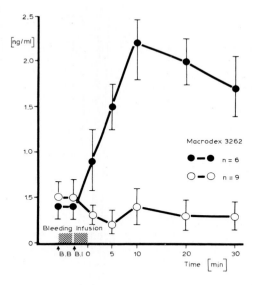

Fig. 6.21. Histamine release in human subjects by rapid infusion of dextran. Mean values ± S.E.M. ● — ●, subjects reacting to dextran by elevated plasma histamine concentrations. ○ — ○, non-reacting subjects. For further conditions see Lorenz et al. (1976).

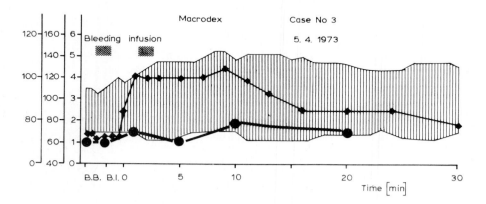

Fig. 6.22. Correlation between plasma histamine concentration, heart rate and arterial pressure in a case of anaphylactoid reaction to dextran-60 (Macrodex(R)). Single values. ● — ●, plasma histamine concentration (ng/ml),   blood pressure (mm Hg); ♦ — ♦, heart rate (beats/min). B.B., before bleeding; B.I., before infusion. For further conditions see Lorenz et al. (1976).

TABLE 6.18

CLINICAL SYMPTOMS AND PLASMA HISTAMINE LEVELS FOLLOWING DEXTRAN INFUSION

Single values for plasma histamine concentrations (time of maximum increase after the end of infusion in round brackets). Two batches of dextran "Fisons" were administered at random to 10 male volunteers (age 20-35 years) in a dose of 500 ml in 3 min after a blood donation of 500 ml according to Lorenz et al. (1976).

Volunteer No.	Clinical symptoms	Plasma histamine levels [ng/ml]	
		before dextran	after dextran
1	0	0.45	0.20 (5)
2	Severe gastrointestinal cramps and pain, nausea	0.20	0.25 (5)
3	Epigastric fullness, straining, flush, erythema on thorax and upper extremity	0.20	0.60 (5)*
4	0	0.15	0.45 (1)*
5	Slight erythema on face and neck, narrowness in the chest	0.10	0.40 (10)*
6	0	0.15	0.10 (5)
7	0	0.15	0.35 (5)*
8	0	0.35	0.75 (10)*
9	0	0.35	0.45 (10)
10	Nausea, almost vomiting, epigastric fullness, increase in heart rate (74→84 beats/min)	0.45	0.50 (10)

* Cases with histamine release according to the criteria of Lorenz and Doenicke (1978b). (See later on in this review article). Assessment of clinical symptoms and determination of blood pressure, pulse rate and plasma histamine according to Lorenz et al. (1972a). Note that there existed no correlation between the only very small increase in plasma histamine levels and the occurrence and severity of clinical symptoms!

release could play any significant role in dextran — induced adverse responses in man — and these reactions are the most life-threatening of all those to plasma substitutes (30 cases of death! See Ahnefeld et al., 1979). In the case of dextran, it is our opinion that unwarranted conclusions based on animal experiments applied to a clinical problem can endanger the patient. For all plasma substitutes investigated so far the present situation is summarized in Table 6.20 demonstrating that histamine release has to be shown to a reasonable extent under clinical conditions before any conclusion can be drwan on the role of histamine in adverse reactions to these drugs.

(b) In adverse responses to intravenous agents many vasoactive substances could be implicated as suitable candidates (Table 6.4). Animal experiments are

TABLE 6.19

ANAPHYLACTOID REACTIONS IN HUMAN SUBJECTS FOLLOWING INFUSION OF DEXTRAN-60

Single values from each of the subjects. The sample for testing the plasma histamine concentration in the patient was obtained 5 min after cardiac arrest when external cardiac massage was already in progress. The sample from patient no. 2 (test subject) was obtained 1 min after the end of the rapid infusion of dextran. For further conditions see Lorenz et al. (1976).

Patient no.	Dextran-60 batch no.	Clinical observations and symptoms	Plasma histamine concentration (ng/ml)	
			Before infusion	After infusion
1 (O. A.)	Dextran-60 Medac R 614	After slow infusion of about 20 ml of dextran (within approximately 3 min): dizziness, feeling of weakness, generalized erythema. *2 min later*: weals on the neck and thorax, cyanosis, bronchospasm. The infusion was stopped. Ringer and bicarbonate solution were administered together with oxygen, cortisone 2 mg/kg, calcium gluconate 10 mg/kg, clemastine 0.03 mg/kg and orciprenaline 0.06 mg/kg. *5 min later* pulse not palpable, arterial pressure not measurable, but e.c.g. normal. *2 min later* cardiac arrest. Despite external cardiac massage, electrical defibrillation, administration of bicarbonate, cortisone, orciprenaline, the patient died	Not tested	0.5
2 (J. D.)	Macrodex 3262/A 3	*3 min after the beginning of infusion* erythema on the face, hot feeling, swelling in the nose. *2 min after the end of infusion* weals on the neck and the thorax, bronchospasm. *5 min later*: oxygen given. *1 min thereafter* prednisolone 1 mg/kg and clemastine 0.025 mg/kg were injected i.v. and the bronchospasm disappeared within a few minutes. *30 min later*: the test subject still complained of pain in the chest and feeling cold. Mild tachycardia but no hypotension	1.2	1.8

TABLE 6.20

ANAPHYLACTOID REACTIONS AND HISTAMINE RELEASE FOLLOWING INFUSION OF
PLASMA SUBSTITUTES IN HUMAN SUBJECTS AND ANIMALS
Gelatin cross-linked by urea = Haemaccel, gelatin cross-linked by glyoxal = Gelifundol S, for further
explanations see Table 6.6. Dextran 75 = Salvia (Boehringer). + = positive result; − = negative result;
n.t. = not tested. According Lorenz and Doenicke (1978a).

Plasma substitute	Anaphylactoid reactions observed in clinics	Histamine release in			Histamine release roughly in agreement to symptoms
		Animals	Test persons	Clinical incidents	
Gelatin					
Cross-linked by urea	+	Dog, monkey	+	+	+
Cross-linked by glyoxal	+	Dog	+	−	−
Cross-linked by succinic acid anhydride	+	Dog	n.t.	n.t.	−
Dextran					
Dextran-75	+	Rat	+	n.t.	n.t.
Dextran-60	+	Rat	+	−	−
Dextran-40	+	Rat	+	n.t.	n.t.
Hydroxyethyl starch					
HES-400	+	Dog	+	n.t.	−
Albumin	+	Dog	n.t.	n.t.*	n.t.

*only one case tested in Table 6.36.

performed in which the species is chosen which is most sensitive to a particular
amine or polypeptide such as rats for serotonin and guinea-pigs for histamine
(Table 6.17). Human subjects, however, are much less sensitive to serotonin
than rats and much less serotonin is released from human mast cells than from
rat and mouse mast cells (for a survey see Erspamer, 1966). Another example is
the histamine release by anaphylatoxin which is shown in guinea-pigs to be very
small (Giertz et al., 1961). In guinea-pigs which are highly sensitive to histamine
this histamine release may contribute to the anaphylactoid reaction, but in man
this is more than uncertain.
(c) Adverse reactions to clinical dextran have usually been linked with findings
obtained in rats which are highly sensitive to dextran and respond immediately
by an anaphylactoid reaction and a tremendous histamine release (Hahn and
Wellmann, 1952). However, one strain derived from Wistar rats was found not
to be susceptible to the effect of dextran and was selected for its non-reactivity
(Harris and West, 1961, 1963; Harris et al., 1963; Harris and West, 1964; West,

1967). In contrast to this opinion we suggest that this strain may possibly be *more* suitable for investigating the anaphylactoid reaction to dextran in man, since unlike rats, human subjects do not suffer tremendous release of histamine and since the adverse reaction to dextran in this strain may not be completely prevented, but only be relatively rare − as in man.

(d) Cremophor E1 injected in a relatively large dose subcutaneously elicited the formation of a typical wheal (Werner and Wolff, 1973). It was assumed that this was due to the release of histamine and other mediators, but usually drugs dissolved in cremophor E1 for intravenous injection never reach such a high concentration of the solvent in the skin as used in those clinical experiments. It is also very unusual to inject d-tubocurarine intraarterially as it has been carried out by Mongar and Whelan (1953). Basic research scientists unfortunately are not sufficiently aware of the tremendous gap between their experimental work in animals or in suspensions of mast cells or basophilic granulocytes and the clinical situations in which the adverse responses to drugs actually occur. It is incorrect logistics to talk first about animal studies and to develop diffuse hypotheses on "mechanisms" before the involvement of a particular mediator in an adverse response has been shown in human subjects and especially in patients under exactly those conditions which occur every day during routine clinical application.

3.3. Free, biologically active histamine?

If alterations in histamine levels of body fluids or tissues have reliable been measured after administration of a particular drug it seems reasonable to accept this as evidence for histamine release and to assume that histamine may in part or predominantly be responsible for the adverse reaction elicited by this particular drug. But again there are examples which show that caution is still necessary to avoid a misleading conclusion: It has to be demonstrated that alterations of histamine levels are caused by the appearance of free, biologically active histamine which in turn causes the adverse reaction to the particular intravenous agent.

Many reports on histamine being involved in several types of asthma, urticarial reactions and angioneurotic oedema are based on the incorrect assumption that changes in whole blood histamine necessarily indicate a change in free vasoactive histamine (for a critical view see Lindell and Westling, 1966). In cases of anaphylactoid reactions to drugs evidence has been presented that changes in white blood cell counts occur which can explain fully the alterations in whole blood histamine content observed after injection of anaesthetic drugs or plasma substitutes (Lorenz et al., 1972a,c; Doenicke et al. 1973; Lorenz et al., 1976; Watkins et al., 1976).

However, even elevated *plasma* histamine levels are sometimes the subject of considerable misunderstanding and in our opinion very often reflect the preconceptions of the investigators more than the unquestionable evidence for the release of free, physiologically and pathophysiologically active histamine. The simplest way to explain many such errors is the unsatisfactory preparation of plasma samples (Table 6.21). Some basophils or thrombocytes may still be suspended in the plasma supernatant following centrifugation of blood or haemolysis may sometimes be responsible for apparently "elevated" plasma histamine concentrations. Analysing our assays over a period of more than 10 years we have collected some examples in which histamine concentrations as high as observed in anaphylactoid reactions to drugs to were produced in association with haemolysis (Table 6.22). However, as findings with promethazine show haemolysis is not necessarily connected with an increase in plasma histamine concentrations.

Techniques for demonstrating free, biologically active histamine in states with altered histamine contents in body fluids or tissues include the concomitant recording of typical histamine-induced biological reactions. Most of these are shown in Table 6.1. They are more or less non-specific for histamine since other mediators elicit just the same symptoms, except stimulation of gastric acid secretion which is fairly specific in adverse responses to intravenous agents (calcium, para-sympathomimetics, gastrin and some related peptides may interfere!). Examples for these techniques were described by Lorenz et al. (1969), Doenicke and Lorenz (1970), Lorenz et al. (1972a,c and 1976) and are shown for the anaesthetic agent

TABLE 6.21

POSSIBLE ERRORS IN SAMPLE-HANDLING WHICH CAN INFLUENCE THE RELIABILITY OF PLASMA HISTAMINE DETERMINATION. From Lorenz (1975).

---

1. Inappropriate time for sample-taking
    Less than 30 min after alcohol desinfection,
    Less than 30 min after anaesthesia or small operations,
    Less than 6 h after a meal,
    Less than 30 min after manual work or other kinds of stress

2. Inappropriate sample-cooling

3. Inappropriate sample-preparing
    Heparin contaminated with histamine
    Syringes or glassware contaminated with histamine or OPT reactive substances
    Haemolysis (not regularly!)
    Plasma contaminated with leucocytes or thrombocytes
    Delay in preparing plasma until precipitation of proteins by perchloric acid

---

TABLE 6.22

INCIDENCE OF "ELEVATED" HISTAMINE LEVELS IN HAEMOLYTIC PLASMA SAMPLES
Series of controlled clinical trials in which prospectively all samples were recorded which showed a visible
haemolysis: Study 1 (year of performance in round brackets): Infusion of Ringer solution published in
Lorenz et al. (1976). Study 2: Injection of a few ml of saline in trial 3 reported in Lorenz et al. (1980).
Study 3: Injection of promethazine into 10 human volunteers in our clinical trials on male, 20-30 years
old subjects in Munich (Table XIII in Lorenz and Doenicke, 1978a). As syringes Injekt 20 and Monovette
were used (See Table 6.21). That haemolysis was associated with "elevated" plasma histamine levels
could be shown by a series of plasma histamine assays *before* and *after* the particular haemolytic sample:
The usual plateau of the plasma histamine level was clearly shown from which the one sample which was
haemolytic performed a *single* exception at an irregular (probably random) point of time during the
experiment. The increase of the plasma histamine level in such cases exceeded by far the 3 S.D. deviation
of the analytical error of our assay. (For definition of it see Lorenz and Doenicke, 1978b in detail). Histamine assay according to Lorenz et al., 1972b, 1974a.

Series	Drug	Typ of syringe	Haemolysis/ total number of samples tested	Number of "ele-vated" histamine levels/haemolytic samples	Plasma histamine level [ng/ml]		
					Before haemolytic sample	Haemolytic sample	After haemolytic sample
1 (1970)	Ringer solution	In	12/140	11/12	0.5 ± 0.2	1.9 ± 0.6	0.6 ± 0.2
2 (1978)	Saline	Sa	3/420	2/3	0.3	1.4	0.5
3 (1974)	Promet-hazine	Sa	50/70	0/50	–	–	–

propanidid in Fig. 6.23. The parallel curves for plasma histamine levels and acid
outputs indicate more than other "philosophies" the presence of free, biologically
active histamine in plasma. Furthermore it can be shown that the determination of
whole blood histamine in adverse responses to drugs is of very limited value.

The best technique for demonstrating free histamine in adverse responses to
intravenous agents is when a randomized controlled clinical trial is performed in
which concomitantly altered histamine contents (increased plasma histamine levels)
are measured, histamineinduced biological reactions and clinical symptoms are
recorded and these reactions are prevented in a treatment group by the application
of H_1 + H_2-receptor antagonists. Using only antihistaminic drugs for
demonstrating histamine involvement in a particular reactions is not enough since
the H_1-receptor antagonists in particular were shown to exert a large spectrum of

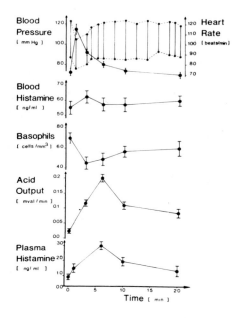

Fig. 6.23. Histamine concentrations in plasma and whole blood, basophils, gastric secretion, blood pressure and heart rate after intravenous injection of propanidid. Mean values ± S.E.M., 5 subjects tested after i.v. injection (20 sec) of 7 mg/kg. In each subject all parameters were studied simultaneously. Note the coincidence of increases in plasma histamine and gastric acid output! For other comments and further conditions see Lorenz et al. (1972a).

"unspecific" effects (Werle and Lorenz, 1970; Lorenz et al., 1973c) which so far have only been partly studied for the H_2-receptor antagonists (Lorenz et al., 1973a).

Unfortunately only two examples exist at present in the literature where these techniques have been applied to studies in man:

(1) In a study of adverse reactions to the plasma substitute Haemaccel[R], saline or the combination of an H_1-blocker and H_2-blocker (dimethpyrindene and cimetidine) was given to 50 human volunteers (Lorenz et al., 1977a; Lorenz et al., 1980). Elevated plasma histamine levels were shown in both groups of test persons with a high incidence (Table 6.23). The case with the highest plasma histamine concentration is shown in Fig. 6.24. However clinical symptoms and biological reactions corresponding quantitatively to the histamine levels were observed only in the control group, not in the subjects being treated by the H_1 + H_2-blocker (Table 6.24).

214

TABLE 6.23

INCREASE IN PLASMA HISTAMINE LEVELS FOLLOWING INFUSION OF HAEMACCEL AND
PREMEDICATION BY H_1- AND H_2-RECEPTOR ANTAGONISTS

A randomized controlled single-blind trial in 50 male volunteers. Saline or the combination of the H_1-receptor antagonist dimethpyrindene (Fenistil[R], Zyma, Nyon-Munich) (0.1 mg/kg) and the H_2-receptor antagonist cimetidine (Tagamet[R], Smith, Kline and Dauelsberg, Göttingen) (10 mg/kg) were applied 10 min before blood donation and subsequent haemaccel infusion. Absolute frequencies are given. $\chi^2 AI/II = 7.04$, $p < 0.01$. For further conditions see Lorenz et al. (1980).

Treatment	Incidence of histamine release	
	< 1 ng/ml (A)	> 1 ng/ml (B)
Saline (I)	11/25	6/25
$H_1 + H_2$ (II)	21/25	7/25

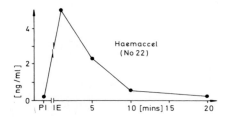

Fig. 6.24. Case with the maximum histamine release observed in test persons after infusion of Haemaccel in the trial on premedication with $H_1 + H_2$-blockers. No. 22 in the series of 50 volunteers. Kl. N., 22, 180, 72 (name, age, height, weight in kg), male, non medical student, no allergy now or previously (more than 9 months earlier in his life-time). The subject had received the H_1- and H_2-receptor antagonists and did not show any clinical symptoms of an anaphylactoid reaction. For further conditions see Lorenz et al. (1980).

(2) Similarly in *mild* adverse reactions to the anaesthetic drug propanidid, saline or the combination of an H_1-blocker and H_2-blocker was given to 32 human volunteers (Doenicke et al., 1980). Elevated plasma histamine levels were shown in both groups, but their extent was relatively small (Table 6.25). It was, however, interesting to note that the "propanidid flush" was to a large extent prevented in the $H_1 + H_2$-group (Table 6.26) and that headache — resembling a hang-over — was more frequently observed in the saline group than in the treatment group. Myocloni, however, occurred more in the treated group than in the control group.

TABLE 6.24

CLINICAL SYMPTOMS AND REACTIONS IN 50 VOLUNTEERS PRETREATED BY $H_1 + H_2$-RECEPTOR ANTAGONISTS OR SALINE FOLLOWING INFUSION OF HAEMACCEL
Anaphylactoid reactions were defined according to the definition given in Section 2. Allergoid reactions were defined by erythema, wheals and itching only. Flush = heat sensation or discomfort in the upper half of the body, associated with reddening, especially at the face and neck. Feeling of heat = feeling at the extremities or the lower part of the body, especially and mostly observed around the genitals and the anus. Feeling of other tastes = sweetish, fruity, peculiar but not comparable to other special ones, spicy, taste like peppermint, beans, ether, plastic material, nitro, vanilla. Significance in the χ^2-test: anaphylactoid reactions $\chi^2 = 4.79$, $p < 0.05$, allergoid reactions (= total, including anaphylactoid reactions which all were associated with wheals) $\chi^2 = 10.94$, $p < 0.01$. For further conditions see Table 6.23. From Lorenz et al. (1980).

Reactions and symptoms	Number of subjects reacting	
	Saline (n = 25)	$H_1 + H_2$-blocker (n = 25)
Anaphylactoid	6*	0
Allergoid (wheals only)	9**	0
Flush	6	1
Feeling of heat	17	12
Metallic taste	5	2
Feeling of other tastes	14	15

Except for preventing of flush these differences, however, were not significant in the small sample of 32 subjects.

The considerable increase in heart rate already in the first min after propanidid was also significantly reduced by the premedication with $H_1 + H_2$-blockers (Table 6.27) whereas the hypotensive response remained the same in the two groups (Table 6.28). The influence of the $H_1 + H_2$-blockers on the propanidid-induced tachycardia is a remarkable finding since at this time the plasma histamine levels have still not reached the highest values (see Fig. 6.23). Like wheals in the skin this may be another example where *local* histamine release is not or not yet associated with an increase in plasma histamine levels and therefore not or not yet with a systemic reaction to the histamine release.

3.4. Exogenous histamine?

If histamine is measured reliably in samples of the most suitable organ system at

216

TABLE 6.25

INCREASE IN PLASMA HISTAMINE LEVELS FOLLOWING INJECTION OF PROPANIDID
AND PREMEDICATION BY H_1- AND H_2-RECEPTOR ANTAGONISTS

A randomized controlled trial in 32 male volunteers, single-blind for clinical investigations, double-blind
for EEG and plasma histamine assays. As in Table 6.22 and 6.24 dimethpyrindene (0.1 mg/kg) and
cimetidine (5 mg/kg) were tested against saline solution. Propanidid (7 mg/kg in 45 sec) was injected in
the morning of each day. Mean values of basal plasma histamine levels 0.3 ng/ml. Subjects ordered by
ranking. Time of maximum increase in round brackets. For further conditions see Doenicke et al. (1980).

Number of subjects reacting	Increase in plasma histamine level (ng/ml)	
	Group I (n = 16) NaCl + propanidid	Group II (n = 16) H_1 + H_2-blocker + propanidid
1	0.5 (1)	0.4 (1)
2	0.6 (1)	0.5 (5)
3	0.6 (5)	0.7 (1)
4	0.9 (1)	0.7 (1)
5	1.0 (2)	0.9 (2)
6	1.1 (5)	1.6 (5)
7	1.1 (10)	1.7 (5)
8	1.4 (5)	–
9	1.8	–
x̄ (range)	1.0 (0.5-1.8)	0.7 (0.4-1.7)

the right time and under the most correct clinical conditions available, there remains
the possibility that the histamine playing a significant role in an adverse reaction is
not endogenous, but simply a more or less important contaminant of the drug. An
example of this surprising clinical finding is heparin, which may cause allergoid or
anaphylactoid reactions in clinical states, and as a constituent of the solution for
plasma histamine assays (Lorenz et al., 1972a) may produce false-positive results of
"histamine release" by a drug following administration of which blood samples
were taken (Table 6.29; Fig. 6.25). The histamine content of the heparin constituent
may be so high to account for an apparent histamine value corresponding to that in
a life-threatening adverse reaction (Table 6.29).

Therefore as a routine procedure all drugs in question for an anaphylactoid
reaction in clinical states should be tested for their contamination with histamine or
any other substance interfering with the histamine assay.

TABLE 6.26

CLINICAL SYMPTOMS IN 32 MALE VOLUNTEERS PRETREATED BY H_1 + H_2-RECEPTOR
ANTAGONISTS OR SALINE FOLLOWING INJECTION OF PROPANIDID
Symptoms evaluated by a EDA questionnaire (Lorenz et al. 1977a). For definitions see also Table 6.24.
Note the increased incidence of myocloni following premedication with H_1 + H_2-receptor antagonists.
Significance in Fisher's exact test (two-sided); Flush A/B; $p < 0.05$; headache A/B, not significant;
myocloni A/B, not significant. For further conditions see Doenicke et al. (1980).

Clinical symptoms	Number of subjects reacting	
	Saline (n = 16) (A)	H_1 + H_2-blocker (n = 16) (B)
Flush	11	4
Headache	3	0
Metallic taste	0	1
Narrowness in throat	2	1
Narrowness in chest	0	3
Respiratory distress	0	0
Epigastric fullness	1	0
Epigastric pain	0	1
Straining	0	1
Myocloni	2	5

TABLE 6.27

INFLUENCE OF H_1 + H_2-RECEPTOR ANTAGONISTS ON THE PROPANIDID-INDUCED
TACHYCARDIA IN VOLUNTEERS
Heart rate measured by ECG (lead II) according to Lorenz et al. (1972a). For further conditions of the
trial see Table 6.25 and 6.26. Statistical significance: Mann-Whitney test (two sided) $p < 0.02$. For further
conditions see Doenicke et al. (1980).

Parameter	Increase in heart rate at first min (beats/min)	
	Saline n = 16	H_1 + H_2-blocker n = 16
Median	45	33
Interquartile range	42-59	29-48
Range	31-73	16-62

TABLE 6.28

INFLUENCE OF $H_1 + H_2$-RECEPTOR ANTAGONISTS ON THE PROPANIDID—INDUCED TACHYCARDIA IN VOLUNTEERS

Blood pressure (systolic) measured by a sphygmomanometric assay according to Lorenz et al. (1972a). For further conditions of the trial see Table 6.25 and 6.26. No significant difference between values obtained after premedication with saline and $H_1 + H_2$-blockers. For further conditions see Doenicke et al. (1980).

Parameter	Decrease in blood pressure (mm Hg)	
	Saline $n = 16$	$H_1 + H_2$-blocker $n = 16$
Median	20	23
Interquartile range	15-25	10-30
Range	5-40	0-35

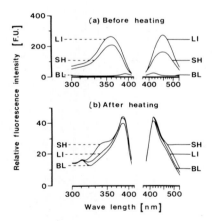

Fig. 6.25. Fluorescence excitation and emission spectra of contaminations in a heparin preparation (Liquemin$^{(R)}$). Identification as histamine. Original registration. Batch No. 1 of Liquemin in Table 6.29. The ampoule content was added to perchloric acid to give a volume of 6 ml and a perchloric acid concentration of 0.5 M as used for plasma preparations. Then the mixture run through the combined procedure (Dowex-50 + butanol extraction) and was analysed after condensation with O-phthaldialdehyde like standard histamine. Before heating = spectra of the condensation mixture at 21°C. After heating = spectra of the same sample, but after heating for 2 h. LI = Liquemin; SH = standard histamine; BL = blank (6 ml 0.5 M perchloric acid running through the whole procedure). For further conditions see Lorenz et al. (1974a).

TABLE 6.29

CONTAMINATION OF HEPARIN PREPARATIONS WITH HISTAMINE AND THEIR INFLUENCE ON THE "PLASMA HISTAMINE LEVEL" MEASURED AFTER ADDITION OF HEPARIN TO WHOLE BLOOD TO PREVENT COAGULATION

Measurement at λ(excitation) = 360 nm and λ(fluorescence) = 450 nm. * 2 mg of dry substance obtained from the company dissolved in our laboratory in 0.5 ml saline (See Lorenz et al., 1972b); ** usage of the ampoule content as described in Fig. 6.25; *** histamine content referring to the ampoule content. Liquemin (purified) = batch obtained from La Roche for biochemical purposes. Syringes which contain sometimes plasticizers interfering with the assay were specified: Inject 20[R] (Braun, Melsungen, F.R.G.), Monovette (R) (Sarstedt, Nümbrecht–Rommelsdorf, F.R.G.). In the Monovette heparin is already added to the syringe by the manufacturer. Note that the increase in plasma histamine levels caused by the particular batch of heparin Novo corresponds to that observed in extremely severe anaphylactoid reactions. For further conditions see Fig. 6.25.

Anticoagulant	Type of syringe	Histamine content (ng/20 ml syringe volume) after addition of heparin		Increase in "plasma histamine level" (ng/ml)
No addition	2 mg* 0.5 ml**			
Heparin, Novo[R]	Glass	270	1800	90.0***
Heparin Roche	Injekt 20	6.7*	57*	3.0***
(Liquemin[R])		2.8**	24**	1.0***
Liquemin[R]	Injekt 20	0		0
(purified)		0		0
Ammonium heparinate	Monovette	0		0
Lithium heparinate	Monovette	0 0		0 0

3.5 Histamine release?

Methods for demonstrating histamine release in man have been compiled in previous reviews (Rothschild, 1966; Lorenz, 1975; Lorenz and Doenicke, 1978a) and include all the direct and indirect techniques summarized in Talbe 6.30. The main difference to items already dealt with in earlier sections of this review are the characteristics which define alterations in histamine levels and physical parameters as histamine release (Table 6.31). The reasons for these definitions were extensively explained by Lorenz et al. (1974c) and Lorenz and Doenicke, (1978b) as far as the plasma histamine levels are concerned. However, it is necessary to emphasize that

TABLE 6.30

METHODS FOR DEMONSTRATING HISTAMINE RELEASE IN MAN
From Lorenz (1975).

---

(1) Direct methods
   Histamine determination in plasma, whole blood, urine or other body fluids
   Histamine determination in isolated cells (basophils) or tissues (lung)

(2) Indirect methods
   Estimation of gastric secretion,
   changes in heart rate (tachycardia),
   delayed depressor response,
   haemoconcentration,
   bronchospasm,
   formation of erythema and oedema
   Inhibition of these biological reactions by histamine
   H_1- and H_2-receptor antagonists

TABLE 6.31

DEFINITION OF HISTAMINE RELEASE IN MAN AND ANIMALS USING PLASMA
HISTAMINE ASSAYS
From Lorenz and Doenicke (1978b).

Criterion concerning augmented plasma histamine levels	Attributes for discrimination
(1) Onset	Shortly after drug application, about 1-5 min after i.v. injection
(2) Velocity of increment	Explosive. Maximum levels about 3-5 min after i.v. injection
(3) Quantity	Peak level significantly higher than basal level (before and after drug administration)
(4) Frequency	More than 1 value. Optimum are 2-3 values before and 4-5 values after drug application
(5) Kinetics	Bateman function. Clearance curves. Half-life time for elimination about 5-10 min
(6) Biological effects	Gastric secretion, increase in heart rate and hypotension corresponding to values with respect to quantity and time-course

such criteria are valid also for the indirect methods, for instance the increase in heart rate, the delayed depressor response of the blood pressure, the increase in respiratory distress and the stimulation of gastric secretion. A sudden tachycardia or respiratory distress may be caused by anxiety. Coughing may be the first symptom of the beginning of an acute cardiac insufficiency as the consequence of a rapid infusion of a plasma substitute in an older patient (which is usually *not* observed in healthy test persons who are engaged in so many trials). Furthermore all the drugs and combination of drugs given before anaesthesia and during operation may imitate anaphylactoid reactions *and* cause some histamine release such as atropine or the muscle relaxants. The only chance to identify such adverse reactions to drugs as anaphylactoid reactions is to measure meticulously the clearance curve of histamine in plasma and to record as exactly as possible the time-course of the physical (heart rate, blood pressure) and the biochemical parameters (haematocrit, acid secretion). Finally, in patients receiving digitalis premedication, it should be noted that true anaphylactoid reactions, especially skin reactions *plus* tachycardia (see definitions of "anaphylactoid" in section 2) may be suppressed by the particular pretreatment. This occurred in at least 4 patients in one of our clinical trials (Schöning and Lorenz, 1980).

3.6. Histamine release specifically caused by the drug itself?

Anaphylactoid reactions and histamine release may be caused — as already mentioned in previous sections — by inserting a needle or injecting and infusing saline or Ringer solution (Lorenz, 1975, Lorenz and Doenicke, 1978b, Lorenz et al., 1976, Lorenz et al., 1980). Only carefully designed randomized controlled clinical trials can exclude those "placebo" effects. Anaphylactoid responses to intravenous agents, however, are relatively rare. Often many patients or test persons have to be included in such trials before the convincing answer to our initial question (Fig. 6.1) "Does histamine play a role in anaphylactoid reactions to a particular intravenous agent in man in clinical condition?" is found: "Yes, histamine plays a definite role in this specific situation".

4. ADVERSE REACTIONS TO INTRAVENOUS AGENTS IN WHICH HISTAMINE WAS SHOWN TO PLAY A DEFINITE AND PREDOMINANT ROLE IN CLINICAL CONDITIONS — THE PLACE OF TYPE I ANAPHYLAXIS

Since the pioneer work of Dale (1920, 1929) and Lewis (1924–1927) histamine is considered and accepted as an active substance (mediator) in immediate hypersensitivity reactions − both of the true anaphylactic (antigen-antibody mediated) and the anaphylactoid type. However, following the first detection of histamine in the literature also other candidates for active substances have been discovered (Table 6.4) which at present make it very difficult to define exactly and quantitatively the role which histamine plays in those reactions. It was Rocha e Silva (1966) who classically described the limitations of the histamine theory in anaphylactic shock (Table 6.32). Recent reviews on this subject unfortunately have not evaluated the importance of this problem and thus have contributed little to its solution (Morrison and Henson, 1978; Orange, 1978; Warrington et al., 1978).

The basic statements which may be helpful for stimulating discussion and a substantial progress in this field are included in Table 6.33. Today a solution of these problems seems to be possible since reliable methods for plasma histamine assay have been developed (Lorenz et al., 1970; Beaven et al., 1972) and new histamine antagonists (H_2-receptor antagonists) are available for clinical use (Black et al., 1972, 1973; Brimblecombe et al., 1975). It is necessary for the clinicians that these problems are solved since undoubtedly some of the adverse reactions to intravenous agents are mediated by antigen-antibody interactions, and for this

TABLE 6.32

LIMITATIONS OF THE HISTAMINE THEORY IN ANAPHYLACTIC REACTIONS ("ANAPHYLACTIC SHOCK")
The table was constructed from Rocha e Silva (1966).

Basic statements favouring the histamine theory	Exceptions and discrepancies disproving or questioning the histamine theory
(1) Histamine reproduces, in certain animal species, the complex of symptoms characteristic of the anaphylactic crisis;	(1) There are differences in degree between the most characteristic symptoms developed after the injection of the antigen and that of histamine;
(2) Histamine is encountered in the so-called shock organs in quantities to explain the most marked effects produced locally, in the event of its liberation;	(2) Histamine sometimes produce an effect just the opposite of the one produced by the antigen;
(3) There is much experimental evidence that histamine is liberated from the tissues after the injection of the antigen;	(3) There are discrepancies regarding the experimental conditions under which the reaction to histamine and to the antigen are brought forward, especially in relation to specific inhibitors, such as anti-histaminics.
(4) There is a general parallelism between the sensitivity of the different animal species to histamine and to anaphylactic shock.	

TABLE 6.33

RELATIONSHIP BETWEEN IMMEDIATE HYPERSENSITIVITY REACTIONS AND HISTAMINE RELEASE IN MAN: NO ANSWER IN TYPE I (IgE OR IgG MEDIATED) ANAPHYLAXIS!

– No convincing evidence for histamine release in man in the course of clinical reactions.
– No correlation between intensity and time-course of clinical reactions and histamine release in man.
– No convincing evidence for a significant effect of histamine antagonists
– Interference of histamine effects with those of other mediators never has been quantitatively estimated in clinical reactions.

reason have to be called "anaphylactic reactions" (Table 6.34). It is necessary for the clinician to know whether histamine or any other mediator is predominantly involved in an anaphylactoid reaction to a particular drug so that he may use rational and specific treatment – rather than symptomatic therapy including a whole battery of drugs. Unfortunately many basic research scientists consider life science as their personal game and consequently do not always strictly aim at the

TABLE 6.34

ANALYSIS OF ADVERSE REACTIONS TO INTRAVENOUS INDUCTION AGENTS
Reproduced with kind permission of J. Watkins

	Cases analysed	C3/C4 anomaly	Sequence studies possible	Complement activation		IgE involved
				Classical	Alternate	
1974						
Althesin	19	9	5	1	4	1/1; 1/4
Thiopentone	1	1	0	0	0	0
Methohexitone	1	0	1	0	1	1
1975						
Althesin	16	9	7	3	4	1/3; 1/4
Epontol	1	1	0	0	0	0
Thiopentone	1	1	1	0	0	0
1976						
Althesin	15	7	12	4	6	0/4; 1/6
Epontol	2	0	2	0	2	0
Thiopentone	2	2	2	1	1	1/1; 1/1

benefit of the patients. For those who are lucky enough to detect an antibody in a serum of a patient suffering from an adverse response to a particular drug and who believe that they have elucidated the whole trouble, the passage written by Gell and Coombs (1975) may be especially useful (Table 6.35). That the generation of antibodies is frequently an epiphenomenon has been pointed out clearly by Dukon et al.) 1980).

TABLE 6.35

STATEMENT PUBLISHED BY GELL AND COOMBS (1975) CONCERNING THE RELATION-SHIP BETWEEN THE OCCURRENCE OF HYPERSENSITIVITY REACTIONS AND THE CONCOMITANT DEMONSTRATION OF IMMUNOLOGICAL PROCESSES

"It is an easy error to assume that when one process is demonstrable (e.g. antibody formation against organ antigens), that this and only this is responsible for the whole trouble, or indeed for any of it"

In our opinion there are only a few adverse reactions to intravenous agents in clinical states in which the role of histamine is defined exactly and quantitatively. These include reaction to polyurea gelatin (Haemaccel[(R)]), propanidid (Epontol[(R)]) and dextran (Macrodex[(R)], Dextran "Fisons"). In Haemaccel- and propanidid-induced clinical incidents histamine release plays a predominant role, in dextran-induced events histamine release very probably does *not* play any significant role. Evidence for these statements will be summarized answering the questions in the decision tree (Fig. 6.1).

(a) *Haemaccel:* Anaphylactoid and/or allergoid symptoms and reactions were observed in clinical states (Table 6.2), human volunteers (Table 6.2) and animals (dogs) (Messmer et al., 1970). During these reactions changes (increases) in peripheral venous plasma histamine concentration were measured in patients (Lorenz et al., 1980, Table 13, Fig. 11; Schöning and Lorenz, 1980) and human volunteers (Lorenz et al., 1971b, 1976, 1977a). In dogs changes in arterial and venous plasma histamine content, in whole blood histamine content and in histamine content of various tissues could be demonstrated (Fig. 6.9 and 6.10; Table 6.12).

The appearance of free, biologically active histamine could be clearly shown by the best technique at present available: randomized controlled clinical trials in which *concomitantly* increased plasma histamine levels were measured, biological reactions and clinical symptoms of anaphylactoid reactions were recorded and in a treatment group these reactions were prevented by the application of $H_1 + H_2$-receptor antagonists (Lorenz et al., 1977a; Lorenz et al., 1980; Lorenz and

Doenicke, 1978a). Pretreatment by antihistaminic drugs was successful even in the most severe reactions to Haemaccel in dogs (Lorenz and Doenicke, 1978a). By various, meticulous investigations it could be shown that Haemaccel was free of contamination with exogenous histamine (Lorenz et al., 1974b, Fig. 3, Table, 6 and 7). All criteria for demonstrating histamine release under in-vivo conditions could be fulfilled for patients (Lorenz et al., 1980; Schöning and Lorenz, 1980, Fig. 11), human volunteers (Lorenz et al., 1976; Lorenz et al., 1980) and dogs (Messmer et al., 1970; Lorenz et al., 1974a, 1974c). In human volunteers (Lorenz et al., 1976) and dogs (Messmer et al., 1970) it could be shown that the drug itself, not Ringer solution, released histamine in conditions which were especially unfavourable for the "placebo" medication (relatively large volume, rapid infusion speed).

Using the verbal formulation in Lusted's book on medical decision making (1968) we have to say: OK, histamine plays a definite and predominant role in adverse reactions to Haemaccel[(R)]. Pretreatment with H_1 + H_2-receptor antagonists is a rational prophylaxis in all patients at risk for anaphylactoid reactions to this drug.

(b) Propanidid. As with Haemaccel the questions in the decision tree can be answered also for propanidid. The facts are included in the various paragraphs in section 3 and need not be repeated here again. Differences to Haemaccel, however, exist since probably not *all* anaphylactoid reactions to propanidid are caused by the same pathomechanism (Watkins et al., 1976; Watkins et al., 1978; Watkins, 1979) and since the drug consists of the anaesthetic agent *plus* the solvent which is responsible for anaphylactoid reactions in dogs (Lorenz et al., 1971a, 1973b, 1977b) and pigs (Glen et al., 1978, 1979).

(c) Dextran. Clinical dextran elicits anaphylactoid reactions, but the path along the decision tree end at the second question node. In patients and in human volunteers suffering from adverse reactions to extran, significant changes in plasma histamine levels have never been shown (Lorenz et al., 1976; for details see Tables 18 and 19 as well as Fig. 6 and Table 11 in Lorenz and Doenicke, 1978b). Despite the overwhelming evidence that dextran is a histamine releaser in rats (Goth, 1972, Kazimierczak and Diamant, 1978) it has therefore to be concluded that histamine does *not* play a definite role in adverse reactions to this drug in clinical conditions. According to Popper's philosophy (1972) this holds true till the refutation of this statement by the first case of an anaphylactoid reaction to dextran associated with a considerable, if not massive histamine release.

5. ADVERSE REACTIONS TO INTRAVENOUS AGENTS WHICH ELICIT INCREASES IN PLASMA HISTAMINE LEVELS INTERPRETABLE AS HISTAMINE RELEASE

A large variety of anaesthetic drugs, muscle relaxants, drugs for premedication in anaesthesia, antihistaminic drugs and plasma substitutes have been investigated for their histamine releasing activity in man using clinical doses and the clinical *route* of application. Table 6.36, as a modification of Table XIII in Lorenz and Doenicke (1978a) shows a survey of the present state of our knowledge. All the drugs mentioned as positive have fulfilled criteria 1–5 for histamine release in Table 6.31 when tested in prospective controlled clinical trials in human volunteers and patients or in a few exceptions in single cases in patients. However, in the medical decision tree (Fig. 6.1) many questions cannot yet be answered and caution seems necessary for many reasons mentioned in section 3. Nevertheless at present it cannot be excluded that histamine plays a definite and qualitatively and quantitatively distinct role in adverse reactions to these intravenous agents.

TABLE 6.36

HISTAMINE RELEASE IN MAN BY DRUGS USED IN ANAESTHESIA AND SURGERY

All assays were performed by the fluorometric assay of Lorenz et al. (1972b). Work in human volunteers if not otherwise stated. All this work (except ranitidine) was performed by A. Doenicke and W. Lorenz in Munich in the years 1968-1979 using techniques described in Lorenz et al., 1972b, 1976 and 1977a. Ranitidine was studied by J. Parkin (Middlesex London) and W. Lorenz (Marburg). Trials in patients or studies in single cases were executed with B. Schöning (Heidelberg), A. Thornton and J. Watkins (Sheffield), H. Lennartz, M. Thermann (Marburg), R. Dudziak (Frankfurt), A. Doenicke (Munich) and W. Lorenz (Marburg). Only significant histamine release (plasma levels more than 1 ng/ml) was evaluated. Dimethpyrindene in this table was given i.v., not orally as in earlier studies.

Substances		Number of subjects	Dose (mg/kg i.v.)	Result of testing
Anaesthetics and hypnotics:				
Propanidid,	volunteers	56	5-7	+
	patients	2	7	+
Althesin,	volunteers	8	0.075	+
	patients	18	0.07	+
Etomidate		43	0.2	−
Thiopentone		15	5	+
Methohexitone		10	2.5	+
Diazepam		10	0.15	−
Flunitrazepam		10	0.02	+
Lormetazepam		10	1.0	+

Substances	Number of subjects	Dose (mg/kg i.v.)	Result of testing
Muscle relaxants:			
Succinylcholine, volunteers	8	0.7	+
patient	1	0.7	+
Alloferin	8	0.15	+
Pancuronium	8	0.1	+
Drug combinations:			
Etomidate − pancuronium	8	0.2, 0.1	(+)
Etomidate − lormetazepam	10	1.5, 1.0	+
Premidication			
Saline	48	0.1-0.2*	+
Atropine	36	0.01	+
Methylprednisolone	7	15	+
Antihistaminic drugs			
Dimethpyrindene	7	0.1	−
Promethazine	10	0.4	−
Chlorpheniramine	7	0.3	+
Cimetidine	12	5, 10	+
Ranitidine	5	1.0	+
Plasma substitutes			
Haemaccel, volunteers	80	6 ml/kg	+
patients	600	6 ml/kg	+
Oxypolygelatin, volunteers	10	6 ml/kg	+
patients	1	ca. 20 ml	+
Dextran-60 (Macrodex),			
volunteers	35	6 ml/kg	+
patients	2	ca. 20 ml	−
Dextran-70 (Fisons)	10	6 ml/kg	+
Dextran-75 (Salvia)	5	6 ml/kg	+
Dextran-40 (Salvia)	5	6 ml/kg	+
Hydroxyethyl starch (400/0.7)	20	6 ml/kg	+
Human albumin, patient	1	3 ml/kg	+
Protease inhibitors			
Aprotinin, volunteers	10	6000 E/kg	−
patient	1	3000 E/kg	+

* Saline is given in ml/kg. (+), only symptoms, no significant increase of histamine levels.

From Table 6.36, studies on contrast media were excluded. Since for the first time in human subjects Seidel et al. (1974) showed increases in plasma histamine levels by a reliable assay following the injection of contrast media this problem became a subject of major interest in the last few years (Ring et al., 1978; Simon et al., 1979; Arroyave et al. 1979). Studies in animals and isolated cells were carefully performed by Lasser and his group (Lasser et al., 1971, 1974), by Rockoff et al. 1970, 1971, 1972), Rockoff and Brasch (1971) and by Rockoff and Aker (1972). However asking the questions in the decision tree (Fig. 6.1) there are in our opinion still too many unanswered questions and until they were answered the role of histamine in adverse responses to contrast media in clinical states remains unclear.

6. SUMMARY

This review is concerned with the problem of whether histamine plays any significant role in adverse reactions to intravenous agents and whether this role can be qualitatively and quantitatively be defined.

First of all, the adverse reactions dealt with in this article were defined as "anaphylactoid" and "allergoid" using functional or operational items. Therefore a decision tree was constructed to define an intravenous agent as histamine liberator in clinical states.

The decision tree included the following questions: Are anaphylactoid symptoms and reactions observed to a particular drug in clinical states and are these reactions caused by the drug itself? Are changes in histamine content of body fluids or tissues measurable during these reactions by a reliable histamine assay in samples of the relevant organ system at the right time under correct in-vivo (clinical) conditions? Are the changes in histamine content caused by free, biologically active histamine? Is the free histamine exogenous histamine, or just a contamination of a drug? Is the free, endogenous histamine released from its storage sites? Is the histamine release specifically caused by the drug itself? After a positive answer to the last question the decision tree ends with the statement: "OK, histamine plays a definite role in adverse reactions to that particular drug".

Adverse reactions to intravenous agents in which histamine was shown to play a definite and predominant role in clinical conditions include only the plasma substitute Haemaccel and the anaesthetic drug propanidid. In adverse reactions to dextran histamine did not have a significant role, and in type I anaphylaxis the role of histamine is uncertain and difficult to define in quantitative terms.

A list of intravenous agents has been compiled which elicit increases in plasma histamine levels interpretable as histamine release. It includes many anaesthetic and hypnotic drugs, muscle relaxants, drug combinations, premedications, antihistaminic drugs, plasma substitutes and protease inhibitors. In addition, contrast media were mentioned since in recent years many studies have been performed on this particular subject. However, in the decision tree many questions cannot yet be answered for these drugs and caution seems necessary. Nevertheless at present it cannot be excluded that histamine plays a definite and distinct role in adverse reactions to all these intravenous agents.

7. ACKNOWLEDGEMENTS

We are very grateful to J.B. West, T.H.V. Hanahoe, J. Watkins and A. Thornton for stimulating discussions and to J. Parkin for help with the English. The assistance of D. Weber, E. Hinterlang, B. Schwarz and A. Schmal is also very appreciated.

6.8. REFERENCES

Adam H.M., Card, W.I., Riddell, M.J., Roberts, M. and Strong, I.A. (1954): The effect of intravenous infusions of histamine on the urinary histamine and on gastric secretion in man. *Brit. J. Pharmacol., 9*, 62-67.

Adam, H.M., Hardwick, D.C. and Spencer, K.E.V. (1957): Method for determination of histamine in plasma. *Brit. J. Pharmacol., 12*, 397-405.

Ahnefeld, F.W., Fischer, F., Frey, R., Kilian, J. and Schöning, B. (1979): Der Infusionszwischenfall nach künstlichen Plasmasubstituten im Meldekollektiv der Arzneimittelkommission. *Anaesthesist, 28*, 207-220.

Alam, M., Anrep, G.V., Barsoum, G.S., Talaat, M. and Wieninger, E. (1939): Liberation of histamine from skeletal muscle by curare. *J. Physiol. (London), 95*, 148-158.

Altura, B.M. and Halevy, S. (1978a): Cardiovascular actions of histamine. In: *Histamine II and Anti-Histaminics, Handbook of Experimental Pharmacology, Vol. 18/2.* Editors: M. Rocha e Silva and H.A. Rothschild. Springer-Verlag, Berlin, Heidelberg, New York. pp. 1-39.

Altura, B.M. and Halevy, S. (1978b): Circulatory shock, histamine, and antihistaminics: therapeutic aspects. In: *Histamine II and Anti-Histaminics, Handbook of Experimental Pharmacology, Vol. 18/2.* Editors: M. Rocha e Silva and H.A. Rothschild. Springer-Verlag, Berlin, Heidelberg, New York. pp. 575-602.

Anrep, G.V. and Barsoum, G.S. (1935): Distribution of histamine between plasma and red blood corpuscles. *J. Physiol. (London), 85*, 36P-37P.

Anrep, G.V., Barsoum, G.S., Talaat, M. and Wieninger, E. (1939): Determination of histamine in blood. *J. Physiol. (London), 95*, 476-484.

Arnoldsson, H., Helander, C.G., Helander, E., Lindell, S.E., Lindholm, B., Olsson, O., Roos, B.-E., Svanborg, A., Söderholm, B. and Westling, H. (1962): Elimination of ^{14}C-histamine from the blood in man. *Scand. J. clin. Lab. Invest., 14*, 241-246.

Arroyave, C.M., Wolbus, R. and Ellis Ph.P. (1979): Plasma complement and histamine changes after intravenous administration of sodium fluorescein. *Amer. J. Ophthalmology, 87*, 474-479.

Barsoum, G.S. and Gaddum, J.H. (1935): The pharmacological estimation of adenosine and histamine in blood. *J. Physiol. (London), 85*, 1-13.

Barth, H., Niemeyer, I. and Lorenz, W. (1973): Studies on the mode of action of histamine H_1- and H_2-receptor antagonists on gastric histamine methyltransferase. *Agents Actions, 3*, 138-147.

Barth, H., Crombach, M., Schunack, W. and Lorenz, W. (1980): Evidence for a less high acceptor substrate specificity of gastric histamine methyltransferase: methylation of imidazole compounds. *Biochem. Pharmacol., 29,* 1399-1407.

Beaven, M.A. (1976): Histamine. *New Engl. J. Med., 294,* 30-36 and 320-325.

Beaven, M.A. (1978): *Histamine: Its Role in Physiological and Pathological Processes. Monographs in Allergy, Vol. 13.* S. Karger, Basel, Mñchen, Paris, London, New York, Sydney. pp. 1-113.

Beaven, M.A. and Horáková, Z. (1978): The enzymatic isotopic assay of histamine. In: *Histamine II and Anti-Histaminics, Handbook of Experimental Pharmacology, Vol. 18/2.* Editors: M. Rocha e Silva and H.A. Rothschild. Springer-Verlag, Berlin, Heidelberg, New York. pp. 153-173.

Beaven, M.A., Jacobsen, S. and Horáková, Z. (1972): Modification of the enzymatic isotopic assay of histamine and its application to measurement of histamine in tissues, serum and urine. *Clin. Chim. Acta, 37,* 91-103.

Beger, H.G., Stopik, D., Bittner, R., Kraas, E. and Roscher, R. (1975): Der Einfluß der Leber auf die Plasmahistaminkonzentration. Messungen im prä- und posthepatischen Blut vor und nach abdominellen Operationen. *Z. Gastroenterologie, 13,* 474-478.

Behrmann, V.G., Schelling, V. and Hartmann, F.W. (1945): Blood histamine levels in experimental burns. *Amer. J. Physiol., 145,* 483-490.

Benke, A., Balogh, A. and Reich-Hilscher, B. (1979): Über die atmungs-spezifische Wirkung des Lösungsvermittlers von Diazepam (Valium[R]). *Anaesthesist, 28,* 24-28.

Bjurö, T., Lindberg, S. and Westling, H. (1961): Observations on histamine in pregnancy and the puerperium. *Acta obst. gynecol. scand., 40,* 152-173.

Black, J.W., Duncan, W.A.M., Durant, C.J., Ganellin, C.R. and Parsons, E.M. (1972): Definition and antagonism of histamine H_2-receptors. *Nature, 236,* 385-390.

Black, J.W., Duncan, W.A.M., Emmett, J.C., Ganellin, C.R., Hesselbo, T., Parsons, M.E. and Wyllie, J.M. (1973): Metiamide – an orally active histamine H_2-receptor antagonist. *Agents Actions, 3,* 133-137.

Blatchley, D. (1977): Allergy to diazepam. *Brit. med. J., 1,* 287-287.

Brimblecombe, R.W., Duncan, W.A.M., Durant, G.J., Emmett, J.C., Ganellin, C.R. and Parsons, M.E. (1975): Cimetidine – a non-thiourea H_2-receptor antagonist. *J. int. med. Res., 3,* 86-92.

Clarke, R.S.J., Dundee, J.W., Garrett, R.T., McArdle, G.K. and Sutton, J.A. (1975): Adverse reactions to intravenous anaesthetics. *Brit. J. Anaesth., 47,* 575- 585.

Clarke, R.S.J., Fee, J.H. and Dundee, J.W. (1978): Hypersensitivity reactions to intravenous anaesthetics. In: *Adverse Response to Intravenous Drugs.* Editors: J. Watkins and A.M. Ward. Academic Press, Grune and Stratton, London, New York. pp. 41-47.

Code, C.F. (1937): The source in blood of the histamine-like constituent. *J. Physiol. (London), 90,* 349-364.

Code, C.F. (1939): The histamine content of the blood of guinea-pigs and dogs during anaphylactic shock. *Amer. J. Physiol., 127,* 78-93.

Code, C.F. and Jensen, J.L. (1941): A comparison of the histamine content of blood and bone marrow. Amer. J. Physiol., 131, 768-775.

Code, C.F. and Mitchell, R.G. (1957): Histamine, eosinophils and basophils in the blood. *J. Physiol. (London), 136,* 449-468.

Cohen, J., Weetman, A.P., Dargie, H.J. and Krikler, D.M. (1979): Life- threatening arrhythmias and intravenous cimetidine. *Brit. Med. J., 2,* 768-768.

Dale, H.H. (1920): The biological significance of anaphylaxis. *Proc. roy. Soc. B., 91,* 126-146.

Dale, H.H. (1929): On some chemical factors in the control of circulation. Croonian Lectures II and III. *Lancet, 216,* 1233-1237, 1285 ff.

Dannemann, H. and Lübke, P. (1970): Komplikationen während Narkosen mit Epontol[R]. *Z. prakt. aesth. Wiederbel., 4*, 273-277.

Doenicke, A. (1974): Propanidid. In: *Proc. IVth Europ. Congr. Anaesthesiol. (Madrid)*. pp. 107-113.

Doenicke, A. (1977): Klinische Pharmakologie. In: *Lehrbuch der Anaesthesiologie, Reanimation und Intensivtherapie*. Editors: H. Benzer, R. Frey, W. Hügin and O. Mayrhofer. Springer-Verlag, Berlin, Heidelberg, New York. pp. 123-183.

Doenicke, A. and Lorenz, W. (1970): Histaminfreisetzung und anaphylaktische Reaktionen bei Narkosen. Biochemische und klinische Aspekte. *Anaesthesist, 19*, 413-417.

Doenicke, A. and Lorenz, W. (1973): Nachweis von Histaminfreisetzung bei hypotensiven Reaktionen nach Propanidid und ihrer Therapie mit Corticosteroiden. *Anaesth. Wiederbel., 74*, 189-199.

Doenicke, A. and Lorenz, W. (1976): Interférences entre libération d'histamine et médicaments utilisés en anesthésiologie. *Ann. Anesth. (France), 17*, 355-364.

Doenicke, A. and Lorenz, W. (1978): Histaminliberierung durch Flunitrazepam. In: *Klinische Anaesthesiologie und Intensivtherapie*. Editors: F.W. Ahnefeld, H. Bergmann, C. Burri, W. Dick, M. Halmagyi, G. Hossli, E. Rügheimer. Springer-Verlag, Heidelberg, Bd. 17. pp. 62-66.

Doenicke, A., Lorenz, W., Beigl, R., Bezecny, H., Uhlig, G., Kalmar, L., Praetorius, B. and Mann, G. (1973): Histamine release after intravenous application of short-acting hypnotics: a comparison of etomidate, althesin (CT 1341) and propanidid. *Brit. J. Anaesth., 45*, 1097-1104.

Doenicke, A., Lorenz, W. et al. (1980): (In preparation).

Domschke, W., Subramanian, N., Mitznegg, P., Baenkler, H.W., Domschke, S. and Wünsch, E. (1977): Gastric mucosal histamine in duodenal-ulcer patients: release by secretin. *Acta Hepato-Gastroenterol., 24*, 444-446.

Dukov, P., Kallós, P., Schlümberger, H.D. and West, G.B. (1980): Introduction in Pseudo-Allergic Reactions Involvements of Drugs and Chemicals. Karger, Basel (in press).

Dundee, J.W. and Wyant, G.M. (1974): *Intravenous Anaesthesia*. Churchill and Livingstone, Edinburgh and London. pp. 1-341.

Emmelin, N., Kahlson, G. and Wicksell, F. (1941): Histamine in plasma and methods of its estimation. *Acta physiol. scand., 2*, 123-142.

Erspamer, V. (1966): 5-Hydroxytryptamine and related indolealkylamines. In: *Handbook of Experimental Pharmacology, Vol. 19*. Editors: O. Eichler, A. Farah. Springer-Verlag, Berlin, Heidelberg, New York, pp. 1-928.

Falk, R.H. (1977): Allergy to diazepam. *Brit. med. J., 1*, 287-287.

Fantozzi, R., Moroni, F., Masini, E., Blandina, P. and Mannaioni, P.F. (1978): Modulation of the spontaneous histamine release by adrenergic and cholinergic drugs. *Agents Actions, 8*, 347-358.

Fisher, M.M. (1975): Severe histamine mediated reactions to intravenous drugs used in anaesthesia. *Anaesth. Intens. Care, 3*, 180-197.

Galen, R.S. and Gambino, S.R. (1975): *Beyond Normality: The Predictive Value and Efficiency of Medical Diagnoses*. John Wiley, New York. pp. 30-40.

Gell, P.G.H. and Coombs, R.R.A. (1975): *Clinical Aspects of Immunology*. Blackwell, Oxford, pp. 1-1754.

Giertz, H. and Hahn, F. (1966): Makromolekulare Histaminliberatoren (Eiklar, Dextran, Polyvinylpyrrolidon, Tween 20, Anaphylatoxin). In: *Histamine and Anti-Histaminics, Part 1, Handbook of Experimental Pharmacology, Vol. 18/1*. Editors: M. Rocha e Silva and H.A. Rothschild. Springer-Verlag, Berlin, Heidelberg, New York. pp. 481-568.

Giertz, H., Hahn, F., Juma, I. and Schmutzler, W. (1961): Vergleichende Untersuchungen über den anaphylaktischen Schock und den Anaphylatoxin-Schock am intakten Meerschweinchen. *Naunyn-Schmiedebergs Arch. exp. Pathol. Pharmakol., 242,* 65-75.

Glen, J.B., Davies, G.E., Thomson, D.S., Scarth, S.C. and Thompson, A.V. (1978): Adverse reactions to intravenous anaesthetics in animals. In: *Adverse Response to Intravenous Drugs.* Editors: J. Watkins and A.M. Ward. Academic Press, London, Grune and Stratton, New York. pp. 129-135.

Glen, J.B., Davies, G.E., Thomson, D.S., Scarth, S.C. and Thompson, A.V. (1979): An animal model for the investigation of adverse responses to i.v. anaesthetic agents and their solvents. *Brit. J. Anaesth., 51,* 819-827.

Goth, A. (1972): Histamine release by drugs and chemical. In: *Histamine and Antihistaminics. Int. Encyclop. Pharmacol. Ther., Vol. 74/1.* Pergamon Press, Oxford. pp. 25-43.

Guggenheim, M. and Löffler, W. (1916): Biologischer Nachweis proteinogener Amine in Organextrakten und Körperflüssigkeiten. *Biochem. Z., 72,* 303-324.

Hahn, F. and Wellmann, A. (1952): Experimentelle Untersuchungen über Histaminfreisetzung durch künstliche Blutersatzmittel. *Klin. Wschr., 30,* 998-999.

Halpern, B.N. (1956): Histamine release by long chain molecules. In: *Ciba Foundation Symp. on Histamine.* Editors: G.E.W. Wolstenholme and C.M.O'Connor. Churchill, London. pp. 92-123.

Halpern, B.N., Briot, M., Liacopoulos, P., Neveu, Th. and Branellec, A. (1956): Propriétés histamino-libératrices d'une butylamine substituée (1935L) chez le chien. *C. R. Soc. Biol. (Paris), 150,* 1302-1306.

Harrfeldt, H.P. (1970): Zum Zusammenhang von Todesfällen und Komplikationen mit Propanidid. *Z. prakt. Anaesth. Wiederbel., 5,* 55-60.

Harris, J.M. and West, G.B. (1961): Anaphylactoid reaction in rats. *Nature, 191,* 399-400.

Harris, J.M. and West, G.B. (1963): Rats resistant to the dextran anaphylactoid reaction. *Brit. J. Pharmacol., 20,* 550-562.

Harris, J.M. and West, G.B. (1964): A new link between the anaphylactoid reaction in rats and human allergy. *Int. Arch. Allergy, 25,* 46-57.

Harris, J.M. Kalmus, H. and West, G.B. (1963): Genetical control of the anaphylactoid reaction in rats. *Genet. Res., 4,* 346-355.

Helander, S.G., Lindell, S.E. and Westling, H. (1965): The renal removal of ^{14}C-labelled histamine from the blood in man. *Scand. J. clin. Lab. Invest., 17,* 524-528.

Hinshaw, L.B., Jordan, M.M., Vick, J.A., Doty, S.O. and Wittmers, L.E. (1961): Mechanism of histamine release in endotoxin shock. *Amer. J. Physiol., 200,* 987-989.

Horáková, Z., Keiser, H.R. and Beaven, M.A. (1977): Blood and urine histamine levels in normal and pathological states as measured by a radiochemical assay. *Clin. Chim. Acta, 79,* 447-456.

Kadykov, B.I. and Federowa, A.V. (1956): (Translated) Über die Bildung der Histaminase und ihren Eintritt in das lymphatische System. *Ber. Acad. Wissensch. UdSSR, 110,* 1038-1040.

Kaplan, A.P., Horáková, Z. and Katz, S.I. (1978): Assessment of tissue fluid histamine levels in patients with urticaria. *J. Allergy clin. Immunol., 61,* 350-354.

Kay, B. (1972): Brietal sodium in children's surgery. In: *Das Ultrakurznarkotikum Methohexital.* Editor: C. Lehmann. Springer-Verlag, Berlin, Heidelberg, New York. pp. 149-158.

Kazimierczak, W. and Diamant, B. (1978): Mechanisms of histamine release in anaphylactic and anaphylactoid reactions. *Progr. Allergy, 24,* 295-365.

Langrehr, D., Arnold, R., Kluge, I., Neuhaus, R. and Singbartl, G. (1977): Zur Frage des per- und postoperativen Risikos in Bezug zur Allgemeinanästhesie. *Med. Welt, 28,* 1033-1035.

Lasser, E.C., Walters, A., Reuter, S.R. and Lang, J. (1971): Histamine release by contrast media. *Radiology, 100,* 683-686.

Lasser, E.C., Walters, A.J. and Lang, L.H. (1974): An experimental basis for histamine release in contrast material reactions. *Radiology, 110*, 49-59.

Levi, R., Zavecz, J.H., Lee, C.-H. and Allan, G. (1977): Histamine-drug-disease interactions and cardiac function. *Philadelphia Physiol. Soc. Meeting, March 20-21, 1977*.

Lewis, T. (1924): Vascular reactions of the skin to injury. I. Reaction to stroking. *Heart, 11*, 119-140.

Lewis, T. (1926): Vascular reactions of the skin to injury. IV. An irresponsive condition of the vessels. *Heart, 13*, 153, ff.

Lewis, T. (1927): *Blood Vessels of the Human Skin and Skin Responses*. Shaw and Sons, London.

Lindberg, S. (1963): [^{14}C]-histamine elimination from the blood of pregnant and non-pregnant women with special references to the uterus. *Acta obst. gynecol. scand., 42, Suppl. 1*, 4-25.

Lindell, S.-E. and Viske, K. (1961): A note on the distribution of [^{14}C]-histamine added to blood. *Brit. J. Pharmacol. 17*, 131-136.

Lindell, S.E. and Westling, H. (1966): Histamine metabolism in man. In: *Histamine and Anti-Histaminics, Part 1, Handbook of Experimental Pharmacology, Vol. 18/1*. Editors: M. Rocha e Silva and H.A. Rothschild. Springer-Verlag, Berlin, Heidelberg, New York. pp. 734-788.

Lorenz, W. (1975): Histamine release in man. *Agents Actions, 5*, 402-416.

Lorenz, W. and Doenicke, A. (1973): Biochemie und Pharmakologie der Histaminfreisetzung durch intravenöse Narkosemittel und Muskelrelaxantien. In: *Intravenöse Narkose mit Propanidid. Anaesthesiologie und Wiederbelebung, Vol. 74*. Editors: M. Zindler, H. Yamamura and W. Wirth. Springer-Verlag, Berlin, Heidelberg, New York, pp. 179-188.

Lorenz, W. and Doenicke, A. (1978a): Histamine release in clinical conditions. *Mount Sinai J. Med., 45*, 357-386.

Lorenz, W. and Doenicke, A. (1978b): Anaphylactoid reactions and histamine release by intravenous drugs used in surgery and anaesthesia. In: *Adverse Response to Intravenous Drugs*. Editors: J. Watkins and A.M. Ward. Academic Press, London; Grune and Stratton, New-York, pp. 83-112.

Lorenz, W., Doenicke, A., Halbach, S., Krumey, I. and Werle, E. (1969): Histaminfreisetzung und Magensaftsekretion bei Narkosen mit Propanidid (Epontol[R]). *Klin. Wschr., 47*, 154-157.

Lorenz, W., Benesch, L., Barth, H., Matejka, E., Meyer, R., Kusche, J., Hutzel, M. and Werle, E. (1970): Fluorometric assay of histamine in tissues and body fluids: Choice of the purification procedure and identification in the nanogram range. *Z. Analyt. Chem., 252*, 94-98.

Lorenz, W., Meyer, R., Doenicke, A., Schmal, A., Reimann, H.-J., Hutzel, M. and Werle, E. (1971a): On the species specificity of the histamine release from mast cell stores by Cremophor El. *Naunyn Schmiedeberg's Arch. Pharmakol., 269*, 417-417.

Lorenz, W., Doenicke, A., Messmer, K. and Reimann, H.-J. (1971b): Histamine release in man and dog by plasma substitutes. *Acta Pharmacol. Toxicol., 29, Suppl. 4*, 31-31.

Lorenz, W., Doenicke, A., Meyer, R., Reimann, H.-J., Kusche, J., Barth, H., Geesing, H., Hutzel, M. and Weissenbacher, B. (1972a): Histamine release in man by propanidid and thiopentone: Pharmacological effects and clinical consequences. *Brit. J. Anaesth., 44*, 355-369.

Lorenz, W., Reimann, H.-J., Barth, H., Kusche, J., Meyer, R., Doenicke, A. and Hutzel, M. (1972b): A sensitive and specific method for the determination of histamine in human whole blood and plasma. *Hoppe-Seyler's Z. Physiol. Chem., 353*, 911-920.

Lorenz, W., Doenicke, A., Meyer, R., Reimann, H.-J., Kusche, J., Barth, H., Geesing, H., Hutzel, M. and Weissenbacher, B. (1972c): An improved method for the determination of histamine release in man: Its application in studies with propanidid and thiopentone. *Europ. J. Pharmacol., 19*, 180-190.

234

Lorenz, W., Boeckl, O., Struck, E., Hell, E., Zimmermann, G., Reimann, H.-J., Tauber, R. and Scheffer, B. (1973a): Significance and causes of histamine release during orthotopic homologous liver transplantation in the pig. *Agents Actions, 3,* 2-11.

Lorenz, W., Thermann, M., Hamelmann, H., Schmal, A., Maroske, D., Reimann, H.-J., Kusche, J., Schingale, F., Dormann, P. and Keck, P. (1973b): Influence of H_1- and H_2-receptor antagonists on the effects of histamine in the circulatory system and on plasma histamine levels. In: *Symposium on Histamine H_2-Receptor Antagonists.* Editors: C.J. Wood and M.A. Simkins. Deltakos Ltd., London, pp. 151-168.

Lorenz, W., Huhnd, A., Kusche, J., Barth, H., Haubensack, G., Hutzel, M., Schmal, A., Gerant, M., Wächter, A., Matejka, E., Hahn, H. and Werle, E. (1973c): Histamine and salivary secretion. In: *Histamine.* Editor: Cz. Maslinski. Dowden, Hutchinson and Ross, Stroudsburg, PA, pp. 187-200.

Lorenz, W., Barth, H., Thermann, M., Schmal, A., Dormann, P. and Niemeyer, I. (1974a): Fluorometric histamine determination in canine plasma under normal conditions, following application of exogenous histamine and during histamine release by Haemaccel(R). *Hoppe-Seyler's Z. Physiol. Chem., 355,* 1097-1111.

Lorenz, W., Barth, H., Karges, H.E., Schmal, A., Dormann, P. and Niemeyer, I. (1974b): Problems in the assay of histamine release by gelatin: O-phthaldialdehyde-induced fluorescence, inhibition of histamine methyltransferase and H_1-receptor antagonism by Haemaccel. *Agents Actions, 4,* 324-335.

Lorenz, W., Thermann, M., Messmer, K., Schmal, A., Dormann, P., Kusche, J., Barth, H., Tauber, R., Hutzel, M., Mann, G. and Uhlig, R. (1974c): Evaluation of histamine elimination curves in plasma and whole blood of several circulatory regions: A method for studying kinetics of histamine release in the whole animal. *Agents Actions, 4,* 336-356.

Lorenz, W., Seidel, W., Doenicke, A., Tauber, R., Reimann, H.-J., Uhlig, R., Mann, G., Dormann, P., Schmal, A., Häfner, G. and Hamelmann, H. (1974d): Elevated plasma histamine concentrations in surgery: causes and clinical significance. *Klin. Wschr., 52,* 419-425.

Lorenz, W., Doenicke, A., Freund, M., Schmal, A., Dormann, P., Praetorius, B. and Schürk-Bulich, M. (1975): Plasmahistaminspiegel beim Menschen nach rascher Infusion von Hydroxy-äthylstärke: Ein Beitrag zur Frage allergischer oder anaphylaktoider Reaktionen nach Gabe eines Plasmasubstitutes. *Anästhesist, 24,* 228-230.

Lorenz, W., Doenicke, A., Messmer, K., Reimann, H.-J., Thermann, M., Lahn, W., Berr, J., Schmal, A., Dormann, P., Regenfuss, P. and Hamelmann, H. (1976): Histamine release in human subjects by modified gelatin (Haemaccel(R)) and dextran: An explanation for anaphylactoid reactions observed under clinical conditions? *Brit. J. Anaesth., 48,* 151-165.

Lorenz, W., Doenicke, A., Dittman, I., Hug, P. and Schwarz, B. (1977a): Anaphylaktoide Reaktionen nach Applikation von Blutersatzmitteln beim Menschen: Verhinderung dieser Neben-wirkung von Haemaccel durch Prämedikation mit H_1- und H_2-Rezeptorantagonisten. *Anaesthesist, 26,* 644-648.

Lorenz, W., Reimann, H.-J., Schmal, A., Dormann, P., Schwarz, B. and Neugebauer, E. (1977b): Histamine release in dogs by cremophor El and its derivatives: Oxethylated oleic acid is the most effective constituent. *Agents Actions, 7,* 63-67.

Lorenz, W., Troidl, H., Barth, H. and Rohde, H. (1978a): Histamine, gastric secretion and peptic ulcer disease: An attempt to define special sources of error and problems in clinical biochemical trials. In: *Cimetidine.* Editor: W. Creutzfeldt. Excerpta Medica, Amsterdam, Oxford. pp. 10-36.

Lorenz, W., Schöning, B., Schwarz, B. and Neugebauer, E. (1978b): Increase in sensitivity of the fluorometric plasma histamine determination: Routine assay in the femtomol range. *Naunyn-Schmiedeberg's Arch. Pharm. Suppl., 302,* 63-63.

Lorenz, W., Doenicke, A., Reimann, H.-J., Schmal, A., Schwarz, B. and Dormann, P. (1978c): Anaphylactoid reactions and histamine release by plasma substitutes: A randomized controlled trial in human subjects and in dogs. *Agents Actions, 8,* 397-399.

Lorenz, W., Doenicke, A., Schöning, B., Mamorski, J., Weber, D., Hinterlang, E., Schwarz, B. and Neugebauer, E. (1980): $H_1 + H_2$-receptor antagonists for premedication in anaesthesia and surgery: A critical view basing on randomized clinical trials with Haemaccel and various anti-allergic drugs. *Agents Actions 10,* 114–124.

Lorenz, W., Neugebauer, E., Schöning, B. and Doenicke, A. (1981): (In preparation).

Lundsgaard-Hansen, P. (1969): Treatment of shock with dextrans and gelatins. *Vox Sang., 17,* 161-193.

Lusted, L.B. (1968): *Introduction to Medical Decision Making.* Editor: Ch.C. Thomas. Springfield, IL, pp. 98-140.

Magazinović, V.D., Hamamdzić, M. and Pavlić, S. (1966): Histamine and the evolution of haemorrhagic hypotension. *Acta physiol. Acad. Sci. Hung., 30,* 269-274.

Marcou, I., Athanasiu-Vergu, E., Chiricéanu, D., Cosma, G., Gingold, N. and Parhon, C.C. (1938): Sur le role physiologique de l'histamine. *Presse Medicale, 46,* 371-374.

Maslinski, C. (1975): Histamine and its metabolism in mammals. Part II: Catabolism of histamine and histamine liberation. *Agents Actions, 5,* 183-225.

Messmer, K., Lorenz, W., Sunder-Plassmann, L., Klövekorn, W. and Hutzel, M. (1970): Histamine release as cause of acute hypotension following rapid colloid infusion. *Naunyn-Schmiedeberg's Arch. Pharmakol., 267,* 433-445.

Meyer-Burgdorff, C., Seidel, G. and Schlüter, F.J. (1973): Freisetzung von Histamin und Serotonin bei extrakorporaler Zirkulation. *Anaesthesist, 22,* 212-216.

Milner, L. (1977): Allergy to diazepam. *Brit. Med. J., I,* 144-144.

Minard, D. (1941): The presence and distribution of histamine in blood. *Am. J. Physiol., 132,* 327-335.

Mongar, J.L. and Whelan, R.F. (1953): Histamine release by adrenaline and d-tubocurarine in the human subject. *J. Physiol. (London), 120,* 146-154.

Morrison, D.C. and Henson, P.M. (1978): Release of mediators from mast cells and basophils induced by different stimuli. In: *Immediate Hypersensitivity, Modern Concepts and Developments.* Editor: M.K. Bach. M. Dekker, New-York, Basel. pp. 431-502.

Mota, I. (1966): Release of histamine from mast cells. In: *Histamine and Anti-Histaminics, Part 1, Handbook of Experimental Pharmacology, Vol. 18/1.* Editors: M. Rocha e Silva and H.A. Rothschild. Springer-Verlag, Berlin, Heidelberg, New York. pp. 569-636.

Mundy, R.L., Demaree, G.E., Jakobus, D.P. and Heiffer, M.H. (1967): β-Mercaptoethylamine and cystamine-induced histamine release in the dog. *Arch. int. Pharmacodyn., 165,* 64-70.

Murphy, P. (1962): Histamine in anaesthesia. *Brit. J. Anaesth., 34,* 397-409.

Orange, R.P. (1978): The mast cell derived pharmacologic mediators of anaphylaxis: histamine and slow reacting substance of anaphylaxis. In: *Immediate Hypersensitivity. Modern Concepts and Developments.* Editor: M.K. Bach. M. Dekker, New York, Basel. pp. 589-607.

Padfield, A. and Watkins, J. (1977): Allergy to diazepam. *Brit. Med. J. I,* 575-576.

Paton, W.D.M. (1957): Histamine release by compounds of simple chemical structure. *Pharmacol. Rev., 9,* 269-328.

Paton, W.D.M. (1958): Release of histamine. *Progr. Allergy, 5,* 79-148.

236

Paton, W.D.M. (1959): The effects of muscle relaxants other than muscular relaxation. Anesthesiology, 20, 453-463.

Pavek, K. and Wegmann, A. (1980): Circulatory shock due to anaphylactoid and anaphylactic reactions: its hemodynamics and treatment. A cooperative study. *Fortschr. Med.* (In press).

Popper, K.R. (1972): Objective Knowledge. The Clarendon Press, Oxford.

Rasche, B. and Harrfeldt, H.P. (1973): Biologische Histaminbestimungen nach Propanididgaben. In: *Intravenöse Narkose mit Propanidid, Anaesthesiology and Resuscitation, Vol. 74.* Editors: M. Zindler, H. Yamamura and W. Wirth. Springer-Verlag, Berlin, Heidelberg, New York. pp. 200-206.

Reinhardt, D. (1979): Herzwirkungen von Histamin. Differenzierung unterschiedlicher Rezeptoren, Physiologie und Biochemie des Wirkungsmechanismus. *Anaesthesist, 28,* 67-77.

Richter, W., Messmer, K., Hedin, H. and Ring, J. (1978): Adverse reaction to plasma substitutes: Incidence and pathomechanisms. In: *Adverse Response to Intravenous Drugs.* Editors: J. Watkins and A.M. Ward. Academic Press, London; Grune and Stratton, New York. pp. 49-70.

Ring, J. (1978): Anaphylactoide Reaktionen. In: *Anaesthesiologie und Intensivmedizin, Vol. 111.* Editors: R. Frey, F. Kern and O. Mayrhofer. Springer-Verlag, Berlin, Heidelberg, New York. pp. 1-202.

Ring, J. (1978): Anaphylactoide Reaktionen. In: *Anaesthesiologie und Intensivmedizin, Vol. 111.* Editors: R. Frey, F. Kern and O. Mayrhofer. Springer-Verlag, Berlin, Heidelberg, New York. pp. 1-202.

Ring, J. and Messmer, K. (1977a): Incidence and severity of anaphylactoid reactions to colloid volume substitutes. *Lancet, 1,* 466-469.

Ring, J. and Messmer, K. (1977b): Infusionstherapie mit kolloidalen Volumenersatzmitteln. *Anaesthesist, 26,* 279-287.

Ring, J., Simon, R.A. and Arroyave, C.M. (1978): Increased in vitro histamine release by radiographic contrast media in patients with history of incompatibility. *Clin. exp. Immunol., 34,* 302-309.

Rocha e Silva, M. (1955): *Histamine. Its role in Anaphylaxis and Allergy.* Ch. C. Thomas, Springfield, IL. pp. 1-249.

Rocha e Silva, M. (1966): Release of histamine in anaphylaxis. In: *Histamine and Anti-Histaminics, Part 1, Handbook of Experimental Pharmacology, Vol. 18/1.* Editors: M. Rocha e Silva and H.A. Rothschild. Springer-Verlag, Berlin, Heidelberg, New York. pp. 431-480.

Rockoff, S.D. and Aker, U.T. (1972): Contrast media as histamine liberators: 6. Arterial plasma histamine and hemodynamic responses following angiocardiography in man with 75% hypaque. *Invest. Radiology, 7,* 403-406.

Rockoff, S.D. and Brasch, R. (1971): Contrast media as histamine liberators. 3. Histamine release and some associated hemodynamic effects during pulmonary angiography in the dog. *Invest. Radiology, 6,* 110-114.

Rockoff, S.D., Brasch, R., Kuhn, C. and Chraplyvy, M. (1970): Contrast media as histamine liberators. 1. Mast-cell histamine release in vitro by sodium salts of contrast media. *Invest. Radiology, 5,* 503-509.

Rockoff, S.D., Kuhn, C. and Chraplyvy, M. (1971): Contrast media as histamine liberators. 4. In vitro mast cell histamine release by methylglucamine salts. *Invest. Radiology, 6,* 186-190.

Rockoff, S.D., Kuhn, C. and Chraplyvy, M. (1972): Contrast media as histamine liberators: 5. Comparison of in vitro mast cell histamine release by sodium and methylglucamine salts. *Invest. Radiology, 7,* 177-181.

Rohde, H., Lorenz, W., Troidl, H., Reimann, H.-J., Häfner, G. and Weber, D. (1980): Histamine and peptic ulcer: Influence of sample-taking on the precision and accuracy of fluorometric histamine assay in biopsies of human gastric mucosa. *Agents Actions 10,* 175-185.

Rose, B. (1940): Production of symptoms by subcutaneous injection of histamine without increase of the blood histamine. *Science, 92,* 454-454.

Rose, B. and Browne, J.S.L. (1938): The distribution and rate of disappearance of intravenously injected histamine in the rat. *Amer. J. Physiol., 124,* 412-420.

Rose, B., Rusted, I. and Fownes, J.A. (1950): Intravascular catheterization studies of bronchial asthma. I. Histamine levels in arterial and mixed venous blood of asthmatic patients before and during induced attacks. *J. clin. Invest., 29,* 1113-1119.

Rothschild, A.M. (1966): Histamine release by basic compounds. In: *Histamine and Anti-Histaminics, Part 1, Handbook of Experimental Pharmacology, Vol. 18/1.* Editors: M. Rocha e Silva and H.A. Rothschild. Springer-Verlag, Berlin, Heidelberg, New York. pp. 386-430.

Schöning, B. and Koch, H. (1975): Pathergiequote verschiedener Plasma-substitute an Haut und Respirationstrakt orthopädischer Patienten. *Anaesthesist, 24,* 507-516.

Schöning, B. and Koch, H. (1980): Die Pathergiequote des Neo-Plasmagels[R] bei orthopädischen Patienten in Abhängigkeit von Prämedikation, Geschlecht und Chargenalter (n = 450). *Anaesthesist* (In press).

Schöning, B. and Lorenz, W. (1980): (in preparation).

Seidel, G., Groppe, G. and Meyer-Burgdorff, C. (1974): Contrast media as histamine liberators in man. *Agents Actions, 4,* 143-150.

Shaff, R.E. and Beaven, M.A. (1979): Increased sensitivity of the enzymatic isotopic assay of histamine: measurement of histamine in plasma and serum. *Anal. Biochem., 94,* 425-430.

Shore, P.A., Burkhalter, A. and Cohn, V.H. Jr. (1959): A method for the fluorometric assay of histamine in tissues. *J. Pharmacol. exp. Ther., 127,* 182-187.

Simon, R.A., Schatz, M., Stevenson, D.D., Curry, N., Yamamoto, F., Plow, E., Ring, J. and Arroyave, C.M. (1979): Radiographic contrast media infusions. Measurement of histamine, complement, and fibrin split products and correlation with clinical parameters. *J. Allergy clin. Immunol., 63,* 281-288.

Schmidt, H. and Rieber, W. (1980): Häufigkeit und Schweregrad amphylactoider Reactionen nach Gelatine-Infusionen. Intensiv Behandlung, *5,* 77-81.

Snyder, S.H., Baldessarini, R.J. and Axelrod, J. (1966): A sensitive and specific enzymatic isotopic assay for tissue histamine. *J. Pharmacol. exp. Ther., 153,* 544-549.

Stopik, D., Beger, H.-G. and Bittner, R. (1974): Über den Einfluß der Leber auf die prä- und posthepatischen Konzentrationen des Plasma-histamins beim Menschen. *Klin. Wschr., 52,* 696-698.

Stopik, D., Hampel, K.E. and v. Kleist, D. (1977): Endogenes Plasma-Histamin und "hepatogenes" gastroduodenales Ulkus bei Leberzirrhose. *Dtsch. med. Wschr., 102,* 932-933.

Stopik, D., Beger, H.-G. and Hampel, K.E. (1978): Untersuchungen über die prä- und post-hepatischen Plasmahistaminkonzentrationen und ihre möglichen pathophysiologischen Aus-wirkungen bei Lebercirrhose. *Klin. Wschr., 56,* 241-246.

Subramanian, N., Schinzel, W., Mitznegg, P. and Estler, C.-J. (1978): Regional levels of histamine in rat brain after microwave irradiation: Evidence for artifacts in the enzymatic isotopic assay. *Agents Actions, 8,* 488-490.

Tauber, R., Maroske, D., Schult, H., Dormann, P., Schmal, A., Häfner, G. and Lorenz, W. (1975): Speicherung von Histamin im Blut nach Freisetzung aus Leber und Antrum durch Trypsin: protektiver Mechanismus oder Faktor in der Genese des pankreogenen Schocks? *Langenbecks Arch. Chir., Suppl. Chir. Forum,* 213-216.

238

Taylor, K.M. and Snyder, S.H. (1972): Isotopic microassay of histamine, histidine, histidine decarboxylase and histamine methyltransferase in brain tissue. *J. Neurochem., 19,* 1343-1358.

Taylor, K.M., Kvilis, S. and Baldo, B.A. (1980): An enzymatic isotopic microassay for measuring allergic release of histamine from blood and mast cells *in vitro. Int. Arch. Allergy appl. Immunol.,* 61, 19-27.

Thermann, M., Lorenz, W., Schmal, A., Schingale, F., Dormann, P. and Hamelmann, H. (1977): Alterations in the circulatory system of anaesthetized dogs following administration of histamine and histamine H_1- and H_2-acceptor antagonists in relation to plasma histamine levels. *Agents Actions, 5,* 450-454.

Thermann, M., Lorenz, W., Schmal, A., Schingale, F., Dormann, P. and Hamelmann, H. (1977): Influence of H_1- and H_2-receptor antagonists on the circulatory system and on the endogenous plasma histamine concentrations in dogs. *Agents Actions, 7,* 97-101.

Thompson, W.L. and Walton, R.P. (1963): Elevation of plasma histamine levels in the dog following administration of muscle relaxants, opiates and macromolecular polymers. *J. Pharmacol. exp. Ther., 143,* 132-136.

Tinel, J., Ungar, G. and Parrot, J.-L. (1938): Sur l'histaminemie plasmatique et globulaire. Son evolution au cours du choc peptonique du chien. *C. R. Soc. Biol., 129,* 267-269.

Walton, B. (1978): Anaesthesia, surgery and immunology. *Anaesthesia, 33,* 322-348.

Warrington, R.J., Tse, K.S. and Sehon, A.H. (1978): Drug hypersensitivities with special reference to penicillin. In: *Immediate Hypersensitivity. Modern Concepts and Developments.* Editor: M.K. Bach. M. Dekker, New York, Basel. pp. 749-798.

Watkins, J. (1979): Anaphylactoid reactions to i.v. substances. *Brit. J. Anaesth., 51,* 51-60.

Watkins, J. and Clarke, R.S.J. (1978): Report of a symposium: adverse responses to intravenous agents. *Brit. J. Anaesth., 50,* 1159-1164.

Watkins, J. and Ward, A.M. (1978): *Adverse Response to Intravenous Drugs.* Editors: J. Watkins and A.M. Ward. Academic Press, London; Grune and Stratton, New York. pp. 1-188.

Watkins, J., Clark, A., Appleyard, T.N. and Padfield, A. (1976): Immune-mediated reactions to althesin (alphaxalone). *Brit. J. Anaesth., 48,* 881-886.

Watkins, J., Udnoon, S. and Taussig, P.E. (1978): Mechanisms of adverse response to intravenous agents in man. In: *Adverse Response to Intravenous Drugs.* Editors: J. Watkins and A.M. Ward. Academic Press, London; Grune and Stratton, New York. pp. 71-82.

Werle, E. and Lorenz, W. (1970): The antikinin action of some anti-histaminic drugs on the isolated guinea-pig ileum, rat uterus and blood pressure of the anaesthetized dog. *Adv. exp. Biol. Med., 8,* 447-452.

Werner, M. and Wolff, E. (1973): Klinisch-experimentelle Untersuchungen zur Frage der Propanidid-Allergie. In: *Intravenöse Narkose mit Propanidid. Anaesthesiology and Resuscitation, Vol. 74.* Editors: M. Zindler, H. Yamamura and W. Wirth. Springer-Verlag, Berlin, Heidelberg, New York. pp. 217-223.

West, G.B. (1967): Reactivity of wild and domesticated populations. *Int. Arch. Allergy, 32,* 396-403.

Wicksell, F. (1949): Observations on histamine and histaminolysis in pregnancy. *Acta physiol. scand., 17,* 395-413.

Wolstenholme, G.W.W. and O'Connor, C.M. (1956): *Ciba Foundation Symp. on Histamine.* J. and A. Churchill, London. pp. 1-472.

Zeppa, R., Grossekreutz, D.C. and Sugioka, K. (1961): Histamine release into the circulation by meperidine (Demerol[R]). *Proc. Soc. exp. Biol. Med., 106,* 794-796.

Thornton (ed.) Adverse Reactions of Anaesthetic Drugs
© Elsevier/North-Holland Biomedical Press, 1981

7

Immunological aspects of adverse reactions to inhalational anaesthetic agents

Bryan Walton

INTRODUCTION

Generalised adverse reactions to a wide variety of intravenous anaesthetic agents are being reported with increasing frequency, and it is clear that both immunological and non-immunological mechanisms may be responsible. Far less clear, however, is the question of whether or not immunological mechanisms are involved in any patient suffering an organ-specific adverse reaction to an inhalational anaesthetic agent. Hepatic damage following exposure to chloroform (Brown et al., 1974), fluroxene (Reynolds et al., 1972; Tucker et al., 1973) and, perhaps, trichloroethylene (Herdman, 1945; Baerg et al., 1970) and renal damage associated with exposure to methoxyflurane (Taves et al., 1970; Young et al., 1976) are apparently dose-dependent phenomena *directly* related to the toxic effects of metabolites of the agents concerned. However, the features of the syndromes seen in rare patients with hepatic damage following exposure to halothane and methoxyflurane (including lack of dose dependency, very variable latent period between exposure and onset of damage and variable histological picture) suggest that *direct* hepatotoxicity is not the mechanism involved.

Much "evidence" has appeared in support of the alternative suggestion that such patients are suffering delayed hypersensitivity reactions either to the drugs themselves or to their metabolites — possibly combined with protein carrier molecules. Three main categories of "evidence" form the basis for this hypothesis:

(1) the clinical stigmata of hypersensitivity reported in some patients; (2) the high incidence of certain auto-antibodies; and (3) reports of evidence for cell-mediated immunity in some cases. Much of this chapter will be devoted to a critical review of the "evidence" allegedly supporting the concept that halothane hepatitis has an immunological basis, and references will be made to organ-specific adverse reactions to other inhalational agents where appropriate.

(1) CLINICAL STIGMATA OF HYPERSENSITIVITY

Many clinical features classically associated with hypersensitivity reactions, including skin rash, arthralgia, bronchospasm and unexplained postoperative fever and leucocytosis, appeared in an early review of halothane hepatitis (Doniach, 1970) and have also been reported in patients with hepatitis following methoxyflurane exposure (Lischner et al., 1967; Joshi et al., 1974). Before accepting such a list of features as valid evidence for hypersensitivity in these patients, one must ask whether they are equally likely either to be mere chance associations or explicable by other non-anaesthetic means. In an attempt to assess the relevance of these and other reported features, frequent references will be made to a recent study of postoperative jaundice in the United Kingdom by the present author and his colleagues (Walton et al., 1976a). This study allowed detailed analysis of 76 patients with probable halothane hepatitis (i.e. patients in whom no alternative aetiological factors could be identified by a panel of hepatologists). In addition, comparisons could be drawn between this group and 66 patients with post-halothane jaundice in whom alternative non-anaesthetic factors (including cardiovascular collapse, septicaemia and cirrhosis) were thought to have caused the postoperative hepatic dysfunction.

(a) Skin rash, arthralgia and bronchospasm

Of the 76 patients in the "halothane hepatitis" group, 11 had a skin rash. In all but three of these patients, however, other drugs such as antibiotics were thought likely to be relevant. Thus, an "unexplained" skin rash was found in only four per cent of cases. Arthralgia was even less common as, once painful infusion sites and referred pain (originally reported as "arthralgia") had been excluded, convincing arthralgia was found in only one of the 76 patients. Bronchospasm was not a feature in any patient in the "halothane hepatitis" group. The very low incidence of these features suggests that their occurrence in any patient with halothane hepatitis is just as likely to be a chance association as to be an acceptable "pointer" to a hypersensitivity response.

(b) Unexplained fever

The suggestion that unexplained fever following previous exposure to halothane might be considered a marker of an adverse reaction and should, therefore, preclude its further use in that patient, formed part of the conclusions of the massive United States National Halothane Study (Summary, 1966). Although in the report unexplained fever *and* jaundice following previous exposure were coupled together, much significance has been attached to the fever alone by many subsequent reviewers (Sharpstone et al., 1971; Moult et al., 1975). Certainly, if such a fever could be considered a reliable indication of an earlier adverse response to halothane, advice against its subsequent use would be unarguable. However, studies of post-operative temperature patterns suggest that the interpretation of temperature elevations during this period is far from easy. For example, one author reported that, of 163 consecutive surgical patients in whom temperature were recorded for at least three postoperative days, only *one* failed to develop a fever! Furthermore, in 55% of these patients, the fever could not be explained by infection or other factors (Dykes, 1971). Other workers have reported a 37% incidence of unexplained post-operative fever, although this occurred much less frequently among patients having minor surgery (Trey et al., 1968). It appears that the frequency and patterns of fever are similar following a variety of anaesthetic techniques. In order to exclude these very common early postoperative fevers, it has been suggested that only fevers during the second postoperative week need be considered relevant (Sherlock, 1971). The value of this distinction between fevers during the first and second postoperative weeks was assessed by the present author and his colleagues by comparing temperature patterns following previous halothane exposure in the two groups of patients mentioned above (Walton et al., 1976a). The results suggested that unexplained fever following previous halothane exposure (occurring during either the first *or second* postoperative week) appeared with similar frequency in both groups of patients with postoperative jaundice – irrespective of whether or not halothane was thought responsible for the jaundice. It seems, therefore, that although such a fever *may* occasionally be a marker of an untoward reaction to previous exposure to halothane, its significance in any patient (in relation to possible re-exposure to the drug) remains in some doubt.

It has also been suggested (Klion et al., 1969; Doniach, 1970) that fever as part of the episode of postoperative jaundice further suggests a hypersensitivity response. Once again, the difficulties involved in the interpretation of postoperative fever apply equally well. One additional point is that fever is a common feature of the prodrome of acute viral hepatitis (Sherlock, 1968), and would appear to be associated *non-specifically* with a variety of hepatic diseases – whether or not hypersensitivity is involved.

(c) Leucocytosis

Any suggestion that postoperative leucocytosis may be considered evidence for a hypersensitivity response to halothane ignores the fact that a rise in white cell count occurs very commonly following exposure to anaesthesia and surgery. Many factors influence white cell counts in the perioperative period with the most important being the hormonal aspects of the "stress" response. The numbers of circulating neutrophils and lymphocytes increase in response to a rise in catecholamine levels and the liberation of ACTH is also accompanied by neutrophilia. Hormone levels vary greatly in response to anxiety, pain and trauma, in addition to the direct effects of anaesthetic and other drugs. Postoperative leucocytosis is, therefore, more likely to be attributable to these non-specific factors (reviewed recently by the present author (Walton, 1978)) than to a hypersensitivity response to a recently administered drug. In any event, a majority of patients with halothane hepatitis have normal white cell counts (Sherlock, 1971; Walton et al., 1976a).

It seems, therefore, that several of these "features" of halothane hepatitis are unlikely to be useful markers of hypersensitivity and, in most cases may more logically be considered chance associations related to other factors. On the other hand, several other features seem more convincing and these include the association with multiple exposures (particularly repeated within a short time), eosinophilia, variations in latent period between exposure to halothane and onset of jaundice, and ostensibly positive "challenge" tests reported in the literature.

(d) Multiple exposures

There is little doubt that "halothane hepatitis" is a syndrome associated with multiple exposures to the drug. This association, reported as a result of the United States National Halothane Study (Summary, 1966), has been confirmed by many subsequent studies (Trey et al., 1968; Moult et al., 1975; Inman et al., 1978). Multiple exposures are also a very common feature of "methoxyflurane hepatitis" (Joshi et al., 1974). Furthermore, "halothane hepatitis" appears to be more common after rapidly repeated exposures, although the time interval to be inferred by the term "rapidly repeated" is far from clear. For example, the results of some studies have implied that repeated exposures within one month are of particular concern (Inman et al., 1975; Moult et al., 1975; Inman et al., 1978), whereas other authors have mentioned three months in this context and have recommended that at least this period should be allowed to elapse between exposures (Lomanto et al., 1970; Carney et al., 1972). Two small prospective studies compared liver function in patients receiving either repeated halothane, halothane followed by non-halothane or, in a few cases, repeated non-halothane anaesthetics within one year and concluded that repeated halothane exposures were more likely to produce abnormalities in liver function (Trowell et al., 1975; Wright et al., 1975). In contrast, however, two subsequent prospective studies have produced somewhat contradictory results (McEwan, 1976; Allen et al., 1977), and it may be that minor elevations of particular live enzymes, seen quite commonly after anaesthesia and surgery, are unrelated to the severe hepatocellular damage seen rarely following exposure to halothane. Comparison between patients with halothane hepatitis and post-halothane jaundice due to other identifiable causes (Walton et al., 1976a) showed that 95% of patients with halothane hepatitis had had previous exposure to halothane (54% within one month), compared with 66% (30% within one month) in the latter group. This latter figure (66%) correlates quite well with the suggestion (Carney et al., 1972) that some 56% of adult surgical patients might be expected to have had previous exposure to halothane.

(e) Eosinophilia

It is widely accepted that eosinophilia is a feature of halothane hepatitis and can be considered a reliable marker of hypersensitivity. On the other hand, the low incidence of eosinophilia in some series (Trey et al., 1968 (2/35); Sharpstone et al, 1971 (0/11)) and the wide diversity of unrelated diseases in which eosinophilia has been reported (Dykes et al., 1972), once again calls into question the significance of this feature. The present author and his colleagues found raised eosinophil counts in 32% patients with halothane hepatitis (Walton et al., 1976a). However, of particular interest was the fact that low order eosinophilia (less than twice the upper limit of normal) was not uncommonly found in patients with jaundice due to identifiable factors (following both halothane and non-halothane anaesthesia) and even as a chance *preoperative* finding, and such minor elevations of circulating eosinophils cannot be considered relevant. Elevations higher than this were seen in 10% of patients with halothane hepatitis.

(f) Variations in latent period

The latent period between exposure to halothane and the onset of jaundice varies widely among patients with "halothane hepatitis". Thus, cases have been reported with jaundice appearing on the first postoperative day (Walton et al., 1976a) and as long delayed as 28 days following exposure (Klion et al., 1969). Analyses of variations in latent period have to some extent supported the concept of hypersensitivity.

Firstly, it has been reported (Klatskin, 1968b); Inman et al., 1974) that the latent period is shorter when the episode of postoperative hepatitis follows multiple exposures to halothane than when the problem follows a single exposure. A more recent report lent guarded support to these findings (Walton et al., 1976a) although the small number of patients in their single exposure group rendered their figures of doubtful statistical significance. In contrast, other workers analysing United States National Halothane Study data reported contradictory findings (McPeek et al., 1974).

Secondly, it has been reported (Inman et al., 1974; Walton et al., 1976a) that in patients with more than one episode of "halothane hepatitis", a gradually reducing latent period with succeeding episodes can be demonstrated. This, together with the previous point, has suggested to some reviewers an accelerating immunological response in patients repeatedly exposed to the same "antigen". A similar picture of reducing latent period has also been reported in a patient with two episodes of "methoxyflurane hepatitis" (Brenner et al., 1971).

(g) Positive "challenge" tests

It is widely believed that the most convincing evidence in favour of halothane hypersensitivity is provided by reports of positive "challenge" tests in two anaesthetists (Belfrage et al., 1966; Klatskin et al., 1969), a laboratory technician anaesthetising animals with halothane (Johnston et al., 1971) and a nurse anaesthetist (Lund et al., 1974). In each of these patients, initially presenting with a virus hepatitis-like syndrome, re-exposure to halothane was followed by a relapse of their hepatic dysfunction. The several anomalies evident on close examination of the history of the most famous of these cases (Klatskin et al., 1969) led to the suggestion (Simpson et al., 1974) that the relapses of hepatitis in that patient may well have been *non-specifically* related to a variety of factors − although follow-up data published subsequently (Dykes, 1977) supports the original contention that this case may well be a valid example of hypersensitivity. On the other hand, several apparently negative "challenges" have appeared in the literature, and these and other anomalies can appropriately be considered here.

(h) Anomalies

It can be seen that, although several of the clinical stigmata allegedly associated with halothane hepatitis are far from convincing, features such as multiple exposures and eosinophilia still suggest that an immunological mechanism is more likely than *direct* hepatotoxicity of either halothane or its metabolites. Nonetheless, there are several anomalies which detract from this view — inasmuch as they are difficult to reconcile with the accepted concepts of drug hypersensitivity.

For example, it is odd that, although the syndrome is associated with multiple exposures to halothane, many cases have been reported following single exposure. A recent analysis of reports submitted to the Committee on Safety of Medicines in the United Kingdom (Inman et al., 1978) indicates that almost 20% of patients have had only one exposure. Similarly, a report of patients with methoxyflurane hepatitis (among whom features such as eosinophilia and reducing latent period with multiple episodes also suggest an immunological basis) included some 30% of patients with hepatitis following a single exposure. In some respects, it is difficult to accept that so many patients can manifest a hypersensitivity response without any apparent preceding "sensitising" exposure to the antigen.

Furthermore, it is difficult to explain how some patients with halothane hepatitis have been re-exposed to halothane without problems (Dykes et al., 1965; Walton et al., 1976a), and other patients have apparently had uneventful exposures to halothane in the interval between two episodes of halothane hepatitis (Walton et al., 1976a). In addition, how can one explain patients who had multiple exposures to halothane without problems some years previously and subsequently develop hepatitis following a further single exposure (Walton et al., 1976a)?

It is of interest that cholestatic hypersensitivity-type reactions to chlorpromazine are said to occur occasionally after one exposure to the drug. Furthermore, the fact that problems often do not recur on subsequent exposure had led to the suggestion that desensitisation may occur (Hollister, 1957). What relevance, if any, this information has to discussions of hepatocellular necrosis following halothane is far from clear.

2. Autoantibodies

The possibility that patients with halothane hepatitis may have altered immune status was raised by early reports of antimitochondrial autoantibodies (AMA) in some patients (Doniach et al., 1966; Rodriguez et al., 1969). This finding, allied to reported predominant mitochondrial changes seen by electron microscopy in the liver in some patients (Keeley et al., 1970; Uzunalimoglu, 1970; Schaffner et al., 1971) led to the hypothesis that AMA were a marker of an immune response to mitochondria damaged during exposure to halothane. However, other authors reported a low incidence of AMA in this syndrome (Klatskin et al., 1972), subsequent workers have been less impressed with mitochondrial changes in these patients (Schatzki et al., 1973; Wills et al., 1978), and the incidence of AMA among patients with halothane hepatitis has recently been shown to be no greater than that in the general population (Walton et al., 1976a).

On the other hand, similar, though distinct, liver kidney microsomal autoantibodies (LKM) have been reported in 25% of patients with this syndrome (Walton et al., 1976a). This autoantibody is present in association with a variety of liver diseases and, very rarely, in patients with presumed viral hepatitis (Smith et al., 1974). The LKM antibodies appear transiently in halothane hepatitis (Walton et al., 1976a) and it has been suggested that such a pattern is in favour of their stimulation by drug hypersensitivity (Smith et al., 1974). On the other hand, it has been suggested that these non-organ-specific autoantibodies are probably not responsible for the initiation of the liver lesions with which they are associated (Rizzeto et al., 1973).

It is of interest that a high incidence of thyroid autoantibodies have also been reported among patients with halothane hepatitis — in the absence of overt thyroid disease (Walton et al., 1976a). This is consistent with the earlier report that thyroid and LKM antibodies are often associated (Rizzetto et al., 1976). The persistence of thyroid antibodies in patients with halothane hepatitis (in contrast with the transient LKM) raises the possibility that patients predisposed to organ specific autoimmunity may be more likely to develop this syndrome. It is well recognised that patients suffering adverse reactions to intravenous anaesthetic agents tend to have a history of atopy and allergy (Clarke et al., 1975; Dundee, 1976) and the concept of predisposition to adverse reactions to inhalational agents is supported by reports that 46% of patients with halothane hepatitis have such a history (Carney et al., 1972) and in 15% of patients a history of *drug* allergy can be elicited (Klatskin, 1968a). On the other hand, the present author and his colleagues have found that some 20% of patients with postoperative jaundice have a history of allergy — irrespective of whether or not the anaesthetic agent was thought culpable (Walton et al., 1976a).

Of minor interest is the 25% incidence of smooth muscle autoantibodies (SMA) in patients with halothane hepatitis (Walton et al., 1976a) — a figure higher than the 12% reported in the general population (Sutton et al., 1974), but far lower than the 87% incidence reported in acute viral hepatitis (Farrow et al., 1970).

(3) IN VITRO EVIDENCE FOR CELL-MEDIATED IMMUNITY

The lymphocyte transformation test and leucocyte migration inhibition test, (LTT) and (MIT), are often considered useful in vitro indices of cell-mediated immune responses. Both of these tests depend on the recognition by previously sensitised lymphocytes of an antigen included in the culture medium. In the LTT, this recognition is followed by transformation into lymphoblasts and the degree of blast transformation is monitored by the uptake of tritiated thymidine by the transforming cells. In the MIT, the lymphocytes, having recognised the antigen, release a group of active substances termed lymphokines. One of these lymphokines is migration inhibition factor (MIF) which inhibits the migration of leucocytes from the open end of a capillary tube in culture.

Several authors have performed these tests on patients with halothane hepatitis in an attempt to demonstrate evidence for cell-mediated immunity, and most results have been disappointing. An early report of lymphocyte transformation in the presence of halothane (Paronetto et al., 1970) has not been supported by several other groups of workers (Mathieu et al., 1973b; Walton et al., 1973; Moult et al., 1975). Ostensibly positive migration inhibition results in two patients (Jones Williams et al., 1972) have recently been followed by additional positive results from the same authors (Price et al., 1977) — once again using halothane as the antigen — and the possibility arises that this may prove a useful diagnostic test.

In some respects, however, it will be surprising if tests such as these, using halothane itself as the antigen, prove reliable. Halothane is a relatively small (mol. wt. 197.4) molecule, unlikely to be capable of antigenicity in its own right. It is more likely that, if halothane is indeed responsible for a hypersensitivity response in rare individuals, antigenic status is achieved by the combination of a metabolite with a carrier protein. There is no doubt that metabolites of both halothane (Uehleke et al., 1973; Hempel et al., 1975) and methoxyflurane (Yoshimura et al., 1976) bind covalently to tissue constituents, and it has been shown (in the rabbit) that trifluoroacetate (TFA the major metabolite of halothane) can act as a hapten (Rosenberg et al., 1973). In guinea pigs, specific antibody responses (Mathieu et al., 1975a) and cellular hypersensitivity (Mathieu et al., 1973a; Mathieu et al., 1974) to TFA-protein complexes have been reported. However, attempts to correlate such reactions with liver damage have proved unsuccessful (Mathieu et al., 1975b; Reves et al., 1976a,b), and the relevance of such experiments to human halothane hepatitis remains in doubt.

Recently, positive LTT results in one patient with carcinoma of the breast have been reported using an unidentified halothane metabolite as antigen (Williams et al., 1977). This patient developed a serum sickness type syndrome (with poly-arthralgia and proteinuria) in association with an episode of post-halothane hepatitis, and the unidentified metabolite was shown to be bound to circulating antigen-antibody complexes. However, the relevance of these findings to halothane hepatitis must be questionable inasmuch as no other patient with a serum sickness syndrome (with renal impairment) associated with halothane hepatitis has ever appeared in the extensive literature on this subject. It seems likely that the immune complexes related to some other aspect of this patient's illness and the binding of a halothane metabolite to the complexes, while being of some interest, did not form part of the mechanism for her postoperative jaundice.

Both the LTT and MIT have been performed in patients with halothane hepatitis using TFA-protein complexes as potential antigen, but results were disappointing (Walton et al., 1976b) and the negative results may reflect an inappropriate choice of either the metabolite or the carrier protein. More encouraging has been a recent study in which, using leucocytes from patients with halothane hepatitis, positive MIT results have been seen on exposure to an "antigen" derived from a liver homogenate obtained from rabbits pretreated with halothane. These results have been interpreted as evidence for sensitisation to halothane-altered liver cell components in these patients (Vergani et al., 1978).

HISTOLOGICAL FEATURES OF HALOTHANE HEPATITIS

As some drug hypersensitivity reactions have been associated with granuloma formation – for example, reactions to sulphonamides (More et al., 1946; Espiritu et al., 1967) and thiouracil (Dalgleish, 1952) – reports of granulomas seen in some patients with halothane hepatitis (Klion et al., 1969); Dordal et al., 1970) have suggested an immunological basis for the syndrome. This suggestion has been supported by features of the mononuclear infiltrate reported in some cases (Uzunalimoglu et al., 1970). However, other workers have been unable to demonstrate granulomas (Wills et al., 1978) and, although the close contact between parenchymal and mononuclear cells seen in halothane hepatitis by some authors (Uzunalimoglu et al., 1970; Wills et al., 1978) may represent a cytotoxic reaction, such features have also been reported in viral hepatitis (Wills, 1968). A recent in vitro study has shown that peripheral mononuclear cells from a patient with halothane hepatitis attack target cells coated with normal liver lipoprotein (Vogten et al., 1976). As such a phenomenon is demonstrable in chronic active liver disease (a disease associated with cytotoxicity), this suggests that cell-mediated cytotoxicity may be a feature of halothane hepatitis. However, whether such a reaction is a causative factor or triggered by the liver damage remains unclear.

CROSS-SENSITIVITY

The choice of a suitable anaesthetic agent for a patient who has previously suffered a possible sensitivity reaction to halothane has raised the question of whether such patients are likely to demonstrate hypersensitivity to alternative halogenated agents. The suggestion that cross-sensitivity may well be a problem (Klatskin, 1969) has been supported by several other reviewers (Carney et al., 1972; Dykes et al., 1972; Joshi et al., 1974). Evidence in favour of the hypothesis that patients may react adversely both to halothane and methoxyflurane includes reports of patients with hepatic problems following both agents (Lindenbaum et al., 1963; Elkington et al., 1968; Judson et al., 1971) and apparent in vitro lymphocyte cross-sensitivity (Paronetto et al., 1970). Patients with syndromes suggesting cross-sensitivity between halothane and enflurane (Sadove et al., 1974) and halothane and fluroxene (Haber et al., 1972) have been reported – although, as mentioned earlier, fluroxene-associated liver damage is probably *directly* related to metabolism. If cross-sensitivity does occur, it is clearly a variable phenomenon, as patients have been reported who have had uneventful exposures to trichloroethylene or methoxyflurane following an episode of halothane hepatitis (Walton et al., 1976a).

CONCLUSIONS

Despite recent evidence showing that, under hypoxic circumstances, potentially toxic halothane metabolites may be formed (Widger et al., 1976), many of the features of halothane hepatitis suggest that *direct* hepatotoxicity is unlikely. Notwithstanding the fact that much of the "evidence" for hypersensitivity is unconvincing, and that many anomalies cannot be satisfactorily explained on immunological grounds, it seems, on balance that an immunological mechanism is responsible for most cases of halothane (and methoxyflurane) hepatitis. It is possible that reactive metabolites of these agents combine with liver proteins and achieve antigenic status. It may be that these antigenic complexes produce hepatic dysfunction in a population predisposed to autoimmune organ specific disease.

Ideally, a screening procedure (perhaps involving migration inhibition tests and an autoantibody profile) might allow predisposed patients to be recognised pre-operatively – although much work remains to be done before results of such tests can be interpreted with confidence. One other disturbing possibility remains. It may be that more than one mechanism can result in halothane hepatitis – with direct toxicity of halothane metabolites being possible under certain perioperative conditions. Such a mechanism may eventually be shown to explain the immunological anomalies which at present weaken the concept that, in most patients, halothane hepatitis is a hypersensitivity phenomenon.

REFERENCES

Allen, P.J. and Downing, J.W. (1977): A prospective study of hepatocellular function after repeated exposure to halothane or enflurane in woman undergoing radium therapy for cervical cancer. *Brit. J. Anaesth., 49*, 1035-1039.

Baerg, R.D. and Kimberg, D.V. (1970): Centrilobular hepatic necrosis and acute renal failure in solvent sniffers. *Ann. int. Med. 73*, 713-720.

Belfrage, S., Ahlgren, I. and Axelson, S. (1966): Halothane hepatitis in an anaesthetist. *Lancet, 4*, 1466-1467.

Brenner, A.I. and Kaplan, M.M. (1971): Recurrent hepatitis due to methoxyflurane anesthesia. *New Engl. J. Med., 284*, 961-962.

Brown, B.R., Sipes, I.G. and Sagalyn, A.M. (1974): Mechanisms of acute hepatic toxicity. *Anesthesiology, 41*, 554-561.

Carney, F.M.T. and Van Dyke, R.A. (1972): Halothane hepatitis: A critical review. *Anesth. Analg. Curr. Res. 51*, 135-160.

Clarke, R.S.J., Dundee, J.W. and Garrett, R.T. (1975): Adverse reactions to intravenous anaesthetics: A survey of 100 reports. *Brit. J. Anaesth., 47*, 575-585.

Dalgleish, P.G. (1952): Polyarteritis after thiouracil. *Lancet, 2*, 319-320.

Doniach, D. (1970): Cell mediated immunity in halothane hypersensitivity. *New Eng. J. Med., 283*, 315-316.

Doniach, D., Roitt, I.M., Walker, J.G. and Sherlock, S. (1966): Tissue antibodies in primary biliary cirrhosis, active chronic (lupoid) hepatitis, cryptogenic cirrhosis and other liver diseases, and their clinical manifestations. *Clin. exp. Immunol., 1*, 237-262.

Dordal, E., Glagov, S. and Orlando, R.A. (1970): Fatal halothane hepatitis with transient granulomas. *New Engl. J. Med., 283*, 357-359.

Dundee, J.W. (1976): Hypersensitivity to intravenous anaesthetic agents. *Brit. J. Anaesth., 48*, 57-58.

Dykes, M.H.M. (1971): Unexplained postoperative fever. Its value as a sign of halothane sensitisation. *J. Amer. med. Ass., 216*, 641-644.

Dykes, M.H.M. (1977): Is halothane hepatitis chronic active hepatitis? *Anesthesiology 46*, 233-235.

Dykes, M.H.M., Gilbert, J.P. and Schur, P.H. (1972): Halothane and the liver. *Canad. J. Surg. 15*, 217-238.

Dykes, M.H.M., Walzer, S.G. and Slater, E.M. (1965): Acute parenchymatous hepatic disease following general anesthesia. *J. Amer. med. Ass. 193*, 339-344.

Elkington, S.g., Goffinet, J.A. and Conn, H.O. (1968): Renal and hepatic injury associated withe methoxyflurane anesthesia. *Ann. Int. Med. 69*, 1229-1236.

Espiritu, C.R., Kim, T.S. and 'Levine, R.A. (1967): Granulomatous hepatitis associated with sulphadimethoxine hypersensitivity. *J. Amer. med. Ass., 202*, 985-988.

Farrow, L.J., Holborow, E.J. and Johnson, G.D. (1970): Autoantibodies and the hepatitis associated antigen in acute infectious hepatitis. *Brit. med. J., 2*, 693-697.

Haber, M.H. and Lau, J.M. (1972): Midzonal liver necrosis associated with fluorinated anesthetic agents. *Hawaii med. J., 32*, 18-20.

Hempel, V. and Remmer, H. (1975): In vivo and in vitro studies on irreversible binding of halothane metabolites to protein. *Experientia, 31*, 680-681.

Herdman, K.N. (1945): Acute yellow necrosis of the liver following Trilene anaesthesia. *Brit. med. J., 2*, 689-690.

Hollister, L.E. (1957): Allergy to chlorpromazine manifested by jaundice. *Amer. J. Med., 23*, 870-879.

Inman, W.H.W. and Mushin, W.W. (1974): Jaundice after repeated exposure to halothane: An analysis of reports to Committee on Safety of Medicines. *Brit. med. J., 1*, 5-10.

Inman, W.H.W. and Mushin, W.W. (1978): Jaundice after repeated esposure to halothane: A further analysis of reports to the Committee on Safety of Medicines. *Brit. med. J., 2*, 1455-1456.

Johnston, C.I. and Mendelsohn, F. (1971): Halothane hepatitis in a laboratory technician. *Aust. NZ J. Med., 2*, 171-173.

Jones Williams, W., Pioli, E. and Horton, J.N. (1972): MIF test in halothane jaundice. *Brit. med. J., 4*, 47.

Joshi, P.H. and Conn, H.O. (1974): The syndrome of methoxyflurane-associated hepatitis. *Ann. int. Med., 80*, 395-401.

Judson, J.A., De Jongh, H.J. and Walmsley, J.B.W. (1971): Possible cross-sensitivity between halothane and methoxyflurane. *Anesthesiology, 35,* 527-532.

Keeley, A.F., Trey, C. and Marcon, N. (1970): Anicteric halothane hepatitis: Histologic and ultrastructural lesion associated with postoperative fever in two patients. *Gastroenterology, 58,* 965.

Klatskin, G. (1968a): Mechanisms of toxic and drug induced hepatic injury. In: *Toxicity of Anesthetics.* Editor: B.R. Fink. Williams and Wilkins, Baltimore, p. 168.

Klatskin, G. (1968b): Mechanisms of toxic and drug induced hepatic injury. In: *Toxicity of Anesthetics.* Editor: B.R. Fink. Williams and Wilkins, Baltimore, p. 169.

Klatskin, G. (1969): Toxic and drug induced hepatitis. In: *Diseases of the Liver*, 3rd edition. Editor: L. Lippincott, Philadelphia, pp. 529-530.

Klatskin, G. and Kantor, F.S. (1972): Mitochondrial antibody in primary biliary cirrhosis and other diseases. *Ann. int. Med., 77,* 533-541.

Klastskin, G. and Kimberg, D.V. (1969): Recurrent hepatitis attributable to halothane sensitisation in an anesthetist. *New Engl. J. Med, 280,* 515-522.

Klion, F.M., Schaffner, F. and Popper, H. (1969): Hepatitis after exposure to halothane. *Ann. int. Med., 71,* 467-477.

Lindenbaum, J. and Leifer, E. (1963): Hepatic necrosis associated with halothane anesthesia. *New Engl. J. Med., 268,* 525-530.

Lischner, M.W., MacNabb, G.M. and Galambos, J.T. (1967): Fatal hepatic necrosis following surgery: possible relation to methoxyflurane anesthesia. *Arch. Int. Med., 120,* 725-728.

Lomanto, C. and Howland, W.S. (1970): Problems in diagnosing halothane hepatitis. *J. Amer. med. Ass., 214,* 1257-1261.

Lund, I., Skulberg, A. and Helle, I. (1974): Occupational hazard of halothane *Lancet, 2,* 528.

Mathieu, A., Dipadua, D.f and Kahan, B.D. (1973a): Lymphocyte transformation, reaginic and complement fixing antibodies in guinea pigs sensitised to a metabolite of halothane and fluroxene. *Anesth. Analg. Curr. Res., 52,* 676-681.

Mathieu, A., Dipadua, D. and Kahan, B.D. (1975a): Humoral immunity to a metabolite of halothane, fluroxene and enflurane. *Anesthesiology, 42,* 612-616.

Mathieu,, A., Dipadua, D. and Kahan, B.D. (1973a): Lymphocyte transformation, reaginic and complebolite of halothane and hepatic lesions after mltiple exposures. *Anesth. Analg. Curr. Res., 54,* 332-39.

Mathieu, A., Dipadua, D. and Mills, J. (1974): Experimental immunity to a metabolite of halothane and fluroxene. *Anesthesiology, 40,* 385-390.

Mathieu, A., Walzer, S. and Dipadua, D. (1973b): Test de transformation lymphocytaire dans deux cas d'hepatite apres anesthesie a l'halothane. *Anesth. Analg. Reanim., 30,* 109-116.

McEwan, J. (1976): Liver function tests following anaesthesia. *Brit. J. Anaesth., 48,* 1065-1070.

McPeek, B. and Gilbert, J.P. (1974): Onset of postoperative jaundice related to anaesthetic history. *Brit. med. J., 2,* 615-617.

More, R.H., McMillan, G.C. and Duff, G.C. (1946): The pathology of sulphonamide allergy in man. *Amer. J. Path., 22,* 703-735.

Moult, P.J.A., Adjukiewicz, A.B. and Gaylarde, P.M. (1975): Lymphocyte transformation in halothane-related hepatitis. *Brit. med. J., 1,* 69-70.

Moult, P.J.A. and Sherlock, S. (1975): Halothane-related hepatitis. *Quart, J. Med., XLIV,* 99-114.

Paronetto, F. and Popper, H. (1970): Lymphocyte stimulation induced by halothane in patients with hepatitis following exposure to halothane. *New Engl. J. Med., 283,* 277-280.

Price, C.D., Gibbs, A.R. and Jones Williams, W. (1977): Halothane macrophage migration inhibition factor test in halothane-associated hepatitis. *J. clin. path., 30,* 312-316.

Reves, J.G. and McCraken, L.E. (1976a): Failure to induce hepatic pathology in animals sensitised to a halothane metabolite and subsequently challenged with halothane. *Anesth. Analg. Curr. Res., 55*, 235-242.

Reves, J.G. and McCraken, L.E. (1976b): Hepatic pathology and skin test reactions to trifluoro-acetylated autologous protein after repeated halothane anaesthesia in the guinea pig. *Brit. J. Anaesth., 48*, 419-424.

Reynolds, E.S., Brown, B.R. and Vandam, L.D. (1972): Massive hepatic necrosis after fluroxene anesthesia − A case of drug interaction. *New Engl. J. Med., 286*, 530-531.

Rizzetto, M., Swana, G. anmd Doniach, D. (1973): Microsomal antibodies in active chronic hepatitis and other disorders. *Clin. exp. Immunol., 15*, 331-344.

Rodriguez, M., Paronetto, F., Schaffner, F. and Popper, H. (1969): Antimitochondrial antibodies in jaundice following drug administration. *J. Amer. med. Ass., 208*, 148-150.

Rosenberg, P.H. and Wahlstrom, T. (1973): Trifluoroacetic acid and some possible intermediate metabolites of halothane as haptens. *Anesthesiology, 38*, 224-227.

Sadove, M.S. and Kim, S.I. (1974): Hepatitis after use of two different fluorinated anesthetic agents. *Anesth. Analg. Curr. Res., 53*, 336-340.

Schaffner, F. and Paronetto, F. (1971): Immunological observations and electron microscopy of halothane induced hepatic injury. In: *Immunology of the Liver*. Editors: M. Smith, R. Williams, Heinemann, London, pp. 186-193.

Schatzki, P.F., Kay, S. and McGavie, J.D. (1973): Ultrastructural pathology of a case of halothane hepatitis. *Digestive Dis., 18*, 905-911.

Sharpstone, P., Medley, D.R.K. and Williams, R. (1971): Halothane hepatitis − a preventable disease? *Brit. med. J., 1*, 448-450.

Sherlock, S. (1968): In: *Diseases of the Liver*. Blackwell, Oxford, p. 328.

Sherlock, S. (1971): Progress report: halothane hepatitis. *Gut, 12*, 324-329.

Simpson, B.R., Strunin, L. and Walton, B. (1974): Evidence for halothane hepatotoxicity is equivocal. In: *Controversy in Internal Medicine II*. Editors: J. Ingelfinger and R.V. Ebert, Saunders Company, Philadelphia, p. 580.

Smith, M.G.M., Williams, R. and Walker, G. (1974): Hepatic disorders associated with liver/kidney microsomal antibodies. *Brit. med. J., 2*, 80-84.

Summary of the National Halothane Study (1966): *J. Amer. med. Ass., 197*, 121-134.

Sutton, R.N.P., Emond, R.T.D., Thomas, D.B. and Doniach, D. (1974): The occurrence of antibodies in infectious mononucleosis. *Clin. exp. Immunol., 17*, 427-436.

Taves, D.R., Fry, B.W. and Freeman, R.B. (1970): Toxicity following methoxyflurane anesthesia II Fluoride concentrations in nephrotoxicity. *J. Amer. med. Ass., 214*, 91-95.

Trey, C., Lipworth, L., Chalmers, T.C. and Davidson, C.S. (1968): Fulminant hepatic failure: Presumable contribution of halothane. *New Engl. J. Med., 279*, 798-801.

Trowell, J., Peto, R. and Crampton Smith, A. (1975): Controlled trial of repeated halothane anaesthetics in patients with carcinoma of the uterine cervix treated with radium. *Lancet, 1*, 821-823.

Tucker, W.K., Munson, E.S. and Holaday, D.A. (1973): Hepatorenal toxicity following fluroxene anesthesia. *Anesthesiology, 39*, 104-107.

Uehleke, H., Hellmer, K.H. and Tabarelli-Poplawski, S. (1973): Metabolic activation of halothane and its covalent binding to liver endoplasmic proteins in vitro. *Arch. Pharmacol., 279*, 39−52.

Uzunalimoglu, B., Yardley, J.H. and Boitnott, J.K. (1970): The liver in mild halothane hepatitis. *Amer. J. Pathol., 61*, 457-470.

Vergani, D., Tsantoulas, D. and Eddleston, A.L.W.F. (1978): Sensitisation to halothane-altered liver compounds in severe hepatic necrosis after halothane anaesthesia. *Lancet, 4*, 801-803.

Vogten, A.J.M., Summerskill, W.H.J. and Shorter, R.G. (1976): Cell mediated cytotoxicity against human hepatocyte membrane lipoprotein in halothane hepatitis. Activation by a serum factor? *Gastroenterology, 71*, 934.

Walton, B. (1978): Anaesthesia, surgery and immunology. *Anaesthesia, 33*, 322-348.

Walton, B., Dumonde, D.C., Williams, C. et al. (1973): Lymphocyte transformation: absence of increased responses in alleged halothane jaundice. *J. Amer. med. Ass., 225*, 494-499.

Walton, B., Simpson, B.R., Strunin, L. et al. (1976a): Unexplained hepatitis following halothane. *Brit. med. J., 1*, 1171-1176.

Walton, B., Hamblin, A., Dumonde, D.C. et al. (1976b): Absence of cellular hypersensitivity in patients with unexplained hepatitis following halothane. *Anesthesiology, 44*, 391-397.

Widger, L.A. Gandolfi, A.J. and Van Dyke, R.A. (1976): Hypoxia and halothane metabolism in vivo. Release of inorganic fluoride and halothane metabolite binding to cellular constituents. *Anesthesiology, 44*, 197-201.

Williams, B.D., White, N., Amlot, P.L. Slaney, J. and Toasland, P.A. (1977): Circulating immune complexes after repeated halothane anaesthesia. *Brit. med. J., 2*, 159-162.

Wills, E.J. (1968): Acute infective hepatitis: Fine structural and cytochemical alterations in human liver. *Arch. Pathol., 86*, 184-207.

Wills, E.J. and Walton, B. (1978): A morphological study of unexplained hepatitis following halothane anesthesia. *Amer. J. Pathol., 91*, 11-32.

Wright, R., Eade, O.E., Chisholm, M. et al. (1975): Controlled prospective study of the effect on liver function of multiple exposures to halothane. *Lancet, 1*, 817-820.

Yoshimura, N., Holaday, D.A. and Fiserova-Bergerova, V. (1976): Metabolism of methoxyflurane in man. *Anesthesiology, 44*, 372-379.

Thornton (ed.) Adverse Reactions of Anaesthetic Drugs
© Elsevier/North-Holland Biomedical Press, 1981

8

Effects of pollution due to inhalational agents used for anaesthesia

T.E.J. Healy

The effect of chronic exposure to chemical agents, on the health and the progress of pregnancy in those exposed, has been a cause for concern for a long time. Attention was probably first drawn to the relation between working conditions and disease by Percival Pott (1775), who described the occurrence of scrotal cancer among chimney sweeps. The embryotoxic, teratogenic and carcinogenic characteristics of many chemical agents have now been distinguished. Identification of the responsible agent has sometimes been possible when an association between a disease and a specific occupation has been recognised. All employees who work in the operating theatre environment are exposed to low concentrations of gaseous and volatile chemical agents which include anaesthetic drugs. Frederick Hewitt (1893) was among the first to report on the unpleasantness of working in unventilated theatres. Others in the early part of the century described the adverse effects of chronic exposure to anaesthetic agents (Hirsch and Kappus, 1929). However the alarm about the "real" dangers to operating theatre staff was raised initially by Vaisman (1967) whose report has been followed by many others which have supported her thesis. Nonetheless there are many claims and reports which refute the arguments supporting a biological hazard associated with the use of inhalational anaesthetic agents. Nitrous oxide in particular, probably because it has been considered to have low potency, is thought to be particularly benign. However a perusal of the literature may suggest a different conclusion. Gormsen (1955) reported that thrombocytopenia and leucopenia occurred following the use of nitrous oxide in combination with oxygen, chlorpromazine and curare used for the treatment of a patient with tetanus. These changes were attributed (Gormsen, 1955) to the use of curare. Leucopenia following the use of nitrous oxide in the treatment of tetanus was not mentioned by Bodman et al. (1955) but in later reports (Lassen et al., 1956; Lassen and Kristensen, 1959; Eastwood et al., 1963; Mollaret, 1965) bone marrow depression, leucopenia, thrombocytopenia and retarded erthro-poiesis were observed. Eastwood et al. (1963) studied the effect of 80% nitrous in oxygen on rats in exposure chambers. A leucopenia developed, polymorphonuclear cells disappeared more rapidly than lymphocytes. Similar findings (Okamoto, 1963) in rats were reported in Eastwood et al. (1963).

Green and Eastwood (1963) in reporting a decrease in the peripheral white count concluded that the prolonged administration of nitrous oxide and oxygen to the rat is toxic to the bone marrow.

A number of attempts have been made to determine the effect of nitrous oxide on cellular metabolism. However contradictory results have been cited in studies using brain slices or brain homogenate. Reduced oxygen consumption has been reported (Quastel and Wheatley, 1932; Bulow and Holmes, 1932; Hosein et al., 1955) on the other hand Pittinger et al. (1951) and Levy and Featherstone (1954) were unable to demonstrate any effect by nitrous oxide on the metabolism of brain homogenate. Schreiner and Gregoire (1963) studied the effects of high concentrations of nitrous oxide on fungal oxygen consumption. A fall in oxygen consumption which was restored when the colony was returned to an oxygen nitrogen mixture was recorded, however some cells were irreversibly damaged.

Rat liver cell mitochondria have been exposed to volatile anaesthetic agents and a dose related reduction in oxygen uptake recorded (Cohen, 1973; Nahrwold and Cohen, 1973). For halothane, the reduction in oxygen uptake commences at concentrations slightly below 1% but increases with increasing concentrations of halothane, until oxygen uptake falls to 25% of the normal value at a halothane concentration of 3%. The effect of halothane on the uptake of oxygen by mitochondria is largely reversible up to the 3% halothane level. The reversible depression of oxygen uptake is also shown by methoxyflurane, enflurane and ether. The effect of the anaesthetic agents on oxygen uptake by mitochondria occurs simultaneously with the inhibition of cell growth and therefore the two effects may be linked.

It was noted (Henderson, 1930) that volatile anaesthetic agents inhibit cell division. Kieler et al. (1957) exposed embryonic mouse heart myoblasts in tissue culture to various concentrations of nitrous oxide in nitrogen and oxygen. Nitrous oxide was judged to be a mitotic poison which frustrated the onset of mitosis by interphase cells leading to spindle destruction and chromosomal abnormalities in dividing cells. Furthermore nitrous oxide even in the presence of high oxygen concentrations was shown to be both cytocidal and cytostatic. A similarity between metaphase inhibition by nitrous oxide and the antimitotic effect of colchicine has been stressed by Anderson (1966). Snegireff et al. (1968) have studied the effect of anaesthetic concentrations of different anaesthetic agents including nitrous oxide on mitotic activity in the chick neural tube. A depressant effect on cell growth was detected after the 12th day of incubation. However, the mitotic index was unchanged i.e. the total number of mitotic cells was found not to vary significantly but more cells were shown to be in metaphase and fewer cells were shown to be in prophase. The results suggested either an increase in the rate of prophase or a retardation in the rate of metaphase. Metaphase arrest by nitrous oxide has previously been reported by Ostergreen (1944) and at high pressure (Rao, 1968).

Chinese hamster fibroblasts have been used (Sturrock and Nunn, 1976) to study the effect of halothane and nitrous oxide separately and in combination on chromosome patterns. The mitotic index was not altered by 75% nitrous oxide but was reduced with increasing concentrations of halothane. This reduction was not influenced by the combination of nitrous oxide with the halothane. The incidence of colchicine type metaphases (c mitoses) was markedly increased by halothane but not affected by nitrous oxide. During interphase halothane was associated with a marked increase in the incidence of nuclear abnormalities including multi nucleate cells and though nitrous oxide alone produced no significant change, the combination of nitrous oxide and halothane further increased the incidence.

The observation (Fink and Kenny, 1966) that nitrous oxide decreases the rate of mammalian cell proliferation in mono-layer culture led Fink et al. (1967) to examine this effect, using the rat embryo and foetus, by continual exposure of pregnant rats singly or in pairs for 2, 4 or 6 days to 45–50% nitrous oxide, 21–25% oxygen and nitrogen. Rats in a control study were exposed to air or to a mixture of 21% oxygen and 79% nitrogen. An increase in death with resorption of the embryos and foetal skeletal abnormalities were the most frequent findings in the study group. The number of survivors and the average foetal weight also was less in the study group, furthermore the male to female ratio among the foetuses was significantly reduced. The authors concluded from their results that there was a selective destruction by nitrous oxide of male rat embryos. The skeletal changes which also occurred following exposure for 2 days to 50% nitrous oxide and 40% oxygen were reminiscent of the effects of gross hypoxia in mice (Ingalls et al., 1972). Inert gases such as nitrous oxide may compete with oxygen for sites within the cell or its nucleus (Ebert and Hornsey, 1958a) and this may form a basis for an explanation of the embryotoxic effect of nitrous oxide. Similar results have been obtained by Ramazzotto et al. (1975) who found a statistically significant increase in the foetal death rate above that of the controls when rats were exposed to 50% nitrous oxide for 25 min per day during either the 1st, 3rd or all trimesters of pregnancy.

Suppression of spermatagenesis without a significant change in testosterone level has been demonstrated (Kripke et al., 1976) after exposure of rats for a maximum of 35 days to 20% nitrous oxide in 20% oxygen and 60% nitrogen. There was evidence in some rats of injury to the seminiferous tubules by the 2nd day of exposure. The toxic effect of nitrous oxide was confined to the spermatogenic cells and the pattern of injury was found to be similar to that following exposure to some other agents (Ribelin, 1963; Reddy and Svoboda, 1967). Though the quality of spermatozoa produced during the exposure to nitrous oxide was not fully determined there was evidence of abnormality.

The inhibition of cell growth by nitrous oxide may be relevant to the finding that nitrous oxide protects against radiation damage (Ebert and Hornsey, 1958a,b,; Evans and Orkin, 1962; Evans et al., 1964).

From the evidence available it must be concluded that nitrous oxide is a cell poison both in man and in animals. Though this information is valuable in terms of the totality of knowledge, the periods of exposure were protracted and the concentrations of nitrous oxide used in the various studies have been high. These facts must be remembered if an attempt is made to relate the toxic effects which have resulted from prolonged exposure of animals other than man to high concentrations of nitrous oxide and the consequences for man of exposure to ultra low concentrations measured in parts per million.

Linde and Bruce (1969) described levels of nitrous oxide in the operating theatre ranging from 130–428 ppm. Whereas Askrog and Peterson (1970) reported average concentrations of 7000 ppm nitrous oxide close to the anaesthetist when a non rebreathing system was used. Corbett (1972) found the concentration of nitrous oxide to be approximately 1000 ppm (range 330 to 9700 ppm) in the vicinity of the anaesthetist and to range from 310 to 550 ppm near to the surgeon. Millard and Corbett (1974) reported than an average peak concentration of 6767 ± 2466 ppm (1%) nitrous oxide was achieved after 60 min in the region of a dental surgeon whereas close to the dental assistants the average peak level was 587 ppm. However, even after 15 min concentrations of 3833 ± 1953 ppm were recovered close to the dentist. Even though some doubt, has been expressed about the value of such measurements (Beynen et al., 1978) due to temporal and spatial gradients, in nitrous oxide concentrations, they are the best estimate we have of the exposure of anaesthetic and operating theatre workers to nitrous oxide. It may, therefore, be more appropriate to consider the results obtained from animal studies in which concentrations of nitrous oxide in the range which has been measured in the atmosphere in the operating theatres have been used.

Corbett et al. (1973) reported a study of the effect on the progress of rat pregnancy of nitrous oxide in concentrations of either 1000 or 15000 ppm, administered continually throughout either days 12 to 19 or 8 to 13 of pregnancy respectively and on the effect of 1000 ppm and 100 ppm nitrous oxide administered for 8 hours per day. There were significantly higher foetal death rates in those groups of rats exposed continually compared with control studies. Increased foetal death rates were also recorded when pregnant rats were exposed to 100 ppm for 8 hours per day.

Vieira et al. (1978) have shown that nitrous oxide (1% in air) administered to pregnant rats for 6 hours per day either for the entire gestation period (i.e. 3 weeks) or for the 1st and 2nd weeks or only for the 3rd week resulted in fewer rats per litter in all the groups compared with a control study and furthermore, the offspring of those exposed during the 1st week of pregnancy were significantly smaller than those obtained from the other two groups. Implantation does not take place until day 5 of pregnancy and small size may therefore relate to exposure of the fertilized ovum before implantation or suggest an increased sensitivity of the ovum at about the time of implantation. The post natal growth of all the rats was also retarded.

In a recent study (Vieira, 1979), pregnant rats have been exposed to 0.5% (5000 ppm) nitrous oxide in air throughout pregnancy and this has been associated with a significant decrease in liter size compared with a control group breathing air. Foetal resorption, an overall decrease in size and skeletal abnormalities were found in the study animals but not in the control animals.

Cleaton-Jones et al. (1977) have administered 1% nitrous oxide for 6 hours per day 5 days per week for six months to rats without evidence of a leucopenia in contrast with the results obtained by Green and Eastwood, 1963 Green, 1964 and Parbrook, 1967 who using higher concentrations demonstrated a leucopenic effect. However, a transient polycythemia developed (Cleaton-Jones et al., 1977). It was postulated that the mechanism for this effect may be induction of hypoxia by nitrous oxide.

In another study (Cleaton-Jones et al., 1975) an increase in the number of mast cells was recorded in rats exposed to 1% nitrous oxide. The mutagenic potential of a number of gaseous and volatile agents has recently been examined (Baden et al., 1979). Nitrous oxide was not shown to be mutagenic.

The chick embryo, which is sensitive to teratogenic agents, was used (Andersen, 1968) to assess the teratogenic property of cyclopropane. Fertilised chicken eggs were exposed for three of twelve hours to different concentrations of cyclopropane on different days of the first third of the incubation period. Cyclopropane significantly increased the mortality and incidence of abnormalities in the treated embryos. Mortality was related to the length of exposure to cyclopropane in addition to the cyclopropane concentration and the timing of treatment. The mean weight in the test groups was always smaller than in the corresponding control groups except groups except that the mean weights of the embryos treated for six hours on the fourth day present an inverse relation to the cyclopropane concentration. The most common abnormality was rumplessness. Rumplessness was found to be the most frequent abnormality when chicken embryos were treated with other anaesthetic agents (Smith et al., 1965).

In an attempt to avoid hypoxia and hypercarbia, which may occur during mammalian anaesthesia and which are know to have a teratogenic effect, Bradley et al. (1965) also chose chick embryos for their experimental model. The anaesthetic agents tested were halothane in air and methoxyflurane in air, 0.25, 0.5, 1.0 and 1.5 per cent and 0.5, 1.0 and 2.0 per cent respectively. The combined risk to the embryo of death or a major non lethal abnormality was increased from a control value of 14.8% to 26.5% and 22.4% after exposure to 2% halothane or 0.5% methoxyflurane respectively. The species difference limits the clinical implications which may be drawn from this work but the results certainly suggests the need for further study.

In studies using mice Bruce (1967) has shown that halothane inhibits motility and phagocytosis by mammalian neutrophils. Nunn et al. (1970) examined the effect of lymphocyte exposure to 2% halothane and demonstrated a dramatic reduction in lymphocyte motility which may explain the reduction in circulating lymphocytes reported by Bruce and Koepke (1966) and the decrease in the number of antibody producing lymphocytes in rats (Wingard and Humphrey, 1968). Halothane has also been shown to inhibit cell division (Bruce and Keopke, 1966). The mechanism for these changes has been explained by assuming an alteration in cytoplasmic structure. Fink and Kenny (1966, 1968) in studies using cell culture have reported a dose dependent inhibition of growth in different strains of mammalian cells. The possibility that the development of an embryo may be altered by exposure to halothane, at a critical stage in development, was therefore examined (Basford and Fink, 1968). Rats were exposed to 0.8% halothane in 25% oxygen for 12-hour periods at different stages of pregnancy. The foetal weight, number of foetal resorptions and the incidence of skeletal anomalies were recorded. No difference in foetal weight was found between the control group and the study group. Some variation in the numbers of foetuses resorbed was recorded and this appeared to be related to the day of pregnancy on which exposure took place, but when the study is considered as a whole the difference in the numbers of resorptions between control and study groups was marginal and is seen to be not significant. The effect of exposure on the numbers of resorptions was subject however to a distinct diurnal variation. More resorptions occurred after exposure of the pregnant rats to halothane during the day than during the night $P < 0.001$. Skeletal changes showed a similar trend but at lower levels of significance. These results correlate with the report (Matthews et al., 1968) that mice are more susceptible to the toxic effects of halothane during the period of normal sleep.

Kennedy et al. (1976) exposed male and female rats and rabbits to halothane (1.34−1.48%). The animals were divided into groups and various exposure permutations were studied. Halothane did not have an adverse effect on the reproductive processes when administered prior to mating nor did it exert a teratogenic effect on rats or rabbits treated during the various stages of foetal development. There were not significant differences between the control and study groups with respect to the numbers of corpora lutea, implantation and resorption sites and viable foetuses. These findings were largely in agreement with the results of other studies. There was no support in this study for the report of an increased abortion rate in rats exposed to halothane (Wittman et al., 1974). Wittman et al. (1974) exposed pregnant rats to halothane 0.8% in oxygen for 12 hours per day on gestation days 6 and 10 and the abortion rate rose from 15% to 44%.

Bruce and Koepke (1969) exposed mice daily to 100 ppm (0.1%) halothane in air and a marked increase in mortality occurred but there was no increase in the effect of simultaneous irradiation at 1.4 R/hour. However liver pathology was identified in all the animals studied up to 4 weeks after exposure. Evans et al. (1964) have shown that sensitivity to irradiation may be reduced by nitrous oxide.

Whitcher et al. (1971) reported that the concentrations of halothane within a 3 foot radius of the exhalation port averaged 8.7 ppm when a non rebreathing circuit was used in an operating theatre where no anaesthetic agent scavenging devices were fitted.

One of the first studies to report the effect of halothane using a concentration similar to that found in unscavenged operating theatre air was reported by Bruce (1973). In order to mimic the lives of many anaesthetists, male and female mice were sexually isolated and exposed to either 16 ppm halothane in air or to air alone for seven hours per day five days per week for six weeks. Animals were then paired such that in each pair either the male, the female, both or neither had been exposed to halothane. The animals were treated, as before pairing, by exposure individually by day to halothane or air, but were caged in pairs at night. Halothane was shown not to reduce fertility nor increase the number of resorptions. Furthermore a numerically greater number of foetuses were found in females exposed to halothane, however the result was not statistically significant.

A number of studies attempting to analyse the effect of subanaesthetic concentrations of halothane on foetal development using the rat model have now been described (Katz and Clayton, 1973; Buzzard et al., 1974). An increase in foetal wastage and malformations have been reported. Lansdown et al. (1976) exposed pregnant rats in groups of 8 to halothane concentrations of 50, 100, 200, 800, 1600 and 3200 ppm in air for 8 daylight hours per day, on gestation days 8 to 12 inclusive. There was neither evidence of increased foetal death nor resorption, furthermore no retardation in growth or increased frequency of skeletal anomalies was recorded, except that foetal growth was retarded when rats were exposed to 1600 ppm halothane for all the 21 days of pregnancy but there was no evidence of an increased foetal loss. In a second study, groups of 8 rats were exposed to 1600 or 3200 ppm for 8 hours each day on days 1 to 21 of pregnancy inclusive. Control groups were exposed to an identical environment but without the addition of halothane. Some skeletal anomalies were seen, but as the anomalies were variable, not treatment related, and present in a control litter they were considered to be a sporadic defect and not halothane related. The occurrence of imperfections in the sternum was felt to be evidence of immaturity. Similar findings in normal rats were construed as evidence of developmental retardation by Fritz and Hess (1970).

There is evidence (Chang et al., 1974a) that inhalation of low concentrations of halothane leads to pathological lesions in the central nervous system. Chang et al. (1974a) exposed pregnant rats to halothane 10 ppm for 40 hours per week throughout pregnancy. Though no gross foetal anomalies were seen, many pathological changes were identified with the use of an electron microscope. These changes which included vacuolation, myelin figure formation, focal accumulation of vesicular structures, disruption of the nuclear envelope of cortical neurones, occasional neuronal necrosis and abnormal synaptic complexes, suggest a teratogenic action. The changes demonstrated in the central nervous system may contribute to the behavioural changes and poorer learning abilities of these animals reported by Quimby et al. (1974). Ultrastructural changes leading to hepatic damage have also been shown (Chang et al., 1974b) following chronic exposure to low levels of halothane. Ultrastructural changes followed exposure of rats to 0.25% halothane for 7 hours per day for 7 days. However these changes were described as normal responses associated with an alteration in the synthesis of enzymes (Ross and Cardell, 1972). In another study mice were exposed up to 4 times to 0.7 to 0.8% halothane. Each exposure lasting three hours. No evidence of hepatoxicity was seen (Stoyka and Havasi, 1977). Chang et al. (1975) demonstrated that the prolonged administration of halothane, in low concentrations, may induce pathological changes in rat kidneys. Pregnant rats were exposed to halothane 10 ppm for 8 hours per day, 5 days per week throughout pregnancy. The ultrastructure of kidneys removed from neonatal rats was studied and a number of pathological changes were identified which are consistent with the conclusion that halothane is toxic to the foetal renal system. Most lesions were found in the proximal convoluted tubule, and these included (1) Flattening or loss of the basal infolding of the epithelial cells. This may be due to either agenesis or degeneration associated with halothane toxicity. (2) Basal accummulation of lipid droplets. This may follow a change in fat metabolism leading to a rise in free fatty acids (Makelainen et al., 1973a,b) and consequent accumulation of lipids in the epithelial cells of the proximal convoluted tubule. (3) Disruption of mitochondria by halothane which has been previously documented (Taylor et al., 1972; Cohen, 1973; Berman et al., 1974). (4) Formation of clusters of smooth endoplasmic reticulum (SER), which may represent a detoxification response by the kidney. (5) Enlargement of apical vacuoles. Extensive enlargement of apical vacuoles can be induced by other agents including fluoroacetic acid which is nephrotoxic. Trifluoroacetic acid is a metabolic product of halothane and a chemical analogue of fluoracetic acid. It is not inconsistent therefore to expect that trifluoroacetic acid may exert a similar toxic effect on the kidney leading to vacuole enlargement. The evidence from studies of the microstructure of the kidneys, brain and liver therefore suggests that halothane in concentrations found in the operating room air, if breathed regularly for long periods, may be toxic.

It has been suggested (Nunn et al., 1970) that general anaesthetics may act as rapidly reversible immunosuppresive agents. Indeed Cullen et al. (1976) measured the inhibition of tumour cell destruction by leukocytes and showed that an increase in halothane concentration from 0.5% to 2.5% leads to an increase in inhibition from 5% to 44.7%. The effects were reversible. In a general review Duncan and Cullen (1976) concluded that anaesthetics inhibit leukocyte multiplication in a dose dependent manner, but that the effect would be unlikely to be important during general anaesthesia.

The remote possbility must also be considered that anaesthetic agents may induce malignant disease. Indeed a carcinogenic activity was predicted on the basis of structure for bis (chloromethyl) ether and chloromethyl methyl ether and subsequently confirmed (Van Duuren et al., 1968; Van Duuren et al., 1972). Marked structural similarities exist between bis (chloromethyl) ether, chloromethyl methyl ether, isoflurane, methoxyflurane and enflurane. Gargus et al. (1969) found a higher incidence of pulmonary adenomata and more tumours per mouse, in those that had received bis (chloromethyl) ether administered subcutaneously than in those receiving chloromethyl methyl ether or in uninjected controls. Industrial exposure to these volatile agents is generally via the respiratory tract and therefore the effect of inhalational exposures was studied using rats (Laskin et al., 1971). Animals were exposed to 0.1 ppm bis (chloromethyl) ether for six hours per day five days per week. A marked increase in pulmonary carcinomata was recorded in animals dying 332 to 463 days after the start of the exposure to bis (chloromethyl) ether. Repeated inhalation of bis (chloromethyl) ether and chloromethyl methyl ether at concentrations of one and two ppm was associated with an increase in the incidence of pulmonary adenomata in mice (Leong et al., 1971). Figueroa and others (1973) reported an increased incidence of lung cancer in men exposed to chloromethyl methyl ether at a chemical manufacturing plant. The α-chloro ether structures of bis (chloromethyl) ether and choromethyl methyl ether may be responsible for the carcinogenicity of these agents (Van Duuren et al., 1972). Isoflurane is also an α-chloro ether and for this reason Corbett (1976) considered the potential value in examining the tumour inducing potency of isoflurane in oxygen. Pregnant mice were exposed to either 0.5% isoflurane in oxygen on days 12, 14, 16 and 18 of pregnancy or to 0.1% isoflurane in oxygen on days 12, 14 and 16 of pregnancy. The progeny of both groups were then exposed twenty five times to 0.1% isoflurane on alternate days from age 5 days. A control group of pregnant mice and their offspring were then exposed to room air only. Post-mortom examination of offspring were carried out at 3, 6, 9 and 15 months after birth. At each age, i.e., 3, 6, 9 months, the incidence of pulmonary adenomata was highest in the study group. However, the difference in the incidence of pulmonary adenomata between the groups though apparent was not significant. At the fifteen months examination of survivors, hepatic neoplasia was found in 10 of 37 males (27%) of the group exposed to 0.5% enflurane and five of thirty males (17%) of the group exposed to 0.1% enflurane. No evidence of hepatic neoplasia was found in the control animals or in the female animals in the study groups. This sex related incidence finds support (Rice, 1972). The results reported in this study therefore suggested the urgent need to examine for tumour induction potency all the inhalational agents which are chemically related to isoflurane. Notwithstanding this, certain reservations regarding this study (Corbett, 1976) must be considered. The control group in this study cannot be regarded as an ideal control group in that the study group was exposed to isoflurane in oxygen whereas the control group was exposed to air, furthermore not all the pregnant females in the control group were peers of the treated females (Eger et al., 1978). Nonetheless the results are disturbing particularly when seen in the light of the similarity in chemical structure between agents with a known potency for tumour induction and agents used to produce anaesthesia.

$$
\begin{array}{ccc}
\text{Cl} & & \text{Cl} \\
| & & | \\
\text{H} - \text{C} - \text{O} - \text{C} - \text{H} \\
| & & | \\
\text{H} & & \text{H}
\end{array}
$$

Bis (Chloromethyl) ether

```
      Cl          H
      |           |
H  —  C  —  O  —  C  —  H
      |           |
      H           H
```

Chloromethyl methyl ether

```
      F     Cl          F
      |     |           |
F  —  C  —  C  —  O  —  C  —  H
      |     |           |
      F     H           F
```

Isoflurane

```
      Cl    F           H
      |     |           |
H  —  C  —  C  —  O  —  C  —  H
      |     |           |
      Cl    F           H
```

Methoxyflurane

```
      F     F           F
      |     |           |
H  —  C  —  C  —  O  —  C  —  H
      |     |           |
      Cl    F           F
```

Enflurane

However, other α-chloroethers such as alpha, α-dichloromethyl methyl ether have been shown (Van Duuren et al., 1969) in rodent studies not to produce neoplasia. Isoflurane differs from chloromethyl methyl ether and bis (chloromethyl) ether and is similar to other α-chloroethers in that it is a stable compound even in the presence of ultra violet light and strong alkali (Vitcha 1971). Furthermore active radicals produced by metabolism are thought to be essential to the alterations in DNA produced by chemical carcinogens. However isoflurane is only minimally metabolised in animals (Halsey et al., 1971) and in man (Holaday et al., 1975). The results obtained by Corbett (1976) would therefore be unexpected. In a more recent study (Eger et al., 1978) pregnant mice have been exposed 4 times, for 2-hour periods on days 11, 13, 15 and 17 of pregnancy, to isoflurane, enflurane, halothane, methoxyflurane or nitrous oxide. After delivery the progeny received twenty four, 2-hour exposures at two to three day intervals. Oxygen concentrations in the exposure chambers were maintained at one of two levels 25–30% oxygen in air or 85–100% oxygen. 25 sets of mice (1973) mice) were exposed to air, oxygen or the anaesthetic in air or in oxygen and examined after 15 months to identify the presence or otherwise of neoplasia. Neoplastic changes which included pulmonary adenomata, lymphomata, hepatocyte lesions and liver vascular lesions occurred in both the study and the control groups and there was no real evidence to support the thesis that isoflurane induces tumour formation, neither were halothane, enflurane, methoxyflurane nor nitrous oxide shown to have tumour inducing potency.

Eger et al. (1978) have postulated that Corbett (1976) demonstrated carcinogenic property, for isoflurane while they did not, because Corbett used mice raised in Michigan at a time when animal food was contaminated with polybrominated biphenyls which are known to be teratogenic (Corbett et al., 1975) and related to compounds known to be carcinogenic (Kimbrough et al., 1975). Indeed the livers of the animals used by Corbett (1976) but not by Eger et al. (1978) were shown to contain polybrominated biphenyls. This exposure may have contributed to the higher average incidence of liver lesions reported by Corbett (1976).

The carcinogenicity of vinyl chloride at concentrations of 50 ppm has been demonstrated (Maltoni and Lefemine, 1975). Vinyl chloride was also shown to possess transplacental carcinogeneity when administered to rats, for 4 hours per day from day 12 to 18 of pregnancy, at a concentration of 6000 ppm. There is a marked structural similarity between vinyl chloride and trichloroethylene.

$$
\begin{array}{c}
\text{H} \diagdown \quad\quad\quad \diagup \text{Cl} \\
\quad\quad \text{C} = \text{C} \\
\text{H} \diagup \quad\quad\quad \diagdown \text{Cl}
\end{array}
$$

Vinyl chloride

$$
\begin{array}{c}
\text{Cl} \diagdown \quad\quad\quad \diagup \text{Cl} \\
\quad\quad \text{C} = \text{C} \\
\text{H} \diagup \quad\quad\quad \diagdown \text{Cl}
\end{array}
$$

Trichloroethylene

Indeed in animal studies large oral doses of trichloroethylene have been shown to be associated with the development of cancer (Saffioti 1975) though not much importance, in the present context, is attached to these findings (Ferstandig 1978) because trichloroethylene is known to be a dose related toxin. This conclusion gains support from the results of a study arranged by Leong et al (1975). Pregnant mice and rats were allowed to inhale 300 ppm trichloroethylene during the period of gestation and no adverse effects on embryonal or foetal development were seen. Healy and Wilcox (1978) exposed pregnant rats to trichloroethylene 100 ppm in air 4 hours per day, 7 days a week from day 6 of pregnancy. The results suggested a definite association between the inhalation of trichloroethylene, reduced foetal weight and increased foetal loss. The foetal weights in the study group were significantly less than the foetal weights in the control group $0.001 < P << 0.01$ and the number of foetuses resorbed in the study group was greater than in the control group $0.001 < P < 0.01$. No doubt there were differences in the experimental technique between these two studies but the results do serve to underline the difficulties one faces in attempting to compare the results obtained in different studies and to draw definitive conclusions, acceptable for all environmental conditions.

The expression of carcinogenicity following exposure to a carcinogenic agent during in utero life may require an interval of months or years (Corbett, 1976), furthermore tumours induced transplacentally are generally not detected until well after the animals have reached sexual maturity (Rice, 1973). It is therefore important to examine this aspect of possible adverse responses to the chronic inhalation of low concentrations of anaesthetic agents by a multiplicity of animal exposure studies.

Albino mice have been exposed to both halothane (0.7%) and methoxyflurane (0.4%) for one hour each day and no carcinogenic effect was found up to 29 weeks (Kunz et al., 1969). However both agents were found to influence the carcinogenic effect of diethylnitrosamine. Survival time, tumour frequency and tumour localization induced by diethylnitrosamine were unaltered by either halothane or methoxyflurane however the type of tumour was influenced by these drugs. The possibility must be considered therefore, that halothane and methoxyflurane may influence the carcinogenic effect of a known carcinogen. These studies were not continued for long enough to rule out a primary carcinogenic effect of halothane or methoxyflurane and further studies are therefore necessary.

An examination, using animal models, of the embryotoxic, mutagenic and tumour induction potencies of the inhalational agents is essential, even though the comparative vulnerability of the different mammalian species and the human embryo is largely unknown. However, if the susceptibility of the human embryo to harm at each stage in development is similar to that of the other animal embryos, then the human embryo is at maximum risk during the time when its existence may be unknown, i.e. from about the second to the seventh week of development. The present evidence drawn from tissue culture and in vivo animal studies is equivacal though some inhalational anaesthetic agents may possess teratogenic, mutagenic and carcinogenic properties in some species and these findings if real may reflect similar properties with respect to the human embryos. However, the first report to connect the health of anaesthetists and their conditions of work awaited a survey which covered 15 per cent of the anaesthetists in the Soviet Union (Vaisman, 1967). In this report it was concluded that the unfavourable conditions, in which anaesthesia was practiced, adversely influenced the progress and completion of pregnancy in female anaesthetists. Though the inhalation of anaesthetic vapours was included among the likely unfavourable factors, consideration was also given to emotional stress, sustained attention to detail and excessive work. Schulze et al. (1969) suggested that there was an increased rate of spontaneous abortion among nurses and female medical staff working in the operating theatre.

Chromosome changes have been shown to occur (Cain, 1979) in cells in peripheral blood culture taken from anaesthetists during the first six months of training in anaesthesia. The mean percentage increase in metaphase cells, in tissue culture, with an abnormally high number of chromosomes was found to be 98% and this represents a highly significant change.

The inhalation of anaesthetic vapours is a tangible entity and probably for this reason has, of all the potentially harmful factors, attracted most interest. Askrog and Harvold (1970) reported the findings from questionnaires sent to 578 anaesthetic department nurses and to 174 female and male anaesthetists. 570 answers were received and these included information on 212 pregnancies started before employment in an anaesthetic department and 392 pregnancies started during employment in an anaesthetic department. Pregnancies which commenced during employment in an anaesthetic department terminated in abortion or premature delivery twice as often as those before such employment. The pregnancies in the wives of male anaesthetists, who had not themselves been exposed to anaesthetic vapours followed a similar pattern. Whitcher et al. (1971) reported that residual concentrations of halothane were detected in the expired air of many operating room workers 16 hours after exposure. Nitrous oxide and halothane have been detected in the expired air of anaesthetists for up to seven and 64 hours respectively (Corbett, 1974a). The relation between male anaesthetists and the higher incidence of unexpected termination of pregnancy among their wives may be associated with inhalation by the wives of their husbands expired air, containing trace amounts of anaesthetic gases. There was no evidence of an increased incidence of congenital malformation in children conceived during employment in an anaesthetic department. The small numbers of children surveyed in the study may, however, have concealed a marginal change.

Cohen et al. (1971) undertook a two part survey to evaluate the possible relations between spontaneous miscarriage and exposure to the operating room. In a first study 67 operating room nurses (average age 34.3 years) and 92 general duty nurses (average age 30.9 years) were interviewed to obtain information including numbers of pregnancies, incidence of spontaneous miscarriage in the first 20 weeks of pregnancy, contraceptive techniques and birth defects occurring during a four year period. The results indicated that 29.7% of pregnancies in operating room nurses ended in spontaneous miscarriage whereas in the control group i.e. the general duty nurses, the number was only 8.8%. In a second study covering a 6-year period, 50 medically qualified anaesthetists (average age 39.6 years) and a control group of 81 medically qualified practitioners (average age 36.8 years) in specialties other than anaesthesia, were asked to complete a questionnaire. The miscarriage rate for the anaesthetists was 37.8% and this compared with 10.3% for the control group. Furthermore in both studies the anaesthetists and the anaesthetic nurses suffered the maximum incidence of miscarriage at an earlier stage (8th week) than did the members of the control groups (10th week). The ages of the women in both study groups were marginally greater than the ages in the control groups. However, this fact was not thought to be responsible for the different miscarriage rates and indeed the age of the control group 2 was greater than the age of the study group 1. The spontaneous miscarriage rate in control group 2 was 10.3% whereas in the study group 1 the rate was 29.7%. Factors including exposure to X-rays, various chemicals, physical demands and stress may be acting in the operating theatre to produce these variations. However, it is difficult to quantify stress and the authors though aware of the other possibilities nevertheless drew attention to the importance of eliminating all waste gases from the operating theatre.

In another study (Knill-Jones et al., 1972) questionnaires were sent to female anaesthetists and to non anaesthetist female medical graduates. Reply rates of 82.1% (563) and 80% (828) were received from anaesthetists and controls respectively. The anaesthetists did not report a greater incidence of unexpected termination of pregnancy than the controls. However when anaesthetists at work were considered, the ratio for those at work (18.2%) in anaesthesia and the control groups (14.7%) were significantly different ($P<0.25$). There was no significant difference in the incidence of termination of pregnancy, between anaesthetists at work and not at work, but the anaesthetists reported a higher incidence of infertility (12%) than did the control group (6%). These results, though the numbers are small, must increase anxiety among those who work in the operating theatre. However, the authors admit that many factors concerning the control study, including the work history in relation to obstetric history, age of subject at each obstetric event and husbands occupation, were not taken into account.

Bruce et al. (1968) examined the cause of death in 441 anaesthetists dying between 1947 and 1966, and identified an increased incidence of reticuloendothelial and lymphoid malignancies. However, in a prospective study (Bruce et al., 1974) the cause of death of 211 anaesthetists was verified and the death rates from different diseases were compared with those of male standard policy holders of an insurance company. The overall death rates and rate in each of the categories of anaesthetists, i.e. junior, active and retired, were shown to be lower than in the control group with the one exception of suicide. There was no confirmation of a high death rate from neoplasia of lymphoid and reticulo-endothelial tissue. However no data was collected from living anaesthetists and furthermore the number of deaths was small. The data does not therefore allow statistically meaningful interpretation, but there is no evidence to support speculation that malignant disease is more common among anaesthetists than among members of the general population. Corbett et al. (1973), however, do speculate on the relation between malignant neoplasia and inhalation of anaesthetic agents. In a survey of all the nurse anaesthetists (621) in Michigan they obtained an 84.5% response. A total of 35 malignancies occurring in 33 anaesthetists was reported. Thirty three of these malignant changes were diagnosed in 31 nurse anaesthetics after they had started training in anaesthesia. The age adjusted incidence of malignant neoplasia was approximately three times the expected rate (Christine et al., 1971).

Corbett et al. (1974b) also questioned the same female nurse anaesthetists (Corbett et al., 1973) to determine the incidence of birth defects among their progeny. 16.4 per cent of the children born to mothers who worked during pregnancy had birth defects and two of them suffered three neoplastic lesions, whereas only 5.7 per cent of the children whose mothers did not work during pregnancy had birth defects but one child suffered a neoplastic lesion.

Cohen et al. (1974) carried out an American National Study among operating room personnel and compared the results with those obtained from two non anaesthetist professional bodies, 15,151 wives of male anaesthetists and female anaesthetists replied. The control group obtained 9037 replies. The results suggest that female staff in the operating theatre have an increased incidence of spontaneous abortion, congenital abnormalities among their children, neoplasia and hepatic and renal disease. Unexposed wives of male operating room personnel also suffered an increase among their children, of congenital anomalies.

If doubts exist concerning the teratogenic, embryotoxic and neoplastic effects resulting from the chronic inhalation of trace concentrations of the different anaesthetic agents, there may be other consequences of working in contaminated atmospheres. Halothane hepatitis among anaesthetists has been reported (Belfrage et al., 1966; Klatskin and Kimberg, 1969; Lund et al., 1974). Other reports describe ophthalmic hypersensitivity to halothane (Boyd, 1974), and halothane sensitivity leading to atrial fibrillation (Latty, 1970). Schwettwrann and Casterline (1974) described a delayed asthmatic response following occupational exposure to enflurane. A nurse anaesthetist is reported to have suffered an exacerbation of myasthenia gravis as a result of exposure to methoxyflurane (Elder et al., 1971).

Vaisman (1967) considered stress to be a possible explanation of the adverse effects on pregnancy of working in an operating theatre. This suggestion finds support in the study (Rosenberg and Kirves, 1973) in which nurses in anaesthesia, accident department, intensive care unit and scrub nurses were studied. The authors considered that stress was the likely cause of the increased rate of spontaneous miscarriages occurring during hospital employment. Indeed a correlation between stress and abnormal pregnancies has been drawn (Ferreira, 1965; Hertz, 1973; Gorsuch and Key, 1974. Furthermore those women who had abnormal pregnancies were seen to have experienced greater anxiety and stress during the first trimester than did a control group who had normal pregnancies (Gorsuch and Key, 1974). Altered neuroendocrine and autonomic activity may explain this phenomena and indeed in a study using the mouse, abnormal osteogenesis in the foetus has been associated with stress and elevated serum steroid levels (Barlow et al., 1974).

In studying the potential hazards of inspiring trace considerations of anaesthetic gases and vapours we have been able to consider the results obtained by controlled experiments in which animal models have been used. The results obtained using anaesthetic concentrations may lead one to conclude that, at high concentrations some anaesthetic gases and vapours possess embryotoxic, teratogenic and even neoplastogenic properties. However the results obtained using trace concentrations are frequently contradictory though the results obtained by Chang et al. (1974a,b, 1975) would, if control studies had been published, add weight to the arguments of those who consider the inhalation of trace concentrations of anaesthetic gases and vapours to be a threat to the health of operating theatre workers. Epidemiological surveys have in the main supported the suggestion that a hazard exists to pregnancy for those working in the operating theatre. However these reports have suffered from the lack of suitable control studies and therefore conclusions which may be drawn from them are entirely speculative. Furthermore the surveys at present published, even though some purport to establish a relation between cause and effect, can at best identify the effect. One must not attempt to draw conclusions such as a real relation between disease and the inhalation of trace concentrations of anaesthetic gases from evidence drawn from studies which are not designed to exclude other possible factors including stress. It is an assumption which cannot be confirmed in human studies until after pollution has ceased, i.e. at a time when efficient anaesthesia scavenging devices are in full use. If the differences presently existing between the control and study group surveys are seen to disappear, we may conclude with less doubt that anaesthetic gases have been the causative agent.

REFERENCES

Anderson, N.B. (1966): The effect of CNS depressants on mitosis. *Acta anaesth. scand. Suppl., 22*, 1.

Anderson, N.B. (1968): The teratogenicity of cyclopropane in the chicken. *Anesthesiology, 29*, 113-122.

Askrog, V. and Harvald, B. (1970): Teratogen effekt af inhalationsanaesthetika. *Nord. Med., 83*, 498-500.

Askrog, V. and Petersen, R. (1970): Forurening af operationstner med luftformige anaestetika og reontgenbestraaling. *Saertryk Nord. Med., 83*, 501-504.

Baden, J.M., Kelley, M., Mazze, R.I. and Simmon, V.F. (1979): Mutagenicity of inhalational anaesthetics: Trichloroethylene, divinyl ether, nitrous oxide and cyclopropane. *Brit. J. Anaesth., 51*, 417-421.

Basford, A.B. and Fink, B.R. (1968): The teratogenicity of halothane in the rat. *Anesthesiology, 29*, 1167-1173.

Belfrage, S., Ahlgren, L. and Axelson, S. (1966): Halothane hepatitis in an anaesthetist. *Lancet, 2*, 1466-1467.

Berman, M.D., Kewley, C.F. and Kench, J.E. (1974): Contribution of inhibition of NADH-dehydrogenase to the cardiotoxic effects of halothane. *J. mol cell. Cardiol., 6*, 39-47.

Beynen, F.M., Knopp, T.J. and Rehder, K. (1978): Nitrous oxide exposure in the operating room. *Anesth. Analg., 57*, 216-223.

Bodman, R.I., Morton, H.J.V. and Thomas, E.T. (1955): Treatment of tetanus with chloropromazine and nitrous oxide anaesthesia. *Lancet, 2*, 230-231.

Boyd, C.H. (1974): Ophthalmic hypersensitivity to anaesthetic vapour. *Anaesthesia, 27*, 456-457.

Bradley, E., Smith, M.D., Gaub, M.L. and Moya, F. (1965): Investigations into the teratogenic effects of anaesthetic agents: The fluorinated agents. *Anesthesiology, 26*, 260-261.

Bruce, D.L. and Koepke, J.A. (1966): Changes in granulopoiesis in the rat associated with prolonged halothane anaesthesia. *Anesthesiology, 27*, 811-816.

Bruce, D.L. (1967): Effect of halothane anaesthesia on extravascular mobilization of neutrophils *J. surg. Res., 7*, 180-185.

Bruce, D.L., Eide, K.A., Linde, H.W. and Eckenhoff, J.E. (1968): Causes of death among anesthesiologists: A 20 year survey. *Anesthesiology, 29*, 565-569.

Bruce, D.L. and Koepke, J.A. (1969): Interaction of halothane and radiation in mice: possible implications. *Anesth. Analg., 48*, 687-694.

Bruce, D.L. (1973): Murine fertility unaffected by traces of halothane. *Anesthesiology, 38*, 473-477.

Bruce, D.L., Eide, K.A., Smith, N.J. Seltzer, F. and Dykes, H.M. (1974): A prospective survey of anesthesiologist Mortality, 1967-1971. *Anesthesiology, 41*, 71-74.

Bülow, M. and Holmes, E.G. (1932): Die sauestoffanfrahme und ammoniakbilding von gehrin bei gengenward markotisch unirkender stoffe. *Biochem Z, 245,* 459.

Buzzard, D.A., Stoelting, R.K., Peterson, C. and Ishaq, M. (1974): Fetal changes in hamsters anesthetised with nitrous oxide and halothane. *Anesthesiology, 41,* 275-278.

Chang, L.W., Dudley, A.W., Martin, H.A. and Katz, J. (1974a): Nervous system development following in utero exposure to trace amounts of halothane. *Teratology, 9,* A-15.

Chang, L.W., Dudley, A.W. and Katz, J. (1974b): Ultrastructural evidence of hepatic injuries by chronic exposure to low levels of halothane. *Amer. J. Pathol., 74,* 103a-104a.

Chang, L.W., Dudley, A.W., Lee, Y.K. and Katz, J. (1975): Ultrastructure changes in the kidney following chronic exposure to low levels of halothane. *Amer. J. Pathol., 78,* 225-242.

Christine, B., Flannery, J.T. and Sullivan, P.B. (1971): Cancer in Connecticut, 1969. *Conn. Health Bull., 86,* 103-114.

Cleaton-Jones, P., Austin, J.C., Banks, D. and Vieira, E. (1975): Does nitrous oxide harm the dentist? *Lancet, 2,* 931.

Cohen, E.N., Weldon Belville, J. and Brown, B.W. (1971): Anesthesia pregnancy and miscarriage. A study of operating room nurses and anaesthetists. *Anesthesiology, 35,* 343-347.

Cohen, P.J. (1973): Effect of anesthetics on mitochondrial function. *Anesthesiology, 39,* 153-164.

Cohen, E.N., Brown, B.W., Bruce, D.L., Cascorbi, H.F., Corbett, T.H., Jones, T.W. and Whitcher, C.E. (1974): Occupational disease among operating room personnel; A national study. Report of an ad hoc committee on the effect of trace anesthetics on the health of operating room personnel, American Study of Anesthesiologists. *Anesthesiology, 41,* 321-340.

Corbett, T.H. (1972): Anesthetics as a cause of abortion. *Fertil. Steril., 23,* 866-869.

Corbett, T.H., Cornell, R.G., Endres, J.L. and Millard, R.I. (1973a): Effects of low concentrations of nitrous oxide on rat pregnancy. *Anesthesiology, 39,* 299-301.

Corbett, T.H., Cornell, R.G., Lieding, K. and Endres, J., (1973b): Incidence of cancer among Michigan nurse anesthetists. *Anesthesiology, 38,* 260-263.

Corbett, T.H. (1974a): Inhalation Anaesthesia; An occupational hazard. *Hosp. Pract. November,* 81-85.

Corbett, T.H., Cornell, R.G., Endres, J. and Lieding, K. (1974b): Birth defects among children of nurse anaesthetists. Anesthesiology, *41,* 341-344.

Corbett, T.H., Beaudoin, A.R., Cornell, R.G. et al. (1975): Toxicity of polybrominated biphenyls (Firemaster BP-6) in rodents. *Environm. Res., 10,* 390-396.

Corbett, T.H. (1967): Cancer and congenital anomalies associated with anesthetics. *Ann. N.Y. Acad. Sci., 271,* 58-66.

Cullen, B.F., Duncan, P.G. and Ray-Keil, L. (1976): Inhibition of cell mediated cytotoxity by halothane and nitrous oxide. *Anesthesiology, 44,* 386-390.

Duncan, P.G. and Cullen, B.F. (1976): Anesthesia and immunology. *Anesthesiology, 45,* 522-538.

Eastwood, D.W., Green, C.D., Lambdin, M.A. and Gardner, R. (1963): Effect of nitrous oxide on white-cell count in leukemia. *New Engl. J. Med., 268,* 297.

Ebert, M. and Hornsey, S. (1958a): Effect on radiosensitivity of inert gases. *Nature, 181,* 613-616.

Ebert, M. and Hornsey, S. (1958b): Effect of nitrous oxide on the radiosensitivity of mouse Ehrlich ascites tumour. *Nature, 182,* 1240.

Eger, E.I., White, A.E., Brown, C.L., Biava, C.G., Corbett, T.H. and Stevens, W.C. (1978): A test of the carcinogenicity of enflurane, isoflurane, halothane, methoxyflurane and nitrous oxide in mice. *Anesth. Analg., 57,* 678-694.

Elder, B.F., Beal, H., De Wald, W. and Cobb, S. (1971): Exacerbation of subclinical myasthenia by occupational exposure to an anesthetic. *Anesth. Analg., 50,* 383-387.

274

Evans, J.C. and Orkin, L.R. (1962): Protective effect of nitrous oxide against total body radiation in the mouse. *Nature, 195*, 822-823.

Evans, J.C., Roberts, T.W. and Orkin, L.R. (1964): Modification of radiosensitivity of mice by inert gases and nitrous oxide. *Radiat. Res., 21*, 243-255.

Ferreira, A.J. (1965): Emotional factors in prenatal environment. *J. nerv. ment. Dis., 141*, 180-198.

Ferstandig, L.L. (1978): Trace concentrations of anesthetic gases: a critical review of their disease potential. *Anesth. Analg., 57*, 328-345.

Figueroa, W.G., Raszkowski, R. and Weiss, W. (1973): Lung cancer in chloromethyl methyl ether workers. *New Engl. J. Med., 24*, 1096-1097.

Fink, B.R. and Kenny, G.E. (1966): Inhibition of cell culture growth by volatile anesthetics. *Fed. Proc., 25*, 561.

Fink, B.R., Shepard, T.H. and Blandau, R.J. (1967): Teratogenic acitivity of nitrous oxide. *Nature, 214*, 146-148.

Fink, B.R. and Kenny, G.E. (1968): Metabolic effects of volatile anesthetics in cell culture. *Anesthesiology, 29*, 505-515.

Fritz, H. and Hess, R. (1970): Ossification of the rat and mouse skeleton in the perinatal period. *Teratology, 3*, 331-338.

Gargus, J.L., Reese, W.H. and Rutter, H.A. (1969): Induction of lung adenomas in new born mice by bis (chloromethyl) ether. *Toxicol. appl. Pharmacol., 15*, 92-96.

Gormsen, J. (1955): Agranulocytosis and thrombocytopenia in case of tetanus treated with curare and chlorpromazine. *Dan. med. Bull., 2*, 87-89.

Gorsuch, R.L. and Key, M.K. (1974): Abnormalities of pregnancy as a function of anxiety and life stress. *Psychosom. Med., 36*, 352-362.

Green, C.D. and Eastwood, D.W. (1963): Effects of nitrous oxide inhalation on hemopoiesis in rats. *Anesthesiology, 24*, 341-345.

Halsey, M.J., Sawyer, D.C., Eger, E.I., Bahlman, S.H. and Impelman, D.M.K. (1971): Hepatic metabolism of halothane, methoxyflurane, cyclopropane, ethrane and forane in miniature swine. *Anesthesiology, 35*, 43-47.

Healy, T.E.J. and Wilcox, A. (1978): Chronic exposure of rats to inhalational anaesthetic agents. *J. Physiol., 276*, 24-25 P.

Henderson, V.E. (1930): The present status of the theories of narcosis. *Psysiol. Rev., 10*, 171-220.

Hertz, D.G. (1973): Rejection of motherhood. A psychosomatic appraisal of habitual abortion. *Psychosomatics, 14*, 241-244.

Hewitt, F.W. (1893): *Anaesthetics and their Administration*. Charles Griffin and Co., London. p. 33.

Hirsch, J. and Kappus, A.L. (1929): Über die mengen des narkoseathers in der luft von operationssalen. *Z. Hyg. Infekt. Kr., 110*, 391-398.

Holaday, D.A., Fiserova-Bergerova, V., Latto, I.P. and Zumbiel, A. (1975): Resistance of isoflurane to biotransformation in man. *Anesthesiology, 43*, 325-332.

Hosein, E.A., Stachiewicz, E., Bourne, W. and Denstedt, O.F. (1955): Influence of nitrous oxide on metabolic activity of brain tissue. *Anesthesiology, 16*, 708-715.

Ingalls, T.H., Curley, F.J. and Prindle, R.A. (1952): Medical progress: experimental production of congenital anomalies; timing and degree of anoxia as factors causing fetal deaths and congenital anomalies in mouse. *New Engl. J. Med., 247*, 758-768.

Katz, J. and Clayton, W., (1973): Fetal mortality in rats chronically exposed to low concentrations of halothane. *Proc. Am. Soc. Anesth. Ann Meeting*, 57-58.

Kennedy, G.L., Smith, S.H., Keplinger, M.L. and Calandra, J.C. (1976): Reproductive and teratologic studies with halothane. *Toxicol. appl. Pharmacol., 35*, 467-474.

Kieler, J., Mortenson, H. and Peterson, C.R. (1957): Cytologic effect of nitrous oxide at different organ tensions. *Acta Pharmacol. Toxicol., 13*, 301-308.

Kimbrough, R.D., Squire, R.A., Linder, R.E., Strandberg, J.D., Montali, R.J. and Burse, V.W. (1975): Induction of liver tumour in sherman strain female rats by polychlorinated biphenyl araclor 1260. *J. Nat. Cancer Inst., 55*, 1453-1459.

Klatskin, G. and Kimberg, D.V. (1969): Recurrent hepatitis attributable to halothane sensitization in an anesthetist. *New Engl. J. Med., 280*, 515-522.

Knill-Jones, R.P., Rodrigues, L.V., Moir, D.D. and Spence, A.A. (1972): Anaesthetic practice and pregnancy controlled survey of women anaesthetists in the United Kingdom. *Lancet, 2*, 1326-1328.

Kripke, B.J., Kelman, A.D., Shah, N.K., Balogh, K. and Handler, A.H. (1976): Reticular reaction to prolonged exposure to nitrous oxide. *Anesthesiology, 44*, 104-113.

Kunz, W., Schaude, G. and Thomas, C. (1969): The effect of phenobarbitol and halogenated hydrocarbons on nitrosamine carcinogesis. *Krebsforsch. Krebsbekaempf., 72*, 291-304.

Lansdown, A.B.G., Pope, W.D., Halsey, M.J. and Bateman, P.E. (1976): Analysis of fetal development in rats following maternal exposure to subanaesthetic concentrations of halothane. *Teratology, 13*, 299-304.

Laskin, S., Kuschner, M., Drew, R.T., Cappiello, P. and Nelson, N. (1971): Tumors of the respiratory tract induced by inhalation of bis (chloromethyl) ether. *Arch. environ. Health*, 23, 135-136.

Lassen, H.C.A., Henriksen, E., Neukirch, F. and Kristensen, H.S. (1956): Treatment of tetanus: severe bone marrow depression after prolonged nitrous-oxide anaesthesia. *Lancet, 270*, 527-530.

Lassen, H.C.A. and Kristensen, S.H. (1959): Remission in chronic myloid leukaemia following prolonged nitrous oxide inhalation. *Dan. med. Bull., 6*, 252-255.

Lattey, M. (1970): Halothane sensitization. A case report. *Canad. Anaesth. Soc. J., 17*, 648-649.

Leong, B.K.J., MacFarland, H.N. and Reese, W.H. (1971): Induction of lung adenomas by chronic inhalation of bis (chloromethyl) ether. *Arch. environm. Health, 22*, 663-666.

Leong, B.K.J., Schwetz, B.A., Gehring, P.J. (1975): Embryo and fetotoxicity of inhaled trichloroethylene, methyl chlorophorm and methlyene chloride in mice and rats. *Toxicol. appl. Pharmacol., 33*, 136.

Levy, L. and Featherstone, R.M. (1954): The effect of xenon and nitrous oxide on in vitro guinea pig brain respiration and oxidative phosphorylation. *J. Pharmacol. exp. Ther., 110*, 221-225.

Linde, H.W. and Bruce, D.L. (1969): Occupational exposure of anesthesiologists to halothane, nitrous oxide and radiation. *Anesthesiology, 30*, 363-368.

Lund, I., Skulberg, A. and Helle, I. (1974): Occupational hazard of halothane. *Lancet, 2*, 528-529.

Makelainen, A., Nikki, P. and Vapaatalo, H. (1973a): Halothane induced lipolysis in rats. *Acta anaesth. scand., 17*, 170-178.

Makelainen, A., Vapaatalo, H. and Nikki, P. (1973b): Halothane induced lipolysis in vitro in the rat. *Acta anaesth. scand., 17*, 179-183.

Maltoni, C. and Lefemine, G. (1975): Carcinogenicity bio assays of vinyl chloride: Current results. Toxicity of vinyl chloride polyvinyl chloride. *Ann. N.Y. Acad. Sci., 246*, 195-218.

Matthews, J.H., Marte, E. and Halberg, F. (1968): Fluothane toxicity in mice studied by indirect periodicity analysis, In: *Toxicity of Anesthetics*. Editor: B.R. Fink. Williams and Wilkins Co, Baltimore.

Millard, R.I. and Corbett, T.H. (1974): Nitrous oxide concentrations in the dental operatory. *J. oral. Surgery., 32*, 593-594.

Mollaret, P. (1956): Treatment of severe tetanus: Report of four cases. *German med. Month, 1*, 338.

Nahrwold, M.L. and Cohen, P.J. (1973): Additive effect of nitrous oxide and halothane on mitochondrial function. *Anesthesiology, 39*, 534-536.

Nunn, J.F., Sharp, J.A. and Kimball, K.L. (1970): Reversible effects of an inhalational anaesthetic on lymphocyte motility. *Nature, 226*, 85-86.

Ostergren, G. (1944): Colchicine mitosis, chromosome contraction, narcosis and protein chain folding. *Hereditas (Lund), 30*, 429-467.

Pittinger, C.B., Featherstone, R.M., Cullen, S.C. and Gross, E.G. (1951): Comparative in vitro study of guinea pig brain oxidations as influenced by xenon and nitrous oxide. *J. Lab. clin. Med., 38*, 384-387.

Pott, P. (1775): Chirugical observations relative to the cancer of the scrotum. *Reprinted in National Cancer Institute Monograph (1963), 10*, 7-13.

Quastel, J.M. and Wheatley, A.H.M. (1932): Narcosis and oxidations of brain. *Proc. roy. Soc. London., 112*, 60-79.

Quimby, K.L., Aschkenase, L.J., Bowman, R.E., Katz, J. and Chang, L.W. (1974): Enduring learning deficits and cerebral malformation from exposure to 10 ppm halothane. *Science, 185*, 625-627.

Ramazzotto, L.S., Katz, A. and Cupiola, R. (1975): Pharmacological effects of nitrous oxide administered during pregnancy. *J. Dent. Res., 54, Special Issue A., IADR Abstract L31.*

Rao, P.N. (1968): Mitotic synchrony in mammalian cells treated with nitrous oxide at high pressure. *Science, 160*, 774-776.

Reddy, K.J. and Svoboda, D.J. (1967): Alterations in rat testes due to antispermatogenic agent. *Arch. Pathol., 84*, 376-392.

Ribelin, W.E. (1963): Atrophy of rat testes an index of chemical toxicity. *Arch. Pathol., 75*, 229-235.

Rice, J.M. (1972): The biological behaviour of transplacentally induced tumours in mice. Transplacental carcinogenesis. *IARC, Sci. Pub. 4*, 71-83.

Rice, J.M. (1973): An overview of transplacental chemical carcinogenesis. *Teratology, 8*, 113-125.

Rosenberg, P. and Kirves, A. (1973): Miscarriages among operating theatre staff. *Acta anaesth. scand. Suppl., 53*, 37-42.

Ross, W.T. and Cardell, R.R. (1972): Effects of halothane on the ultrastructure of rat liver cells. *Canad. Anaesth. Soc. J., 24*, 243-251.

Saffioti, U. (1975): Memorandum alert. *J. nat. Cancer Inst.* March 1975.

Schreiner, H.R. and Gregoire, R.C. (1963): The effect of nitrous oxide on cellular growth. *Presented 47th Annual Meeting Fed. Amer. Soc. Exp. Biol., Atlantic City, NJ.*

Schulze, H.H., Kastner, D. and Lange, P. (1969): Zur Frage der chronischen toxizitaet von halothan. Konzentrationen in der operationssaalluft. *Anaesthetist, 18*, 378-381.

Schwettwann, R.S. and Casterline, C.L. (1976): Delayed asthmatic response following occupational exposure to enflurane. *Anesthesiology, 44*, 166-169.

Smith, B.E., Gaub, M.L. and Moya, F. (1965): Investigations into the teratogenic effects of anaesthetic agents (Abstr.). *Anesthesiology, 26*, 260-261.

Snegireff, S.L., Cox, J.R. and Eastwood, D.W. (1968): The effect of nitrous oxide, cyclopropane or halothane on neural tube mitotic index, weight mortality and growth anomaly rate in the developing chick embryo. From: *Toxicity of Anaesthetics.* Editor: B.R. Fink, Williams and Wilkins, Baltimore, pp. 279-292.

Stoyka, W.W. and Havasi, G. (1977): The effects of repeated 14C halothane exposure in mice. *Canad. Anaesth. Soc. J., 24*, 243-251.

Sturrock, J.E. and Nunn, J.F. (1976): Synergism between halothane and nitrous oxide in the productions of nuclear abnormalities in the dividing fibroblast. *Anesthesiology, 44*, 461-471.

Taylor, C.A., Williams, C.A., Wakabayashi, T., Valdivia, E., Harris, R.A. and Green, D.E. (1972): The effect of halothane on energized configurational changes in heart mitochondria in situ. In: *Cel-*

lular Biology and Toxicology of Anaesthetics. Editor: B.R. Fink. Williams and Wilkins, Baltimore, pp. 117-127.

Vaisman, A.I. (1967): Work in surgical theatres and its influence on the health of anaesthesiologists. *Ekspkhir, Anesteriol., 3*, 44-49.

Van Duuren, B.L., Goldschmidt, B.M. and Langseth, L. (1968): Alpha-halo ethers: A new type of alkylating carcinogen. *Arch. environm. Health, 16*, 472-476.

Van Duuren, B.L., Sivak, A. and Goldschmidt, B.M. (1969): Carcinogenicity of halo-ethers. *J. nat. Cancer. Inst., 48*, 481-486.

Van Duuren, B.L., Katz, S.C., Goldschmidi, B.M., Frenkel, K. and Sivak, A., (1972): Carcinogenicity of halo-ethers. II Structure activity relationships of analogs of bis (chloromethyl) ether. J. nat. Cancer Inst., *48*, 1431-1439.

Vieira, E., Cleaton-Jones, P.E., Austin, J. and Fatti, P.L. (1978): Intermittent exposure of gravid rats to 1% nitrous oxide and the effect on the post natal growth of their offspring. *S.Afr. med. J. 53*, 106-108.

Vieira, E. (1979): Effect of the chronic administration of nitrous oxide 0.5% to Gravid Rats. *Brit. J. Anaesth., 51*, 283-287.

Vitcha, J.F. (1971): A history of Forane. *Anesthesiology, 35*, 4-7.

Whitcher, C.E., Cohen, E.N. and Trudell, J.R. (1971): Chronic exposure to anesthetic gases in the operating room. *Anesthesiology, 35*, 348-353.

Wingard, D.W. and Humphrey, L.J. (1969): Depression of antibody production by halothane: a dose response. *Anesthesiology, 30*, 353.

Wittman, R., Doenicke, A., Heinrick, H. and Pausch, H. (1974): Abortive effect of halothane. *Anaesthetist, 23*, 30-35.

the agglutination test as a diagnostic aid for typhoid fever. The agglutination test has remained widely applicable in clinical bacteriology and has been extended, by the use of red cell as antigen, to haemagglutination reactions. Although of foremost importance in blood grouping, the red cell lends itself as a carrier of other substances such as aggregated immunoglobulins, DNA and thyroglobulin. This has, in the last few year, given rise to a thriving commercial industry for diagnostic kits for autoantibodies associated with rheumatoid arthritis, systemic lupus erythematosus and thyroiditis respectively. Despite the fact that immunoprecipitation of soluble antigen extracts and specific antiserum (to typhoid and cholera bacilli) had been discovered by Kraus at approximately the same time as the agglutination reaction, little use appears to have been made of this valuable analytical technique until the discovery almost 50 years later by Ouchterlony and other workers that serological precipitation tests could be carried out in gels. In 1953 Grabar and Williams described immunoelectrophoresis, still one of the most powerful tools for resolving complex mixtures of antigens and this was followed in 1957 by the first of the practical, simple, immunochemical quantitation tests, the "Mancini" radial immunodiffusion technique, associated with both Feinberg and Mancini. Unlike the simple Ouchterlony technique in which antigen and antibody diffuse together from wells cut in gel, producing a line of precipitation at optimum combining capacity, the Mancini tests depends on antigen diffusing radially from a circular well cut into a slab of gel already *containing* antiserum. A ring of precipitate is produced, the area of which is directly proportional to the antigen concentration in the test specimen. Other important variants of immunoelectrophoresis such as the Laurell technique have particular application to the study of adverse (anaphylactoid) response to intravenous substances (see page 149). It is interesting to note that within the last 10 years considerable interest has been shown in adaptation of Kraus' original liquid precipitation technique. This "new" technique, the automated immunoprecipitation method (AIP) depends on light scattering of *soluble* complexes formed between antigen and antibody. Practical developments were associated with Ritchie (1974) and a commercial apparatus is now available for the assay of several plasma proteins including the immunoglobulins themselves (Technicon Instruments Corp, New York).

We cannot leave immunoprecipitation techniques without mention of the elegant fluorescent antibody method developed by Coons in 1942 which led to the proof of the role of lymphocyte in antibody production. The test requires the binding of fluorescein isothiocyanate to the antibody molecule as a marker for locating antigens in tissue preparations. Labelled antibody bound to tissue antigen is then located by use of the ultraviolet microscope, a technique perhaps 100 times more sensitive than that of Ouchterlony.

On the structural chemistry side, the 1930's saw a marked increase in physico-chemical techniques of protein fractionation. Using the analytical ultracentrifuge developed in Sweden, Kabat in 1939 conclusively identified antibodies as being in the gamma globulin fraction of serum. The realization that the gamma globulin fraction housed several distinct classes and subclasses of immunoglobulin was yet to come and necessitated further advances in protein fractionation technology. Indeed, the term "immunoglobulins" was not used until 1959 (Heremans). Until pure proteins could be isolated little progress could be made on the structure of the immunoglobulins but in 1934 Marrack proposed a model of antigen-antibody reactions based on the multivalence of each. He postulated that a lattice would be created of alternating antigen and antibody molecules joined through their specific reactive groups: a situation we now know to be true. The basic biochemical structure of the immunoglobulin molecule followed from the work of Porter and Edelman in the 1960s. Using enzymatic and chemical degradation respectively of the immunoglobulin we now know as IgG, both men confirmed the now familiar tetra-peptide structure and the presence of two antigen combining sites.

The clinical phenomenon of anaphylaxis had first been reported in 1902 by the French scientists Portier and Richet using sea anemone toxins to immunize dogs. They found to their surprise that sublethal quantities injected into a *previously sensitized* dog caused convulsions and collapse, terminating in death. Aside from being an important phenomenon this was the first demonstration of the potential harmful nature of antibodies. Their discovery coincided with the vaccination period and reports of serum sickness. This we know to be due to circulating soluble immune complexes of antigen and antibody caused by the introduction of large amounts of foreign antigen into the patient's body. Prausnitz and Küstner published their findings in 1921 on reagin, a serum antibody-like substance associated with allergic disease and hypersensitivity. The immunoglobulin nature of the reagin, now designated IgE, was discovered by Ishizaka and by Bennich and Johansson in the late 1960s. For the most part this antibody exerts a destructive role in man and is associated with Type I hypersensitivity reactions (See page 296). The original Prausnitz-Küstner test (PK test) has recently received a new lease of life in testing patients following adverse (anaphylactoid) response to various intravenous agents. Against this general background of immunobiology and immunochemistry we can now examine areas of more specific interest to the anaesthetist.

MOLECULAR BIOLOGY OF THE IMMUNOGLOBULINS

Immunoglobulin structure

Electrophoretically these proteins show a unique range of heterogeneity and are found in the γ, β, and α fraction of normal plasma. Predictably, this very heterogeneity has made characterisation of *polyclonal* immunoglobulins a difficult task and our knowledge of structure and amino acid sequences of the five major immunoglobulin classes largely derives from studies of monoclonal proteins secreted in the plasma of the myeloma patient.

Structurally, all five immunoglobulins, IgG, IgA, IgM, IgD and IgE are built on a common pattern, two (light) L polypeptide chains and two (heavy) H polypeptide chains bonded together with interchain disulphide bridges (Fig. 9.1). Although IgG, IgA, IgD and IgE exist as monomers of this structure, IgA, particularly in secretions, and IgM exist in dimeric and pentameric forms respectively (Fig. 9.2). Immunoglobulins in some patients with collagenosis may precipitate in the peripheral circulation in cold weather: these cryoglobulins may reflect both a tendency to aggregate and also immune complex formation. Their presence in patients receiving intravenous anaesthetic drugs may increase the risk of anaphylactoid response by acting as micelles for complement activation.

The H chains are antigenically distinguishable by both chemical and immunological methods for all five classes of immunoglobulin. "L" chains are common to all immunoglobulins but exist in Kappa ($\varkappa$) and Lambda (λ) forms. Both L and H chains are composed of constant and of variable amino acid sequences. The variable regions occur in the antigen binding sites and are responsible for antibody specificity. The variable regions from both H and L chain appear to take part in antigen binding but common sense dictates that not all the diversity expressed by the amino acid sequences will be necessary for antibody diversity. We find areas where the amino acid transitions occur frequently in the binding sites and these "hypervariable regions" presumably describe the strongest binding sites in the antibody. The variable region comprises one of the two homology regions of the light chain (V_L) and one of the four homology regions of the heavy chain (V_H) in IgG and IgA molecules. The homology regions are demarked by loops produced by intrachain disulphide linkages (Fig. 9.1) enclosing some 110 amino acid residues. In IgG there are three homology regions in the constant part of the molecule $C_\gamma 1$, $C_\gamma 2$, $C_\gamma 3$. Each region is associated with some specific biological property e.g. complement binding by the $C_\gamma 2$ region (Edelman, 1970).

Even in its genetics the immunoglobulin differs from other proteins in that the component peptide chains are each coded by not one, but by two genes, a variable and a constant gene.

Biological functions of the immunoglobulins

The more obvious physico-chemical parameters and biological functions of human immunoglobulins are compared and contrasted in Tables 9.1 and 9.2.

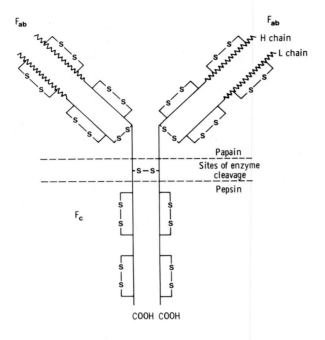

Fig. 9.1. Diagramatic Fig. 9.1. Diagramatic representation of the four chain structure of immunoglo-bulin IgG. The antigen binding sites are made up from the variable regions of each heavy-light chain pair. Inter and intra chain desulphide bridges are shown. The fragments produced by papain digestion of the molecule, two Fab and one Fc fragment, include the antigen bonding sites and the whole molecule "membrane" and complement binding sites respectively.

TABLE 9.1

PHYSICOCHEMICAL CHARACTERISTICS OF THE IMMUNOGLOBULIN

	Previous nomenclature	Mol. wt	Heavy chain type	Molecular formula
IgG	γG, 7Sγ-globulin	160,000	α	$\gamma_2\varkappa_2 : \gamma_2\lambda_2$
IgA	γA, A-globulin	170,000	$\varkappa$	$(\alpha_2\varkappa_2)n : (\alpha_2\lambda_2)n$
IgM	γM, 19S globulin	900,000	μ	$(\mu_2\varkappa_2)5 : (\mu_2\lambda_2)5$
IgD	γD	184,000	δ	$\delta_2\varkappa_2 : \delta_2\lambda_2$
IgE	γE, reagin	188,000	ϵ	$\epsilon_2\lambda_2 : \epsilon_2\lambda_2$

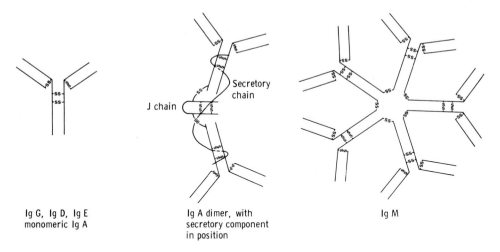

Fig. 9.2. Diagramatic representation of the comparative structures of the five major classes of immuno-globulin, illustrating polymerization via "J" chains and disulphide bridges. Dimeric IgA also exists without the protective "secretory piece" and high concentrations of monomeric IgM may be found in pathological conditions.

TABLE 9.2

BIOLOGICAL FUNCTIONS OF THE IMMUNOGLOBULINS

	Serum concentration (g/l)	Classical complement activation	Placental transfer	Mast cell binding	Biological half-life (days)
IgG	6–14	+[a]	+ +	−[b]	20–28[c]
IgA	1–3	−	−	−	6
IgM	0.5–1.5	+ + +	−	−	10
IgD	≤0.1	−	−	−	3
IgE	$\leq 0.5 \times 10^{-3}$	−	−	+ +	2

[a]not IgG4 subclass. [b]evidence of IgG4 involvement.
[c]IgG3 subclass T½ <10 days.

IgG: Plasma IgG (normal range 6–14 g/l) actually comprised four antigenically distinct subclasses IgG1, IgG2, IgGs and IgG4. The subclass IgGl comprises the bulk of the IgG fraction (some 70%) and IgG4 only 2–3%.

The immunoglobulin is synthesised by the fetus but the majority of fetal IgG is transferred from the maternal circulation during the last trimester of pregnancy. The major functions of IgG are the neutralization of bacterial exotoxins and the stimulation of the complement cascade, providing the manifestations of the inflammatory response. The subclasses do not respond equally to antigenic stimulation: most anti Rh-antibodies belong to the IgG1 and IgG3 subclasses while those produced in response to dextran infusions are of the IgG2 subclass. The Fc regions of IgG1, IgG2 and IgG4 bind the whole molecule to staphylococcal protein A. Such binding may be highly significant in triggering complement mediated anaphylactoid reactions to intravenous substances in patients suffering from acute or chronic infections (Watkins et al., 1978). Despite its relatively low concentration, IgG4, alone of the IgG subclasses, has molecular binding sites for mast-cells and can function, like IgE, as a reagin (Parish, 1970; Berrens et al., 1977). This has important genetic implication since the molecule, unlike IgE, has complement fixiation sites. This means that a relatively minor reagin antibody mediated reaction, initially releasing minimum quantities of histamine, may trigger a grossly exaggerated histamine release via the complement pathways (described later in this chapter).

IgA: This immunoglobulin exists in monomer and dimeric forms, the latter occuring in the secretions from mucous membranes. The normal plasma concentration range lies between 1 and 3 g/l. In the dimeric form the two molecules are linked by a small polypeptide chain (mol.wt 15,000), "J" chain near the C terminal ends of the molecule (Fig. 9.2). In the exocrine secretions a further polypeptide chain (mol.wt approximately 70,000) is linked to the dimer: the function of this secretory piece appears to involve protection against proteolysis from the individuals own enzymes (as in the gut) and in transmission of the molecule into the secretion. There is now good evidence that IgA provides a protective immune cover for mucosal surfaces, thereby excluding potentially harmful antigens. In the gut, IgA antibodies to ingested antigens may prevent further absorption of antigen. It is interesting to note that low plasma IgA are associated with extrinsic asthma and other allergies, particularly to milk. This suggests that if the "first order" immune defence provided by IgA is deficient, then the "second order" involves the highly detrimental IgE response. IgA antibodies appear to be highly effective against viruses and other "replicate" antigens.

IgM: The presence of ten potential antibody combining sites on the pentameric molecule (of which only five are sterically available) is the most probable reason why this antibody is programmed to be the first to respond following the host's exposure to antigen. Its structure gives rise to good complement fixation, agglutination and predominatly intravascular location. There are ideal characteristics for an immunoglobulin which plays a special role in the elimination of particulate antigens and microorganisms from the body. IgM is synthesised by the fetus but high levels in the new-born are indicative of intra-uterine infection. Normal adult levels range between 0.5–1.5 g/l.

IgD: This occurs in microgram quantities in normal plasma (0.19/l). Our knowledge of iets structure derives essentially from the work of Rowe and Fahey (1965) on paraproteins of this class. Structurally the protein is closely related to IgE with which in terms of amino acid sequences it has 41% homology. Very little is known about iets exact function (but see review, Bargellesi et al., 1978). However, its presence on a high proportion of circulating B lymphocytes has suggested a role in the control of the immune response (Rowe et al., 1973) Work in the author's laboratory indicates a particular involvement of IgD in anaphylactoid response to Althesin and some linkage of inheritance of the genes expressing high levels of IgE (atopy and IgD (Watkins et al., 1978).

IgE: This immunoglobulin, like IgA, is produced in lymphoid tissues with close association with mucous membranes. It exists only in trace amounts in normal plasma (0–480 μg/l; 2.4 ng is regarded as 1 I.V.). The IgE class is responsible for the majority of reaginic antibody mediated hypersensitivity reactions (Bennich and Johansson, 1971; Ishizaka and Ishizaka, 1967). The reason lies in the peculiar affinity of both the $C_\epsilon 3$ and $C_\epsilon 4$ homology regions for mast cell membranes. Interaction of (preformed) cell bound reagenic antibody with antigen results in direct histamine release from the mast cell. The correlation between elevated IgE levels and atopic disease is now well established.

LEUCOCYTES, LYMPHOID TISSUE AND ANTIBODY FORMING CELLS

Cells of the body which respond to antigens are variously categorized as belonging to the haematopoietic, reticuloendothelial, phagocytic or the lymphoid system. Cells which will become differentiated for these functions arise and mature in the bone marrow of the haematopoietic system.

Phagocytic cells

The reticuloendothelial system is a collection of cells of diverse morphology united by their common phagocytic activity and is now probably better known as the mononuclear phagocytic system. The macrophages are represented in blood by the circulating monocytes which are also found fixed to specific tissues, e.g. Kupffer cells in liver. The blood granulocyte cells, or microphages, arise from the myeloid series of the haematopoietic system and comprise the neutrophilic leucocytes, basophils and eosinophils. The neutrophils make up some 60% of the blood white cells and are the most phagocytic of the granulocyte series. Because of their large, characteristically lobular nuclei, neutrophils are also referred to as polymorphonu-clear leucocytes − or more simply polymorphs. Both microphagic and macrophagic cells contain lysosomal granules and are consequently highly destructive to ingested material.

Phagocytosis is not the result of random collision between cell and foreign material. The phagocytic cells respond both to chemotactic stimuli and to the presence of immunoglobulins and complement on their surface. The chemotactic stimuli are normally provided by activation and release of complement components following immune response, or from bacteria, or from necrotic tissue or indeed from the products (lymphokines) secreted by other leucocytes. Artificial situations such as the injection of intravenous drugs or inhalation anaesthetic agents may also produce, or interfere with, ongoing chemotaxis. The presence of specific antibodies on the surface of the macrophage encourages binding to the appropriate, particulate, antigen. The antigens are engulfed and hydrolized within the macrophage to molecules evidently possessing characteristic antigenic determinant sites. Information regarding these determinants is passed over the the lymphoid system.

Lymphoid system

The lymphoid system can be considered in terms of the central and of the peripheral lymphoid tissues (Weiss, 1972). The central lymphoid tissues of mammals are bone marrow and thymus: avian species have a third lymphoid organ, the bursa of Fabricius. The peripheral lymphoid tissues include the lymphocyctes themselves, lymph nodes and gut associated lymphoid tissues (GALT).

The bone marrow provides the source of precursor cells which will become differentiated in late fetal and early neonatal life into two distinct lines of lymphocytes, T and B cells following processing by thymus and bursa tissues respectively (See Katz, 1977). The T and B cells are morphologically similar but differ very considerably in their specific functions. Although mammals do not have a bursa they do produce B lymphocytes and it seems probably that the GALT provides a bursal equivalent. Although T and B cells arise from a common precursor stem cell it seems probable that some differentiation occurs before the precursor cells make their way to their respective processing organs. The T cells posses the characteristics of antigen recognition and in addition to providing a tissue for cell maturation the thymus also acts as a filter, removing the majority of those cells with the ability to respond to antigens of the host's own tissues (i.e. self antigens). Unlike the B cells, the T cells do not possess surface bound immunoglobulins as surface receptors. When the T lymphocyte contacts antigen it passes through a phase of growth and cell division known as lymphocyte transformation. The B lymphocyte is programmed to respond to a specific antigen and is transformed into an antibody producing plasma cell. The plasma cell is approximately the same size as the small lymphocyte but in the electron microscope the cytoplasm can be seen to be filled with endoplasmic reticulum laden with protein synthesising ribosomes.

Lymphocytes from the central lymphoid tissues pass along the lymphatic ducts and ultimately enter the circulating system through the thoracic duct at the point at which the vessels enter the heart. In their passage along the lymphatic ducts they encounter the lymph nodes, irregular spheres of spongy tissue whichf act as central collecting points for the lymph from a particular anatomical region. The lymph node also functions as a filter bed for antigenic material, e.g. bacteria, also draining in from the surrounding rissues and these are phagacytosed by macrophages. For the most part lymphocytes form follicles within the cortex of the lumph node. These become germinal centres following antigenic stimulation. The spleen provides a similar service to the circulating system lymphocytes as that provided by the lymph node for the lymphatic system. The organ is vital to the animal in early life but may be removed in the adult with little significant effect upon the established immune system.

Cell interactions and the immune response

Although there is evidence that low molecular weight antigens may activate B and T cells directly, for the most part antigens are first degraded by the macrophage. The B lymphocytes may be then stimulated to produce IgG immunoglobulin by transfer of an RNA-antigen complex or IgM by a specific RNA alone. The transfer of these messages to the T-lymphocytes is less understood but probably results in lymphokine secretions having specific functions in the immune response. The T-lymphocyte polulation is know to contain both helper cells and suppressor cells. The helper effect can be demonstrated more readily with certain antigens, termed T cell dependent antigens, than with T cell independent antigens. Antigens of the former group are usually complex antigens such as viruses, foreign cells and proteins. The helper effect is not confined to primary immune response and experiments in animals show that secondary response in sensitized animals may be lost following experimental removal of T cells. The helper activity may be expressed through hormone like secretion: several thymic factors have been isolated from calf thymus which have a stimulating effect on lymphoid cells in vitro and in vivo. Two of these factors, thymopoietin I and II, have unusual features in that they block normal neuromuscular transmission and increase T cell numbers.

The development and inter-relationship of the cells involved in the immune response are summarized in simple fashion in Fig. 9.3.

The lymphokines: These are a family of low molecular weight proteins secreted by T-cells with highly specific activity on other cells (Dumonde et al., 1969). The antigen sensitized T cell may act as a "suppressor cell" by secretion of a specific lymphokine which inhibits B cell antibody synthesis. This is seen as an important modulator of the extent of immune response. T cells undergoing transformation also exude a lymphokine with mitogenic properties on other lymphocytes. Use of this has been made in the laboratory in the mixed lymphocyte culture technique (MLC), to identify closely related lymphocyte populations from different individuals. Several lymphokines are chemotactic to macrophages, attracting them to areas where the T cell has come in contact with an antigen which its surface receptors indicate is "non-self". Excessive amounts of these chemotactic lymphokines prevent the movement of the macrophages from the antigen site (migration inhibition factor, MIF, Bloom and Bennett, 1966). Interferon is a unique lymphokine of T cells which confers resistance to host cells to infection by viruses. Although the virus may still enter interferon sensitized cells it is no longer able to interfere with the DNA codes.

The unique role of the T lymphocyte: In many ways the T lymphocyte can be seen to provide the overall control of the immune response. Initially in providing a blue print as to what constitutes a foreign antigen and then to stimulate macrophagic processing, leading to B lymphocyte sensitization and ultimately humoral antibody synthesis. Despite its own inability to synthesise specific antibody, the production of interferon confers resistance to viruses on host cells and its ability to recognise non-self antigen leads to immune rejection of allografted tissue. This rejection does not involve humoral antibody but only secretion of a cytolytic lymphotoxin which ultimately causes the target cell to rupture (See Type IV hypersensitivity reactions).

THE COMPLEMENT SYSTEM

The antibody has a primary function in the identification and combination with invading foreign cells or macromolecules. While such reaction neutralises bacterial toxins and may constrain bacterial growth, the main function served by antigen-antibody combination is the activation of the secondary effector systems of the

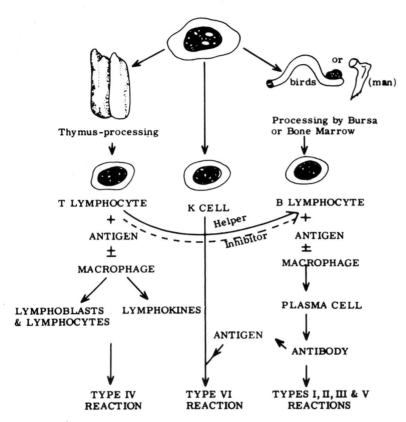

STEM CELL

(bone marrow and fetal liver)

or

birds (man)

Thymus-processing

Processing by Bursa
or Bone Marrow

T LYMPHOCYTE   K CELL   B LYMPHOCYTE

+   Helper   +

ANTIGEN ------ Inhibitor ------ ANTIGEN

±   ±

MACROPHAGE   MACROPHAGE

LYMPHOBLASTS   LYMPHOKINES   PLASMA CELL
& LYMPHOCYTES

ANTIGEN

ANTIBODY

TYPE IV   TYPE VI   TYPES I, II, III & V
REACTION   REACTION   REACTIONS

Fig. 9.3. Role and development of T lymphocytes, B lymphocytes and K cells in immunological responses. The helper and (converse) inhibitor interaction of the T and B cells in memory (antibody) response is illustrated together with the role of macrophages in actually processing antigens for recognition by the lymphocytes. T lymphocytes are essential for the delayed Type IV immunological reactions. Type VI reactions are referred to in the text, Type V reactions involve cell stimulatory mechanisms which are the converse to the Type II cytotoxic reactions. (Reproduced with permission from Irvine (1974). Proc. roy. Soc. Med., 67, 548).

immune response, most particularly the complex group of proteins which comprise the plasma complement. "Complement" was discovered by Bordet at the end of the 19th century. He showed that the lysis of red cells and bacteria by human serum required the interaction of two factors, one thermostatic and specific – the antibody, the other thermolabile and non-specific. The latter was originally called alexine but this is now called *complement*, because it acts in a "complementary" fashion to the antibodies. We now know that complement is not a single substance but comprises a complex system of nine major proteins which represent nearly 10% of the glubulins in the human. It is not surprising that complement participates in several important biological functions (Ruddy et al., 1972). The complement system is triggered in two well defined pathways.

Classical pathway: Conventionally we denote the complement system by the letter C and its components in the classical pathway from Cl to C9. The first component Cl is actually a trimolecular complex, the integrity of which requires the presence of Ca^{2+} ions. The three sub-units are Clq, Clr and Cls of which the Clr acts principally to bind the other two "reactive" entities. Initially the combination of antigen with antibody results in a conformational change in the antibody molecule causing the binding of Cl through the Clq component and the activation of the esterase component Cls. This in turn activates C4 and C2 producing an active enzyme, designated $\overline{C4,2}$ which in turn acts on C3 releasing a small fragment, C3a, or anaphylatoxin. The reaction proceeds through to C9 and is of the cascade type, that is to say, the first step activates more molecules in the next, and so on, and is analagous to the clotting mechanisms. The scission products of complement "activation" have specific biological functions and these, and the cascade sequence, are summarized in Table 9.3.

The products C3a and C5a are both known as anaphylatoxins. Not only are they responsible for histamine release from mast cells but they also intrude into the blood clotting system, causing aggregation of platelets. Complements C3 and C4 exist in plasma in relatively high concentration, C3 in excess of $1 \text{ g} \cdot \text{litre}^{-1}$ and C4, perhaps $0.5 \text{ g} \cdot \text{litre}^{-1}$. Normally, when the target of antibody activity is the surface of a foreign cell, lysis of the cell proceeds both though the activation of components C5 to C9 and also through phagocytosis induced by the chemotactic stimulus of the C3 fragments (Fig. 9.4).

Alternative pathway: The existence of a second pathway of complement activation which was independent of antibody and conferred non-specific resistance to infections was postulated by Pillemer in 1954. This system is activated at the C3 point by variety of substances including bacterial cell wall lipo-polysaccharide, aggregated immunoglobulins (or immune complexes) and cobra venom factor. The activation may involve an initiating factor also present in plasma.

It is important to realise that all the plasma proteins exist in dynamic equilibria and are not static entities. The equilibria are defined by several factors including metabolic processes and vascular-extravascular pool distribution. Potential enzyme

TABLE 9.3

HUMAN COMPLEMENT COMPONENTS. CLASSICAL SEQUENCE (ANTIGEN-ANTIBODY COMPLEX AS TRIGGER)

	Mol. wt	Fragment released	Function
C1(q,r,s)	400,000		Fixes to Ag/Ab complex activates C4, C2
C4	240,000		Immune adherence serotin release
C2	100,000	$\overline{C4C2}$ kinin-like peptide	Activates C3
C3	185,000	C3a (anaphylatoxin)	Vasoamine release chemotactic factor platelet aggregation
		$\overline{C3b}$	Opsonization activates C5 or C3 alternative pathway
C5	170,000	C5a (anaphylatoxin)	Vasoamine release opsonization
C6	100,000	$\overline{C56}$	
C7	110,000	$\overline{C567}$	Chemotactic factor
C8	160,000		
C9	70,000		Total complex C56789 leads to target cell lysis

systems, such as the blood coagulation and the complement systems are further restrained by inhibitor proteins. Complement C3 provides a central point of both the classical and the alternate pathways. It probably breaks down more or less spontaneaously as follows:

C3 $\longrightarrow$ C3a (anaphylatox in) $\overline{C3b}$

The active molecule $\overline{C3b}$ is normally harmlessly inactivated by a specific protease, C3b inactivator (KAF), into a large molecule C3c and a smaller fragment C3d, while the tissue can comfortably absorb the small amount of histamine released by the anaphylatoxin. However, if by blocking of $\overline{C3b}$ inactivator, or by sudden excessive breakdown of C3 itself, the highly active C3b molecule exceeds some predetermined threshold, then a feedback mechanism takes place through C3 proactivator (C3PA or GBG) and thence C3 activator, converting more and more C3 (Fig. 9.5): the reaction is ultimately modulated by C3b inactivator. Magnesium ions (Mg^{2+}) are involved in the reaction. The involvement of metal ions in complement reactions explains why plasma samples taken for subsequent complement studies are best

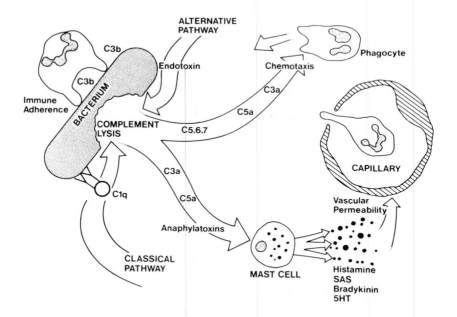

Fig. 9.4. Classical and alternative pathways of complement activation, illustrating both target cell (bacterium) lysis and the products released by both pathways, giving rise to the manifestations of inflamkmatory response. (Reproduced with permission from Whicher and Evans, Notes on Diagnosis, No. 3 complement, Hoechst Pharmaceuticals, U.K.).

taken into EDTA and not heparin: the chelating properties of the former chemical effectively "freeze" the complement system.

The positive feedback loop of the alternative pathway can occur in both solution and on cell surfaces. On the the bacterial cell surface the alternative pathway enzymes activate the classical membrane attack units C5 to C9 and amplify the effects of classical activation.

In addition to natural activators of the alternate pathway, a number of substances administered intravenously have a particular tendency to this type of non-immunological activation. These include the intravenous induction agents Althesin and propanidid, plasma substitutes such as dextrans, and radiocontrast media (See review, Watkins, 1979).

In the laboratory, complement C3 conversion can be readily demonstrated in sequential samples of patients' plasma taken after reaction (Watkins et al., 1976), either by conventional single dimension immunoelectrophoresis or by the two dimensional Laurell (1965) technique which desplays C3 and the conversion product

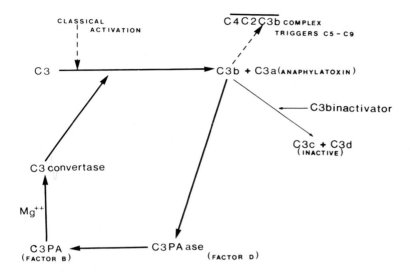

Fig. 9.5. Diagramatic representation of the enzymes involved in the alternative pathway mechanism of complement activation.

C3c in the form of peaks of precipitate, the relative areas of which indicate the degree of conversion. It is necessary to demonstrate C3 activation in the absence of appreciable C4 activation in order to establish involvement of the alternative pathway.

The principal features and overlap of the two major complement pathways are summarised in Fig. 9.4. This account of the complement system has been grossly simplified. The reader seeking greater detail and an extensive bibliography is referred to the excellent text-book by Glynn and Steward (1977).

Miscellaneous activation mechanisms: These result from inherited deficiencies of complement inhibitors. The most important is the C1 esterase inhibitor defect: 80% of cases exhibit low levels of this inhibitor in plasma. Patients with this disease, hereditary angioneurotic oedema (HANE), exhibit recurrent episodes of facial oedema due to increased vascular permeability to fluids, (Donaldson and Evans, 1963). The intestinal tract is frequently involved with abdominal pain, diarrhoea vomiting. Attacks are associated with activation of C1 and consumption of C4 and C2 with the production of a kinin-like polypeptide from C2, which causes increased vascular permeability. Although the author has seen only one Althesin reaction which appeared to utilise C2 activation, low plasma levels of C1 esterase inhibitor, in the absence of HANE, may be associated with reactions to radiocontrast media (Lasser, personal communication).

Relatively few cases of *inherited* C3b inactivator defect have been described, mainly in association with Klinefelters syndrome and grossly impaired "immunity" (Alper et al., 1970). In contrast, the *temporary* blocking of this inhibitor by intravenous substances may well be responsible for a high proportion of adverse reactions.

HYPERSENSITIVITY REACTIONS

Hypersensitivity reactions have a somewhat different meaning to the anaesthetist than tot the immunologist. Many of the clinical manifestations of adverse drug response, cutaneous (urticaria) pulmonary (bronchospasm) and cardiovascular (hypotension), resemble those produced by immediate, antibody mediated, hypersensitivity response. This is because the chemical mediators of all such reactions, predominantly histamine, are identical. The clinical manifestations may arise from true antibody-mediated reactions, complement mediated reactions or direct pharmacological release of histamine. It was suggested at the symposium on Adverse Response to Intravenous Agents held in Sheffield, 1978, that the term *anaphylactoid* would be used to describe reactions where clinical manifestations resembling those of hypersensitivity were observed but for which no collaborating laboratory evidence of antibody involvement was available, (See Watkins and Clarke, 1978). The term *anaphylactic* or *allergic* was reserved for reactions in which antibody involvement could be proven. To the clinician observing an anaphylactoid response to an administered drug it is the Type I immediate hypersensitivity reaction which first springs to mind as the mechanism of the response. In actual fact, antibody mediated reactions are probably the least likely cause of anaphylactoid response. Equally, even the immune mediated hypersensitivity reactions to drugs are not necessarily Type I reactions.

Four *major* types of hypersensitivity are recognised by the immunologist. These are designated Types I to IV (See Table 9.4) and are admirably described in a number of text books (Barrett, 1977; Roitt, 1978). Nevertheless, the four reaction mechanisms are open to slightly different interpretation to the anmaesthetist than to the theoretical immunologist: I should like to summarise them.

The Type I reaction most resembles that exhibited by patients showing anaphylactoid response to i.v. substances since it is by definition, immediate. This immunological reaction is for the most part restricted to a genetically prone individual who produces reagin antibody, in response to antigens or allergens which are well tolerated by the population as a whole. In order to produce anaphylaxis these

TABLE 9.4

IMMUNOLOGICAL MECHANISMS

Type I	(Immediate, anaphylactic, reagin (IgE) mediated)
Type II	(Antibody-dependant cytotoxic hypersensitivity responses)
Type III	(Involve "soluble" antigens, unlike Type II. Tissue damage by antigen-antibody complexes)
Type IV	(Delayed, cell mediated)

unfortunate patients still require previous antigenic challenge in order to achieve a passive sensitization state. If we are considering allergies which result from natural oral, or respiratory, immunization then it is not usually necessary to speculate on the mechanism but only on the specific allergen, but reactions which occur to compounds that the individual has never seen before are most unlikely to be Type I hypersensitivity reactions. Unlikely, but not impossible, since some administered i.v. substances may closely resemble natural antigens such as bacterial proteins and polysaccharides, so that immunological cross-reactions may occur. We should point out, however, that even when "preformed antibodies" to dextran occur, evidence for their involvement in the anaphylactoid response mechanism remains equivocal.

Once produced the reaginic antibodies adhere to mast cells. Subsequent antigen challenge causes a physico-chemical reaction upon the surface of the cell which leads to degranulation (Fig. 9.6). The resulting histamine release causes either local cutaneous phenomena or systemic anaphylaxis.

The reaginic antibodies are for the most part the IgE class of immunoglobulins. However, IgG reagins are also known (Parish, 1970; Berrens et al., 1977); these, unlike IgE, may involve complement proteins for the release of histamine. The patient with high IgE concentration (>400 ng·litre^{-1}) in the plasma is probably hypersensitive. It must be observed, however, that this is still a somewhat crude classification, since we should be considering specific IgE antibodies and normal or even decreased concentrations of plasma total IgE may conceal important allergies. Actually it is the cellbound IgE which is of importance in the Type I reaction: the parallelism between humoral antibody and cellbound antibody may not hold for certain individuals.

The mast cell: Although the mast cell (and the basophil) provide an essential part of the Type I hypersensitivity mechanism, it is, of course, not the sole prerogative of this system (See Baxter, 1973). Histamine and other mediators associated with the

300

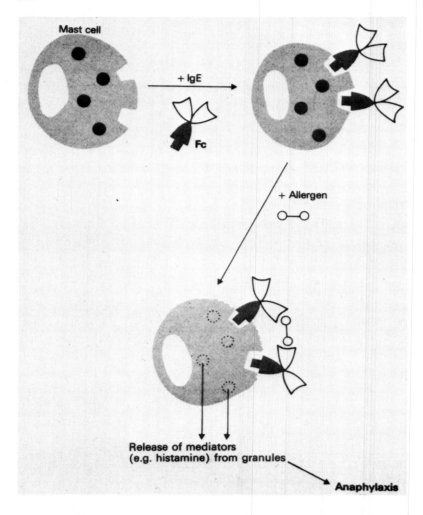

Fig. 9.6. Anaphylactic-hypersensitivity. Mast-cell degranulation following interaction of antigen with bound homocytotropic (reaginic) antibodies. (Reproduced with permission from Roitt, Essential Immunology (1977), Blackwell, Oxford, p. 152).

anaphylactoid response may be released from these cells by mechanisms other than the IgE response, most particularly by anaphylatoxins and by the direct chemical (pharmaceutical) action of drugs on the cells themselves. This is illustrated diagramatically (Fig. 9.7). It is also apparent that the release process involves the cyclic

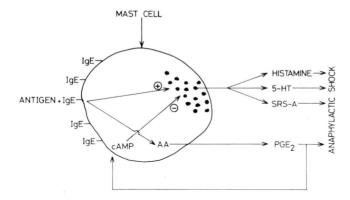

Fig. 9.7. Schematic view of mast cell active substance release, the involvement of cyclic AMP in their release and its possible control by prostaglandins. (Reproduced with permission from Atkins and Russell in Adverse Response to Intravenous Drugs (1978), Academic Press, London, New York, p. 119).

AMP system. β-Stimulants such as isoprenaline and phosphodiesterase inhibitors (Kaliner and Austen, 1975) inhibit the release process and, as expected, isoprenaline and aminophylline are potent inhibitors of immediate allergic bronchospasm. In contrast, alpha adrenergic drugs which might seem the obvious choice for combating histamine release may actually enhance the release mechanism by reducing the cell content of cyclic AMP.

Type II reactions are also described as antibody-dependent cytotoxic hypersensitivity responses. Again, the patient requires previous antigenic challange to produce antibodies, but the antigens in this case are present on the surface of either host or foreign cells. Combination of antibody with cellular antigens encourages demise of that cell either by phagocytosis or by activation of the full classical complement pathway up to C8 and C9, producing lysis. Adverse reactions invoking this type of mechanism include transfusion reaction, rhesus incompatibility and long-standing organ transplants. Autoimmune conditions such as Hashimot's thyroiditis and Goodpasture's syndrome proceed through this mechanism and so may certain types of drug reaction. In the latter, drugs with simple molecular structure may be bound to cell membranes, thus undergoing conversion from haptensf to full antigens. The resulting complex may then evoke autoantibodies, for example haemolytic anaemias to penicillin. However, the majority of small-molecule drugs are more likely to couple to plasma proteins, giving rise to complex-mediated (Type III) reactions.

The formation of excessive amounts of soluble complexes of (non-particulate) antigen and antibody may fix complement, releasing anaphylatoxins which cause histamine release, vascular permeability changes and an influx of polymorphs, which in turn release further factors contributing to the inflammatory response. Two types of complexes may be found, those with antibody excess and those with antigen excess. Classically, antigen excess gives rise to manifestations of serum sickness. In antibody excess (Arthus − type immune vasculitis) the complexes may give rise to diseases such as Farmer's lung or be rapidly precipitated and deposited in the site of (test) specific antigen introduction. Soluble complexes of both types may give rise to nephrotic syndromes, either temporary or permanent (e.g. immune complex disease) in nature. Although the Arthus test may be exploited as a test for antigen sensitization, this should not be confused with the intradermal tests now in vogue for drug hypersensitivity testing. These tests rely on cytotropic antibodies. Their use for testing pharmacologically active substances is equivocal and may carry some risk to the patient unless carried out under carefully defined conditions (Fisher, 1976). Many patients are likely to have infections which may give rise to (harmless) circulating immune complexes. The anaesthetist should remember that these complexes may be "activated" by intravenous agent administration to the critical point for complement C3 (alternative pathway) activation (Watkins et al., 1978), an underlying immune mediated event, totally unrelated to drug activity!

The final hypersensitivity scheme, Type IV, cell-mediated (delayed), is encountered in allergic reactions to bacteria and the like and in the rejection of transplanted tissues. Comparable reactions to soluble proteins are obtained when sensitization is induced by incorporation of the protein into Freund's adjuvant. This raises interesting possibilities regarding the use of detergents or solubilizers for several anaesthetic drugs (for example propanidid, Althesin, etomidate). The effector mechanism is essentially the T lymphocyte.

It should be clear to the reader that these hypersensitivity reactions do not represent abnormal mechanisms. In themselves, they are extremely important in the control of numerous disease processes. It is the magnitude of their involvement in a particular reaction which defines their abnormality. Perhaps not so obvious is the fact that few, if any, hypersensitivity reactions involve specifically one particular mechanism. A Type I reaction may act as a trigger for a Type III, the influence of the former being hidden by the magnitude of the secondary response. Likewise, an apparently insignificant immune reaction may trigger complement non-classically, producing large quantities of anaphylatoxin and systemic anaphylaxis.

CHEMICAL MEDIATORS OF ANAPHYLAXIS

Several important pharmacologically active compounds are discharged from cells during anaphylaxis. Histamine is the most important of these and the only one proven to be essential to the anaphylactic response (Lorenz et al., 1972, 1975, 1978). The other substances of putative significance are serotonin, bradykinin and other kinins, slow reacting substance-anaphylaxis (SRS-A), and prostaglandins.

The prostaglandins (PG) are a family of prostanoids derived from arachidonic acid (AA) by the enzyme cyclo-oxygenase. Experimentally it can be shown that PGE1 and E2 inhibit antigen release of histamine from leucocytes (Bourne et al., 1972) and the IgE and anaphylatoxin mediated release of histamine from mast cells (Kaliner and Austen, 1974). Prostaglandin E2 appears to play an important role in the control of hypersensitivity reactions. (Fig. 9.7), and additionally some of the signs of hypersensitivity response, such as localized pain, leucocyte chemotaxis and platelet aggregation, may involve these substances. Such reactivity may be modified in patients taking prostaglandin synthesis inhibitors e.g. aspirin (Gryglewski et al., 1976). Indeed, it could be argued that such individuals if triggered by i.v. agents might exhibit very severe anaphylactoid response.

The mechanisms and magnitude of anaphylactoid response are likely to involve many inter-related complex processes. In assessing hypersensitivity responses the anaesthetist would be well advised to consider and note not only the premedication prior to anaesthesia and surgery but also any other medication, prescribed or otherwise, taken immediately prior to admission.

THE IN VIVO AND IN VITRO ASSESSMENT OF IMMUNITY

Cell-mediated immunity may be defined as the portion of the specific immune response brought about by T lymphocytes. Processing of antigen introduced into the body occurs for the most part by macrophages and leads through the co-operation of T lymphocyte to B lymphocyte sensitization and ultimate humoral antibody production. The activated T lymphocyte has an additional important role to play in the immune response in the production of lymphokines which attract microphages to the site of antigenic stimulation and amplify their function. Most antigens lead to a response of both cell-mediated and of humoral immunity although the relative involvement of these two limbs of the immune system may vary considerably. Cell mediated immunity is mainly responsible for defence against bacterial and viral infections. One subgroup of the T lymphocytes population, the K cell, provides direct cytolysis against allogeneic target cells. K cell activity is sometimes described as the Type VI immune reaction (See Fig. 9.3.). Other T lymphocytes regulate the humoral response with either helper or suppressor activity. It is not surprising, therefore, that the clinical assessment of immunity should involve in vivo and in vitro tests of T cell numbers and activity and the quantitation of both B lymphocytes and the highly specific products of their progeny plasma cells, the antibodies. The tests employed may be briefly summarized as follows:

  (a) Quantitation of immunoglobulins in plasma and assessment of *specific* antibody. IgE has particular relevance.
  (b) Relatively crude quantitations of T and B cell numbers.
  (c) Lymphocyte transformation with mitogens specific for B and T cells respectively.
  (d) T lymphocyte transformation in response to specific antigens.
  (e) Measurements of the effect of lymphokines e.g. migration inhibition tests (MIF)
  (g) Antibody response of the host in vivo to specific test antigens.

These tests were originally employed in the investigation of either hereditary or disease induced defects of the immune system where the patient exhibited an obvious clinical syndrome, for example, the Wiskott-Aldrich syndrome (a sex-linked genetic disease with combined loss of T and B lymphocytes and of IgM production) and the importance to the prognosis of chronic lymphocytic leukaemia of B or of T lymphocyte deficiency.

Tests of immune function

Serum immunoglobulin concentrations: Severe defects in antibody production, either T or B cell mediated, or both, will be revealed by lowered levels of the plasma immunoglobulin. Accurate quantitations of these may be carried out either by standard Mancini immunodiffusion techniques or by automated nephelometric methods. It is most unlikely that significant changes in these proteins will be observed following the administration of the substances employed in anaesthetic practide although significant changes in IgE humoral levels, reflecting their involvement in anaphylactic reactions, may be observed by careful testing in the period immediately following clinically significant adverse response. Nevertheless, these tests are so simple to do that they should be carried out.

The next step is to proceed with *test* immunization: vague comments that groups of patients following a certain treatment show a greater incidence of infections should be avoided: however, there are ethical problems in choosing safe antigens for human use. "Synthetic" polysaccharides such as dextrans have been used as immunogens in man but this is potentially dangerous in view of their use as plasma substitutes. Since antigens may be either T cell dependant or independent, current practice is to immunize with both a protein and a bacterial polysaccharide antigen and to compare the two antibody responses.

Analysis of lymphocytes in blood: lymphocyte preparations.

This section might well be entitled, "first catch your lymphocyte". Several techniques are in use using heparinised blood. Gelatin and dextran sedimentation under gravity, and gradient centrifugation on Ficoll-Triosil gradients are employed most frequently. The former techniques yield preparations signficantly contaminated with polymorphs and red cells, the latter preparations show minimal contamination with these particular cells but include more monocytes and may show selective loss of part of the B cell population. Whatever technique is decided upon, the separation conditions must be rigidly adhered to, particularly the washing conditions which may paralyse the lymphocyte response for several hours. It cannot be stressed too highly that anyone wishing to embark on lymphocyte work should take himself to a specialized laboratory engaged in this type of work and carry out parallel analyses until his results match those of the laboratory.

Lymphocyte populations

Having obtained a lymphocyte preparation and checked cell viability using Trypan Blue, the next step is to determine the relative T and B cell populations. For T cells use is made of the peculiar property of these cells to form spontaneous rosettes with sheep red cells (E rosettes, see Fig. 9.8). The reaction has no obvious immunological importance but provides a useful analytical tool. B lymphocytes can be identified by detection of their surface membrane immunoglobulin using fluorescein confujated antisera to whole immunoglobulin. The antiserum treated cells are then viewed and counted with a fluorescence microscope.

Mitogenic stimulation of lymphocytes: Lymphocytes may be stimulated to undergo mitotic division in culture. These responses are conveniently monitored by measurement of the incorporation of tritiated thymidine into the stimulated cells. Antigens provoking mitosis can be divided into: (a) allogeneic transplantation-antigens (e.g. mixed lymphocyte reaction, MLR); (b) antigens providing a specific response in sensitized persons; and (c) non-specific antigens such as phytohaemagglutinin (PHA), concanavalin A and pokeweed mitogen. PHA and concanavalin A essentially stimulate T lymphocytes while pokeweed mitogen stimulates both B and T lymphocytes. The division is by no means as clear as much of the literature would suggest (See Phillips and Roitt, 1973; Greaves et al., 1974).

The PHA response is widely used and can be carried out with either whole blood or with lymphocyte preparations. The latter has advantage in that the effect of stimulants or inhibitors (drugs or natural substances) in the plasma may be eliminated but conversely it may not represent the real population of active cells. Cells ($2-15 \times 10^6$/ml) or whole blood samples are set up in triplicate in

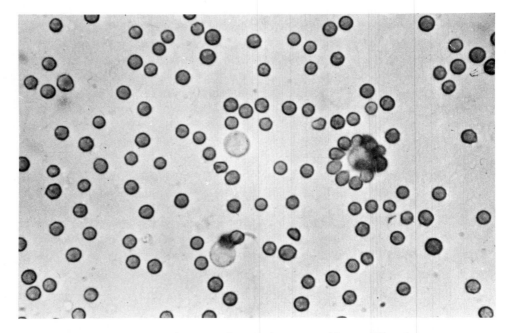

Fig. 9.8. E-rosettes. Formation of sheep erythrocyte cluster around human T lymphocyte.

microculture with two predetermined concentrations of PHA designed to descriminate between high and low "response". After culture for three days, tritiated thymidine is added to the transformed cells and allowed to incubate for a few hours before harvesting of cells. The radioactive uptake of the harvested test samples is then compared directly to controls. For the anaesthetist interested in effects of specific drugs on the lymphocytes of "sensitized" patients then the PHA incubation is omitted and replaced by the drug dissolved at physiological concentration in plasma.

The reader will by now have spotted a major flaw in such investigations, the pharmacological activity of the drug itself. Such activity, particularly with hypnotic agents including the inhalational ones, will severely modify lymphocyte response by direct effect on the cell itself. In general, active drugs should not be used in such analyses and where possible the antigen should consist of the patient's own plasma taken after the pharmacological activity of the drug has been destroyed. Equally, the assumption that thymidine uptake by the cells is synonymous with mitotic division should be checked with all "anaesthetic drugs". This requires microscopic examination of the cells to estimate blast transformation and correlation of this with radioactive uptake since the latter may simply represent a change in the cells synthetic rates as a result of the pharmacological activity of the drug. Such effects *may* be particularly evident in PHA response studies of theatre personnel exposed to anaesthetic gases and not in any way related to significant change in immune function.

Lymphocyte migration inhibition: These tests are based on the assessment of lymphokines production by activated lymphocytes. The most useful practical test is based on peripheral blood leucocyte migration inhibition (Søborg and Bendixen, 1967). The test makes good use of the "cruder" lymphocyte preparations obtained by gelatin or dextran sedimentation. The contaminating polymorphs in these preparations act as the indicator cells which are inhibited by the lymphokines from the responder T lymphocytes. Briefly, lymphocyte preparations are packed into short capillary tubes, (a few mm long and sealed at one end) and these placed horizontally into special "Sterilin" micro culture plates containing tissue culture medium. Upon incubation at 37°, under normal conditions the cells fan out from the open end of the tube (Fig. 9.9). In the presence of lymphokines generated by adding antigen at appropriate dilution to the cultures the migration is impaired and a smaller fan is produced. By comparing the areas of control and test fans the degree of migration inhibition can be estimated.

For the anaesthetist investigating possible response to drugs this technique carries the same problems as PHA response and will require careful design of control experiments.

For practical details of this and other lymphocyte handling techniques the reader is referred to the literature (e.g. Thompson, 1977).

An excellent evaluation and bibliography of the relevant findings in anaesthesia and surgery can be found in a recent review by Walton (1979).

ANTIGENS AND ANTIGENICITY

Most naturally occuring macromolecules, particularly proteins and polysaccharides, induce an immune response when injected into vertebrates to which these materials are foreign. The quality and degree of the immune response varies considerably from antigen to antigen and it is necessary to accept that such substances exhibit two destinct reactivities:

(i) immunogenicity, its capacity to stimulate at immune response either cellular or hormonal, or both,

(ii) antigenic specificity which describes the specific combining capacity of characteristic (determinant) sites on the macromolecule with synthesised antibodies.

An interesting example to the anaesthetist of the distinction between these two

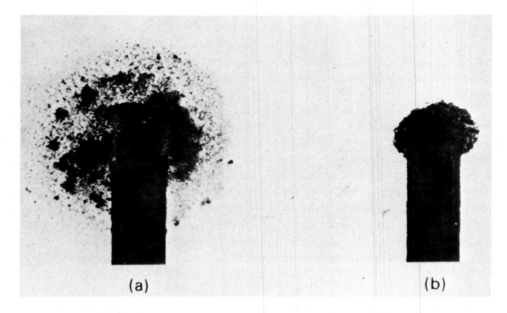

Fig. 9.9. Leucocyte migration inhibition test. Immunologically activated T lymphocytes produce lymphokines on exposure to the specific antigen(s). These substances inhibit polymorphonuyclear leuco- cyte migration in preparations of peripheral white blood cell preparations. The illustration shows (a) migration of cells from a capillary tube (see text) under normal circumstances, as a fan from the end of the tube and (b) inhibited migration in the presence of specific antigen (Photograph by kind permission of Dr. R. Jennings, Department of Virology, Sheffield University).

factors is provided by gelatin. This material is now widely used, following chemical modification (e.g. Haemaccel), as a plasma substitute. Whereas gelatin itself is a poor immunogen and provokes little antibody response (Haurowitz, 1950) it reacts readily with antibodies produced against a tyrosylated derivative (Arnon and Sela, 1960).

Several molecular requirements are now thought to be associated with the mani- festation of immunogenicity. These may be summarised as follows:

(a) molecular size;
(b) accessibility of specific antigenic determinants;
(c) degree of foreigness (non-self) to the animal producing the immune response.

(a) Molecular size effects: Although by definition antigens are macromolecules, quite small proteins and peptides in the 4000 to 5000 molecular weight range are able to elicit an immune response. Similar considerations apply to natural and synthetic,

or modified polysaccharides. With the exception of the plasma substitutes, the substances available to the anaesthetist, hypnotics, neuromuscular blocking agents, analgesics etc., are very low molecular weight compounds, far below the lower size limit of the "antigenic macromolecule". It has long been realized that these small molecules (haptens) cannot themselves stimulate the immune system unless they are coupled to antigenic carriers such as proteins or polysaccharides (Landsteiner, 1945). The coupling of small molecules in vitro by chemical means in the laboratory is a very different matter to the situation in vivo, where for the most part we must assume that they bind in relatively non-specific fashion to cell envelopes and to proteins. Having bound physicochemically in this fashion we can now postulate their role as haptens in Type II or Type III hypersensitivity reactions, as in, for example, penicillin induced haemolytic anaemia: here classically, if one stops administering the drug, haemolysis stops since any existing antibody can no longer couple correctly to the eythrocyte membrane. However, this is not always true and haemolysis may persits. The warning is again clear, we cannot simply consider pharmacologically active drugs as inert immunogens: the pharmacological action of the drug on cells must be considered. Certain drugs may actively depress a selective part of the T cell population, removing the repressor effect on existing T cell subsets which are reactive with self and thus initiating autoimmune situations. Conversely, actively bound drugs because of their charge or polarity may so disturb the surface environment on which they are fixed that immune response takes place directly against modified "self" determinants and not the intruding hapten at all.

Inhalational agents pose particular problems, not least in the interval between exposure of the individual and the appearance of untoward symptoms. The vexed discussion on jaundice after repeated exposure to halothane (Inman and Mushin, 1978) continues unabated. Although altered liver components can be demonstrated in severe hepatic necrosis in patients who have received halothane (Vergani, 1978) the cause-effect relationship to many people remains unproven, particularly since the considerable contribution of surgical trauma cannot be excluded. The adverse mode of action of this simple chloro fluoro ethane molecule is generally considered to lie in its tendency to form toxic metabolites in the liver. Whether such reaction is only severe in certain genetically disposed individuals remains unanswered.

An interesting parallel to halothane occurs with vinyl chloride monomer (VCM) disease, an occupational hazard for workers involved in the manufacture of PVC polymers. The vinyl chloride molecule is superficially similar to halothane but more reactive because of its ethylenic structure. Although there is some incidence of liver involvements the majority of syndromes are of the vascular type, the victims exhibiting sclerodema-like symptoms, suggesting the initiation of autoimmune disease (Ward et al., 1976).

(b) Accessibility of specific antigenic determinants: Substances may not be particularly immunogenic simply because their specific determinants lie hidden within the molecular conformation making contact with T lymphocytes a matter of low probability. We have already mentioned gelatin in this respect but perhaps we should also consider the effect of drug formulation upon molecular conformation, particularly when drugs are administered i.v. in high bolus concentration. Denaturation or random super coiling with hydrogen bonding, is an irreversible process which usually destroys protein function. Such molecules, e.g. heat aggregated IgG, are more powerful immunogens than the "native" molecule. There are, of course, varying degrees of denaturation and thus rheumatoid factor (an IgM autoantibody) may arise from limited unfolding of the IgG molecules of the rheumatoid patient (Johnson et al., 1975). It should be remembered that the extreme point of this particular unfolding is caused by antigen-antibody combination which acts as a trigger to complement activation. The cremophor of Althesin and propanidid may be particularly effective in changing specific protein conformations and we have direct evidence of short term immunological memory involving this powerful detergent in the minipig model (Glen et al., 1978).

(c) Degree of foreignness: This is somewhat linked to the accessibility of specific antigenic determinants. Under normal circumstances animals do not show an immune response to self components but we have already suggested ways in which this might be by-passed by pharmacologically active compounds. In general, the proteins of phylogenetically related species are poorly immunogenic when tested in each other, a situation which reflects the considerable structural homology in the proteins of these animals. Despite the fact that 23 allotypic varieties albumin occur in man (Weitkamp et al., 1973) cross reactions of the transfusion type are rare and this remains one of the safest of the plasma substitutes available. Nevertheless, upon long storage albumin fractions undergo denaturation and aggregation and may either trigger immediate anaphylactoid reactions or produce antibodies which may enhance immune response when albumin is administered on a subsequent occasion.

Finally, we should not overlook the route of antigen or hapten administration, the intravenous, the intraperitoneal or the ingested/inhalational routes. These all have specific immunological surveillance systems immediately associated with them. Thus even the extremely safe drug disodium cromoglycate, which is widely used in the treatment of extrinsic asthma and acts as an inhibitor of bronchospasm and bronchoconstriction when administered by inhalation, itself causes a high incidence of (minor but clinically significant) anaphylactoid phenomena when administered intravenously (Walker et al., 1972). Not only may the route of administration affect the relative immunogenicity (and the degree of foreignness) of a substance but it may also decide the type of response, whether an immediate anaphylactoid response or delayed autoimmune manifestations and febrile reactions.

REFERENCES

Alper, C.A., Abramson, N., Johnson, R.B., Jandl, J.H. and Rosen, F.S. (1970): Increased susceptibility to infection associated with abnormalities of complement mediated functions and of the third component of complement (C3). *New Engl. J. Med., 282*, 349-354.

Arnon, R. and Sela, M. (1960): Studies on the chemical basis of the antigenicity of protein. Antigenic specificity of polytryosyl gelatines. *Biochem. J., 75*, 103-109.

Bargellesi, A., Corte, G., Cosulich, E., Ferrani, M., Sitia, R. and Viale, G. (1978): Recent trends in IgD. *Ric. Clin. Lab., 8*, 195-200.

Barrett, J.T. (1978): *Textbook of Immunology*. C.V. Mosby Co., St. Louis, MO, 505 p.

Baxter, J.H. (1973): Role of Ca^{2+} in mast cell activation, desensitization and histamine release by dextran. *J. Immunol., 111*, 1470-1473.

Bennich, H. and Johansson, S.G.O. (1971): Structure and function of immunoglobulin E. *Adv. Immunol., 13*, 1-55.

Berrens, L., Koers, W.J. and Bruynzeel, P.L.B. (1977): IgE and Ig4 antibodies in specific allergies. *Lancet, 2*, 9.

Bloom, B.R. and Bennett, B. (1966): Mechanism of a reaction in vitro associated with delayed type hypersensitivity. *Science, 153*, 80-82.

Bourne, H.R., Lichtenstein, L.M. and Melmon, K.L. (1972): Pharmacological control of allergic histamine release in vitro: evidence for the inhibitory role of 3, ''5''-adenosine monophosphate in human 'leucocytes. *J. Immunol., 108*, 695-705.

Donaldson, V.H. and Evans, R.R. (1963): A biochemical abnormality in hereditary angioneurotic oedema. Absence of serum inhibitor of C̄1-esterase. *Amer. J. Med., 35*, 37−44.

Dumonde, D.C., Wolstencroft, R.A., Panayi, G.S., Matthew, M. Morley, J. and Howson, W.T. (1969): Lymphokines. *Nature, 224*, 38-42.

Edelman, G.M. (1970): The covalent structure of human γG immunoglobulin. XI. Functional implications. *Biochemistry, 9*, 3197-3205.

Fisher, M.McD. (1976): Intradermal testing after severe histamine reactions to intravenous drugs used in anaesthesia. *Anaesth. intens. Care., 4*, 97-104.

Glen, J.B., Davies, G.E., Thomson, D.S., Scarth, S.C. and Thompson, A.V. (1978): Adverse reactions to intravenous anaesthetics in animals. In: *Adverse Response to Intravenous Drugs*. Editors: J. Watkins and A.M. Ward. Academic Press, London, New York, pp. 129-135.

Glynn, L.E. and Steward, M.W. (Eds.) (1977): *Immunochemistry: An advanced textbook*. John Wiley, Chichester, New York, Brisbane.

Greaves, M.F., Janossy, G. and Doenhoff, M. (1974): Activation of human T and B lymphocytes by polyclonal mitogens. *Nature, 248*, 698-701.

Gryglewski, R., Szezeklik, A. and Nijankowska, E. (1976): Aspirin sensitive asthma: its relationship to inhibition of prostaglandin biosynthesis. In: *Prostaglandins and Thromboxanes*. Editors: F. Berti, B. Samuelsson and G.P. Velo. Plenum Press, New York, London, pp. 191-203.

Haurowitz, F. (1950): *Chemistry and Biology of Proteins*, Academic Press, New York, London.

Inman, W.H.W. and Mushin, W.W. (1978): Jaundice after repeated exposure to halothane: a further analysis of reports of the Committee on Safety of Medicines. *Brit. med. J., ii*, 1455-1456.

Ishizaka, K. and Ishizaka, T. (1967): Identification of γE antibodies as a carrier of reaginic activity. *J. Immunol., 99*, 1187-1198.

Johnson, P.M., Watkins, J. and Holborow, E.J. (1975): Antiglobulin production to altered IgG in rheumatoid arthritis. *Lancet, 1*, 611-614.

Kaliner, M. and Austen, K.F. (1975): Immunological release of chemical mediators from human tissues. *Ann. Rev. Pharmacol., 15*, 177-189.

Kaliner, M. and Austen, K.F. (1974): Hormonal control of the immunological release of histamine and slow-reacting substance of anaphylaxis from human lung. In: *Cyclic AMP, Cell Growth and Immune Response.* Editors: W. Braun, L.M. Lichtenstein and C.W. Parkes. Springer-Verlag, Heidelberg, pp. 164-175.

Katz, D.H. (1977): *Lymphocyte Differentiation, Recognition and Regulation.* Academic Press, London, New York, 749p.

Landsteiner, K. (1945): *The Specificity of Serological Reactions.* Harvard University Press, Cambridge, MA.

Laurell, C.B. (1975): Antigen-antibody crossed electrophoresis. *Anal. Biochem., 10*, 358-361.

Lorenz, W. (1975): Histamine release in man. *Agents Actions, 5*, 402-416.

Lorenz, W. and Doenicke, A. (1978): Anaphylactoid reactions and histamine release by intravenous drugs used in surgery and anaesthesia. In: *Adverse Response to Intravenous Drugs.* Editors: J. Watkins and A.M. Ward. Academic Press, London, New York, 188p.

Lorenz, W., Doenicke, A., Meyer, R., Reimann, H.J., Kushe, J., Barth, H., Geesing, H., Hutzel, M. and Weissenbacher, B. (1972): Histamine release in man by propanidid and thiopentone: pharmacological effects and clinical consequences. *Brit. J. Anaesth., 44*, 355-369.

Parish, W.E. (1970): Short term anaphylactic IgG antibodies in human sera. *Lancet, 2*, 591-592.

Phillips, B. and Roitt, I.M. (1973): Evidence for transformation of human B lymphocytes by PHA. *Nature New Biol., 241*, 254-256.

Pillemer, L., Blum, L., Lepow, I.H., Ross, O.A., Todd, E.W. and Wardlaw, A.C. (1954): The properdin system and immunity. I. Demonstration and isolation of a new serum protein properdin and its role in immune phenomena. *Science, 120*, 279-285.

Ritchie, R.F. (1974): Theory and practice of automated nephelometry. In: *Protides of the Biological Fluids.* Editor: H. Peeters. Pergamon Press, Oxford pp. 569-577.

Roitt, I.M. (1977): *Essential Immunology.* Blackwell, Oxford, 342p.

Rowe, D.S. and Fahey, J.L. (1965): A new class of human immunoglobulins II Normal serum IgD. *J. exp. Med., 121*, 185-189.

Rowe, D.S., Hug, K., Forni, L. and Pernis, B. (1973): Immunoglobulin D as a lymphocyte receptor. *J. exp. Med., 138*, 965-972.

Ruddy, S., Gigli, I. and Austen, K.F. (1972): The complement system of man. *New Engl. J. Med., 297*, 489, 545, 592, 642-646.

Søborg, M. and Bendixen, G. (1967): Human lymphocyte migration as a parameter of hypersensitivity. *Acta med. scand., 181*, 247-256.

Thompson, R.A. (1977): *Techniques in Clinical Immunology.* Blackwell, Oxford, 241p.

Vergani, D., Tsantoulas, D., Eddleston, A.L.W.F., Davis, M. and Williams, R. (1978): Sensitization to halothane − altered liver components in severe hepatic necrosis after halothane. *Lancet, 2*, 801-803.

Walton, B. (1979): Effects of anaesthesia and surgery on immune status. *Brit. J. Anaesth., 51*, 37-43.

Walker, S.R., Evans, M.E., Richards, A.J. and Paterson, J.W. (1972): Then fate of (^{14}C) disodium cromoglycate in man. *J. Pharm. Pharmacol., 24*, 525-531.

Ward, A.M., Udnoon, S., Watkins, J., Walker, A.E. and Darke, C.S. (1976): Immunological mechanisms in the pathogenesis of vinyl chloride disease. *Brit. med. J., 1*, 936-938.

Watkins, J. (1979): Anaphylactoid reactions to i.v. substances. *Brit. J. Anaesth., 51*, 51-60.

Watkins, J. and Clarke, R.S.J. (1978): Report of a symposium. Adverse responses to intravenous agents. *Brit. J. Anaesth., 50*, 1159-1164.

Watkins, J., Padfield, A. and Alderson, J.D. (1978): Underlying immunopathology as a cause of adverse responses to two intravenous agents. *Brit. med. J., 1*, 1180-1181.

Watkins, J., Udnoon, S., Appleyard, T.N. and Thornton, J.A. (1976): Identification and quantitation of hypersensitivity reactions to intravenous anaesthetic agents. *Brit. J. Anaesth., 48*, 457-461.

Weiss, L. (1972): *The Cells and Tissues of the Immune System.* Prentice-Hall, New Jersey.

Weitkamp, L.R., Salzano, F.M., Neel, J., Porta, F., Geerdinf, R.A. and Tanoky, A.L. (1973): Human serum albumin: twenty-three genetic variants and their population distribution. *Ann. hum. Genet., 36*, 381-392.

Glossary of immunological terms

Like most subjects Immunology has its own specific jargon. This is a very incomplete glossary of terms in immunology but it may provide a rapid reference to several chapters within this volume, as well as in interpreting the literature.

Adjuvant: A substance injected together with antigen to improve the immune responses, e.g. Freund's adjuvant.

Adjuvant therapy: A means of therapeutic manipulation of the immune response in patients possessing impaired T lymphocyte function or certain malignant diseases, amied at a general improvement of cellular immunity by injection of adjuvants e.g. B.C.G.

Adrenergic drugs: Drugs such as adrenaline which function in opposition to histamine.

Agglutination: Aggregation of cells or particulate antigens by antibodies directed against the surface antigen(s).

Aggregate anaphylaxis: Anaphylactoid manifestations resulting from the presence of circulating immune or non-immune complexes accumulating in the capillaries of the lung. The mechanism of effector release (e.g. histamine) is obscure.

Aggregated immunoglobulin: Aggregates or polymers of various immunoglobulin proteins, *not* combined with antigen. May be generated in vitro by heating monomeric IgG preparations for short periods at 56°.
The aggregates, like *immune complexes*, are potent activators of complement C3 in vitro and in vivo.

Allergen: Any substance tolerated by the population as a whole which combines with reaginic (IgE) antibody to produce an allergic reaction in atopic subjects.

Allergy:	Hypersensitivity of "immediate" type to a defined allergen.
Allogeneic:	Same species but different genetic type.
Allotype:	Generally refers to protein molecules within a single species which have identical function but differ structurally (i.e. antigenically).
Anaphylactoid reaction:	Acute general clinical manifestation of a release reaction due to a non-immunological course (e.g. insect stings, snake venom).
Anaphylatoxin:	The specific peptides C3a and C5a which are generated from complement and liberate histamine from mast cells and basophils.
Anaphylactic shock:	An acute generalised histamine-release reaction of immediate hypersensitivity type usually involving reaginic (IgE) antibody.
Antibody:	An immunoglobulin with specific combining capacity for antigen through its Fab receptors, not quite synonymous with immunoglobulin.
Antigen:	Any macromolecule or particle which will elicit specific cell mediated and/or humoral immunity when introduced into the tissues.
Arthus reaction:	A necrotic dermal reaction developing several hours after intradermal injection of antigen into a previously immunized animal. The reaction results from immune complex formation with precipitating antibody and involves complement and neutrophils.
Atopy:	Spontaneous tendency to produce high levels of IgE antibodies to one or more common antigens in association with antigen-provoked disorders due to a reaginic mechanism.
Autoantibody:	Antibody reactive with "self" antigens either cellular or humoral, or both.
Autoimmune disease:	Disease where the autoantibody or cell mediated immunity is demonstrably related to its immunopathogenesis.

Avidity:	The strength of the bond between antigen and antibody molecules.
Bence Jones protein:	A free light chain of $\varkappa$ or λ type found, frequently in high concentration, in the serum and urine of some patients with myeloma or certain other neoplastic diseases. Traces of $\varkappa$ chain proteins are also found in *normal* urine.
Cell-mediated immunity:	T-lymphocyte mediated reactions such as allogeneic graft rejection.
Complement system:	The nine major proteins, C1 or C9 and their supporting enzymes and inhibitors which, by interaction with antigen and antigen-antibody complex produce anaphylactic, chemotactic and cytolytic effects.
Complement activation:	*Classical Pathway.* Activation of the complement system as a cascade from C1 to C9 as a result of antibody combination with antigen: terminates in target cell lysis and produces the clinical manifestations of inflammatory response.
Complement activation:	*Alternative Pathway.* Activation of the complement system from C3 onwards by endotoxin, polysaccharides and other substances *without* involvement of a specific immune process: may occur on cell surface or in free solution. Essentially a useful enhancement of classical pathway but if activated excessively liberates a harmful shock wave of histamine (anaphylactoid reaction).
Cryoglobulins:	Immunoglobulins which tend to precipitate from blood on cooling from 37° and to redissolve on warming. Associated with immune complex disease and connective tissue diseases in general, where clinical manifestation occur in vivo. Somewhat similar effects may occur in patients with mono-cloncal gammopathies of the IgA and IgM classes.
Cytophilic antibody:	Antibody attaching to cell surfaces by Fc receptors, leaving its specific combining sites free to react.
Cytotropic antibody:	Antibody attaching non-specifically to mast cells and baso-phils. The term homocytotropic is usually reserved for IgE antibodies.

Endotoxin:	Lipopolysaccharides present in the cell wall structure of gram negative bacteria.
Fluorescent antibody:	Immunoglobulins with specific antibody activity conjugated to fluorescein or other fluorochrome for use in microscopy as tracers to detect serum antibodies and tissue or cell antigens.
Genome:	The set of different chromosomes found in the nucleus of cells of any given species. The haploid gamete has only one genome. Relevant to theories of inheritance of antibody specificity.
Germinal centre:	Discrete cellular structure within follicles of lymphoid tissues of antigenically stimulated animals, containing macrophages and T and B lymphocytes.
Haemolytic plaque forming cell assays:	PFC techniques make use of antigens present (either naturally or otherwise) upon red blood cells. These are mixed with lymphocyte preparations and a complement preparation in a gel so that the cells remain in a fixed, dispersed environment. Antibody when released attaches to red cell lysis by complement. The cell producing antibody then stands out clearly upon microscopic examination in a plaque of lysed red cells.
Hapten:	Small molecules which are not in themselves antigenic but which elicit specific antibody response when covalently bound in vitro or in vivo with the normal proteins or cells (i.e. tolerogens) derived from the immunized animal itself.
Helper cell:	A subclass of T lymphocytes required to assist B lymphocytes to produce antibody to most protein antigens.
HLA complex:	The major histocompatibility complex in man, located on chromosome 6, responsible for coding the lymphocyte activating determinants (D); most strongly expressed on B lymphocytes and macrophages. The various HLA *antigens* constitute a basis for tissue typing.
Immediate hypersensitivity:	Type I hypersensitivity reactions including allergies and involving reaginic antibodies (IgE).

Immune complex: A term used somewhat vaguely but which really implies the specific combination of antibody with antigen and the "polymerization" of such structures until the point of precipitation is reached. Immune complexes may therefore be soluble and circulating in the plasma or insoluble and deposited in tissues. Complement may, or may not, be involved with these complexes.

Immune complex disease: Pathology resulting from the persistence of immune complexes in the circulation. Usually associated with connective tissue diseases, e.g. systemic lupus erythematosus but transient effects (serum sickness) may follow infection and immunization. The immune complexes may be deposited in skin, kidney or central nervous system producing the appropriate syndromes.

Immunoelectro-phoresis: A development of zone electrophoresis applied to biological fluids in which the electrophoretogram is developed, not by conventional protein staining, but by allowing antiserum (either polyvalent or monovalent) to diffuse from a well or wick applied parallel to the original electrophoretic migration. A series of fine arcs of precipitate define the proteins, as selected by the appropriate choice of antisera. This valuable technique, associated with Grabar and Williams, 1953, has undergone various modifications for even greater degrees of resolution of protein mixtures and their *quantitation* (e.g. Laurell technique).

Immunoglobulins, monoclonal: The products of the progeny of a single plasma cell clone giving rise to molecules of restricted electrophoretic mobility: generally associated with myeloma although "benign" situations, notably rheumatoid arthritis may give rise to similar "monoclones". Despite the high concentrations of the monoclone proteins encountered in malignancy, an associated antibody activity is very rarely encountered, in contrast to the benign situations. Electrophoretically these proteins exhibit a characteristic sharp band in the plasma, and sometimes the urine, of patients with multiple myeloma.

Immunoglobulins, polyclonal: Immunoglobulin molecules exhibiting a wide range of electrophoretic mobilities within the same class or subclass. This is the pattern of normal health with immunoglobulin and antibody synthesis arising from a wide range of unrelated clones of plasma cells. The greatest heterogeneity is expressed by IgG which runs as a "streak" rather than a sharp band upon zonal electrophoresis.

Immunoglobulins, Structure:

Constant region: The constant amino acid sequence regions of immunoglobulins involving the C terminal sections of the H and L polypeptide chains, coded by C_H and C_L genes respectively. The sequences define the various immunoglobulin classes and subclasses.

Fab fragment: In vitro proteolysis of the IgG immunoglobulin with papain produces three peptides of equal molecular weight, two Fab fragments and one Fc. Each Fab fragment contains one of the two antigen combining sites of the intact molecule.

F(ab¹)₂ fragment: The corresponding in vitro peptide from the IgG molecule obtained by pepsin hydrolysis. This is bivalent in antigen combining capacity and forms a useful reagent in fluorescent antibody techniques.

Fc fragment: The second peptide fragment obtained by in vitro hydrolysis of IgG with papain and represents the C terminal (COOH) end of the molecule. Contains the membrane attachment sites (and associated functions) of the intact molecules. No antigen combining capacity.

Heavy chain: The large (H) polypeptide chain of the immunoglobulin molecule. There are two of these chains in the tetrapeptide structure of the molecule.

Homology region: Regions of some 110 amino acid residues which have a striking (repeating) homology with each other. They are also demarked by intra-chain disulphide bridges. The variable region of the immunoglobulin comprises one or the two homology regions of the L chain and one of the four homology regions of the H chain in IgG and IgA molecules.

J chain: The polypeptide chain linking the molecules of secretory IgA and IgM.

Light chain: The small (L) polypeptide chain of the immunoglobulin molecule. There are two of these chains in the tetrapeptide structure of the molecule. They exist in either Kappa or in Lambda form, never mixed within the same molecule. Synonymous with Bence Jones protein.

Variable region: The amino acid sequences delineated by both the V_L and V_H genes coding for antibody diversity and comprising the antigen combining sites of the intact molecule.

Immunological tolerance: Specific failure to produce antibodies on exposure to antigen, frequently dose related.

Immunosuppression: Suppression of immunological response by chemical or biological means.

Kinins: Peptides released during anaphylaxis which cause vasodilation and smooth muscle contraction.

K-lymphocytes: Target cells (e.g. bacteria) coated with antibody become a centre not only for complement and phagocytic cell activity but also for a direct antibody dependent cell mediated cytotoxicity produced by the K-cell.

Lymphocyte transformation: Nuclear activity (DNA synthesis) of lymphocytes induced by contact with antigen, or by mitogens.

Lymphokines: Proteins secreted by antigen-stimulated T lymphocytes with specific biological functions.

Lymphotoxin: A lymphokine with cytolytic activity on target cells.

Migration inhibition factor (MIF): A lymphokine secreted by T lymphocytes during inflammatory response which prevents macrophages leaving the site of the response.

Mixed lymphocyte reaction (MLR): Transformation of T lymphocytes in culture with those from another donor. Transformation denotes histoincompatibility.

Non-immune complexes:	Protein aggregates in vivo not involving immunoglobulin proteins. They, like immune complexes may liberate vaso-active substances from peripheral leucocytes and activate complement, possibly generating *aggregate anaphylaxis.*
Null cells:	Immature T lymphocytes, predominantly associated with the thymus.
Opsonin:	An antibody which by attachment to a particulate antigen aids phagocytosis. Complement C3 possesses a similar opsonin role.
Passive cutaneous anaphylaxis (PCA):	An in vivo localised "test" anaphylaxis produced by dermal injection of cytotropic antibody followed by systemic injection of antigen.
PBA (Polyclonal B cell activators):	A general name for the various mitogens used to stimulate T and B lymphocytes in culture (see PHA response). As distinct from specific antigen stimulation which would only activate a few clones of cells these substances activate all lymphocytes, producing a more sensitive assay of "immune responsiveness". The flaw is that the mechanism of activation is *not typically antigenic.*
Phytohaemagglutin (PHA) response:	Transformation of (essentially) T lymphocytes by this plant mitogen.
Plasma cell:	A transformed B lymphocyte actively synthesising immuno-globulin and or specific antibody.
Prausnitz-Kustner (P-K) test:	An in vivo immediate hypersensitivity test in a normal subject or primate passively sensitized with serum IgE from an allergen-sensitive individual.
Prostaglandins (PGs):	A family of unsaturated fatty acids derived from arachi-donic acid widely distributed in most tissues of the body. Their actual mechanism of involvement with immune processes is a little speculative but PGs E1 and E2 inhibit both the IgE and complement mediated release of vaso-active substances from rat peritoneal mast cells.
Reagin:	Antibodies with specific affinities for mast cells and baso-phils, mainly synonymous with IgE but may also include IgG4 antibodies.

Rosette technique:	An identification test for T lymphocytes involving their ability to form spontaneous rosettes with sheep erythrocytes.
Suppressor cell:	A subclass of T lymphocytes which suppress B lymphocyte response to antigenic stimulation.
T Lymphocyte:	A lymphocyte processed by the thymus that is responsible for cell mediated immunity.
Transfer factor:	A soluble (extractable) ribonucleotide which can transfer the cell mediated hypersensitivity of lymphocytes.

Subject Index